LEADERSHIP IN

 W9-CUA-245

INTERPROFESSIONAL HEALTH EDUCATION

AND PRACTICE

Charlotte Brasic Royeen, PhD, OT, FAOTA
Dean, Edward and Margaret Doisy College of Health Sciences
Professor, Department of Occupational Science and Occupational Therapy
Saint Louis University

Gail M. Jensen, PhD, PT, FAPTA
Dean, Graduate School and Associate Vice President in Academic Affairs
Professor, Department of Physical Therapy
Faculty Associate, Center for Health Policy and Ethics
Creighton University

Robin Ann Harvan, EdD
Special Projects Associate, Offices of the Vice Chancellor and Dean for Health Affairs
at the School of Medicine
Associate Professor, Department of Family Medicine
University of Colorado Denver

JONES AND BARTLETT PUBLISHERS
Sudbury, Massachusetts
BOSTON   TORONTO   LONDON   SINGAPORE

World Headquarters

Jones and Bartlett Publishers
40 Tall Pine Drive
Sudbury, MA 01776
978-443-5000
info@jbpub.com
www.jbpub.com

Jones and Bartlett Publishers
Canada
6339 Ormindale Way
Mississauga, ON L5V IJ2
Canada

Jones and Bartlett Publishers
International
Barb House, Barb Mews
London W6 7PA
United Kingdom

Jones and Bartlett's books and products are available through most bookstores and online booksellers. To contact Jones and Bartlett Publishers directly, call 800-832-0034, fax 978-443-8000, or visit our website www.jbpub.com.

Substantial discounts on bulk quantities of Jones and Bartlett's publications are available to corporations, professional associations, and other qualified organizations. For details and specific discount information, contact the special sales department at Jones and Bartlett via the above contact information or send an email to specialsales@jbpub.com.

Copyright © 2009 by Jones and Bartlett Publishers, LLC

All rights reserved. No part of the material protected by this copyright may be reproduced or utilized in any form, electronic or mechanical, including photocopying, recording, or by any information storage and retrieval system, without written permission from the copyright owner.

The authors, editor, and publisher have made every effort to provide accurate information. However, they are not responsible for errors, omissions, or for any outcomes related to the use of the contents of this book and take no responsibility for the use of the products and procedures described. Treatments and side effects described in this book may not be applicable to all people; likewise, some people may require a dose or experience a side effect that is not described herein. Drugs and medical devices are discussed that may have limited availability controlled by the Food and Drug Administration (FDA) for use only in a research study or clinical trial. Research, clinical practice, and government regulations often change the accepted standard in this field. When consideration is being given to use of any drug in the clinical setting, the health care provider or reader is responsible for determining FDA status of the drug, reading the package insert, and reviewing prescribing information for the most up-to-date recommendations on dose, precautions, and contraindications, and determining the appropriate usage for the product. This is especially important in the case of drugs that are new or seldom used.

Production Credits

Publisher: David Cella
Editorial Assistant: Maro Asadoorian
Production Director: Amy Rose
Production Assistant: Julia Waugaman
Associate Marketing Manager: Lisa Gordon
Manufacturing and Inventory Control Supervisor:
  Amy Bacus

Composition: ATLIS Graphics & Design
Cover Design: Kristin E. Ohlin
Cover Image: © Brian Tan/ShutterStock, Inc.
Printing and Binding: Malloy Incorporated
Cover Printing: Malloy Incorporated

Library of Congress Cataloging-in-Publication Data
Royeen, Charlotte Brasic.
  Leadership in interprofessional health education and practice / by Charlotte Brasic Royeen, Gail M. Jensen, and Robin Ann Harvan.
     p. ; cm.
  Includes bibliographical references and index.
  ISBN-13: 978-0-7637-4983-5 (pbk.)
  ISBN-10: 0-7637-4983-4 (pbk.)
  1. Rural health services. 2. Interdisciplinary approach in education. 3. Interprofessional relations.
  4. Leadership. I. Jensen, Gail M. II. Harvan, Robin Ann. III. Title.
  [DNLM: 1. Education, Professional--Congresses. 2. Rural Health Services--Congresses.
  3. Community Health Services--Congresses. 4. Interprofessional Relations--Congresses.
  5. Leadership--Congresses. WA 18 R889L 2009]
  RA771.R62 2009
  362.1'04257--dc22
                                                                        2008033360
6048

Printed in the United States of America
12 11 10 09 08   10 9 8 7 6 5 4 3 2 1

Contents

Contributing Authors   xi

Acknowledgments   xvii

Foreword   Interprofessional Education and Practice in Health Care:
              International Perspectives   xix
              Hugh Barr, John H.V. Gilbert, Madeline H. Schmitt

Section 1: Introduction to Interprofessional Education and Practice   1

Chapter 1:   **Interprofessional Education: Context, Complexity, and Challenge**   3
              Gail M. Jensen, Robin Ann Harvan, Charlotte Brasic Royeen

              Introduction   3
              Interprofessional Education in the United States: Key Events   4
              Interprofessional Education Conference and Book Creation: Key Events   9
              Book Overview   11
              References   13

Chapter 2:   **Interprofessional Education and the Common Good:**
              A Reflective Analysis   15
              Gail M. Jensen, Teresa M. Cochran, Caroline Goulet,
              Brenda M. Coppard

              Introduction   15
              Organizational Ethics Framework for Analysis   16
              IPE and Individuals   18
              IPE and Organizations   21
              IPE and Society   23
              Conclusion   25
              References   26

Chapter 3:   **Interprofessional Education: History, Review, and Recommendations**
              for Professional Accreditation Agencies   29
              Charlotte Brasic Royeen, Sarah R. Walsh, Elizabeth Terhaar

              Introduction   29
              Recommendations for Interprofessional Education   42
              Conclusion   42
              References   43

Chapter 4:   **Grounding Interprofessional Education and Practice in Theory**   45
              Robin Ann Harvan, Charlotte Brasic Royeen, Gail M. Jensen

              Introduction   45
              Key Definitions   47
              Establishing the Evidence   50
              Exploring Theoretical Models   52

Health Care Team Training Assumptions   55
Conclusion   58
References   60

Chapter 5: Issues Related to Interprofessional Assessment   63
Brenda M. Coppard, Gail M. Jensen, Teresa M. Cochran, Caroline Goulet

Introduction   63
IPE and Scholarship of Engagement   64
IPE Assessment Quandary   64
Conclusion   73
References   73

Chapter 6: Shaping the Future: Strategies for Promoting Interprofessional Health
Professions Practice in Rural and Underserved Communities   77
Victoria F. Roche

Introduction   77
Strategies for Promoting Practice in Rural and Underserved Communities   80
Conclusion   91
References   92

Chapter 7: Interprofessional Collaboration: Addressing the Needs of the
Underserved Geriatric Population   95
Ann Ryan Haddad, Joy D. Doll

Introduction   95
Geriatric Population as Underserved   96
Community Dwelling Elders   97
Addressing Health Needs of Older Adults   99
Current Geriatric Models   100
Faculty Development in Geriatrics   102
Best Practices for Academic Settings   105
Conclusion   106
References   106

Section 2: Community Context   109

Chapter 8: The Librarian Is Out: Role of the Librarian in Rural Health Outreach   111
Siobhan Champ-Blackwell, Teresa L. Hartman

Introduction   111
Background: The Rural Setting   112
Information Needs of Rural Health Care Professionals   112
Barriers to Access   114
Role of the Medical Librarian   114
Access to a Medical Librarian   116
Collaboration Is the Answer   116
Expanded Example   117
Global Reach   120

Academic Settings 121
Conclusion 122
References 122

Chapter 9: Addressing Culture While Building the System: Leadership Challenges in Interprofessional, Interagency Rural Health Networks 125
Jane Hamel-Lambert, Caroline Murphy

Introduction 125
Background 126
Regional Cultural 129
Corporate Culture and Climate 132
Participatory Leadership: Structure and Strategy 133
Link to Interprofessional Education and Leadership Development 137
Conclusion 138
References 139

Chapter 10: Community Organization Principles and Sustainable Interprofessional Health Care Practices 141
Mary Ann Lavin, Deborah E. Bust, Brenda Le, David C. Campbell,
Marvin Bostic, Margaret M. Herning, Elaine Wilder,
Claudia List Hilton, Patricia D. Miller

Introduction 141
The Bolivian Story 143
Story of Health Outreach and Preventive Education and the
    Great Mines Health Center 145
James House Health Center 156
Limitations of Report 162
Conclusions 163
References 163

Chapter 11: Connecting Interprofessional Education to the Community Through Service Learning and Community-Based Research 167
Pamela J. Reynolds

Introduction 167
Context of Community Engagement 168
Development of Principles-Based Partnerships 176
Conclusions 184
References 184
Resources for Faculty to Document Community
    Engaged Scholarship 187

Chapter 12: Social, Environmental, and Occupational Justice: Too Many High Sounding Words and Not Enough Action 189
Beth P. Velde

Introduction 189
Interprofessional Rural Health Research and Health Services
    Framed in Justice: Putting the Big Words into Action 191

Conclusions   195
References   196

Section 3: Practice Context   199

Chapter 13: Building a Health Care Workforce That Reflects the People We Serve   **201**
Terry K. Crowe, Patricia Burtner, Theresa A. Torres

Introduction   201
Strategies for Creating a More Culturally Diverse Health Care Workforce   205
Increasing Diversity Begins with Recruitment   207
Adjusting the Curriculum to Student Lifestyles   208
Integrating Cultural Experiences into Curricula   209
Identifying Conflicts in Traditional Curriculum Content with
    Cultural Beliefs   209
Respecting Cultural Responsibilities and Rituals   210
Incorporating Faculty Mentorship for Additional Educational Support   210
Project Escuela: A Personnel Preparation Model to Increase
    Diversity at UNM   211
Increased Recruitment of Students from New Mexico Native Cultures   212
Evaluating Graduates' Impact on Outcomes in Children
    with Disabilities   213
How Does Financial Support Assist Individual Students?   214
Conclusions   215
References   215

**Chapter 14: The AHEC Advantage: Campus–Community Partnerships for
Rural Health Education**   **219**
Robin Ann Harvan

Introduction   219
Campus–Community Partnerships   222
AHEC Experiences in Rural America   224
Health Careers Recruitment and Preparation   226
Health Professionals Training and Placement   227
Health Professionals Retention   228
Community Health Education and Development   229
AHEC Collaborations in Colorado   230
Leadership to Leverage the Benefits   233
Conclusions   236
References   236

**Chapter 15: Professionalization and the Ethic of Care: From Silos to
Interprofessional Moral Community**   **237**
Laura Lee (Dolly) Swisher

Introduction   237
Justice and Care   238
Sample Vignette   242

Professionalization   243
Creating an Interprofessional Moral Community Grounded in
    Care and Justice   245
Conclusions   246
References   247

**Chapter 16: "Against the Current": Strategies for Success in Health Care—A Case
Example of a Rural, Native American Community**   249
Joy D. Doll, Wehnona Stabler

Introduction   249
Overview of Omaha Tribe   251
Demographic Data from Omaha Tribe   253
Overview of Tribal Health Care Delivery System   254
History of Carl T. Curtis Health Education System   258
Lessons Learned   259
Conclusions   261
References   261

Section 4: Educational Context   263

**Chapter 17: Improving Diabetes Outcomes in Rural Practices: Power of
Collaborative Care**   265
Doyle M. Cummings, Paul Bray, Maria C. Clay

Introduction   265
Diabetes in Rural America   266
Redesigning Systems of Care   268
Redesigned Systems of Care in Rural Practices   269
New Model of Care Delivery   270
Interprofessional Collaboration   272
Eastern North Carolina Chronic Care Pilot Project   274
Conclusions   277
References   278

**Chapter 18: Developing Health Professional Students into Rural Health
Care Leaders of the Future Through Best Practices**   281
Patrick S. Cross, Joy D. Doll

Introduction   281
Educational Design   284
Conclusions   293
References   293

**Chapter 19: Interprofessional Education and Multicultural and
Community Affairs**   297
Omofolasade "Sade" Kosoko-Lasaki

Introduction   297
Background   297

Health Professions Partnership Initiative   303
Conclusions   308
References   308

**Chapter 20: Interprofessional Curriculum: Preparing Health Professionals for
Collaborative Teamwork in Health Care   311**
*Irma Ruebling, Judith H. Carlson, Karen Cuvar, Jeanne Donnelly,
K. Jody Smith, Nina Westhus, Rita Wunderlich*

Introduction   311
Interprofessional Curriculum   312
The Curriculum Plan   317
Evaluation   325
Conclusions   326
References   327

**Chapter 21: Interprofessional Training in Telehealth Technologies for Service
Delivery and Development of Rural Communities of Practice   329**
Darlene M. Sekerak, Linn Wakeford, Keith M. Cochran, Joshua J. Alexander

Introduction   329
Background   330
Description of the Project   332
Outcomes   341
Discussion   343
Conclusions   344
References   344

Section 5: Best Practice   347

**Chapter 22: The View From 30,000 Feet: Rural Interprofessional Education
at the Academic Health Center Level   349**
Barbara F. Brandt, Gwen Wagstrom Halaas

Introduction   349
Rural Minnesota: Changing Demographics and Health Disparities   350
The University of Minnesota Academic Health Center   354
Lessons Learned: Strategies for Building the Next Generation
    of Community–Campus Partnerships   362
Conclusions   364
References   365

**Chapter 23: Training for Interprofessional Services to Appalachian Adolescents
with Mental Health Needs: Lessons Learned from PRISYM   367**
*Doris Pierce, Amy Marshall, Stephanie W. Adams, Carol W. Cecil,
Brent Garrett, Marlene Belew Huff, Carmilla Ratliff*

Introduction   367
Lesson One: Defining a Strong Service Team for Appalachian
    At-Risk Youth   370

Lesson Two: Appreciating and Providing Services Within
    Appalachian Culture   375
Lesson Three: The Challenges of Serving an Underserved Rural Area   378
Lesson Four: Addressing Justice and Power at Many Levels   383
Conclusions: A Success and Take Home Lessons   386
References   389

**Chapter 24: The Forgotten Population: Health Communication with
    Rural Racial/Ethnic Communities**   **391**
Shirley A. Wells

Introduction   391
Literacy   393
Health Literacy   396
Impact of Culture   397
Communication Strategies   400
Community Health Communication Project: Health Literacy
    Educational Symposium   404
Health Communication Strategies   408
Conclusions   410
References   410

Chapter 25: Health Report Card Project: Building Community Capacity   **413**
Marlene Wilken

Introduction   413
Building Community Capacity   414
Need for Building Community Capacity   415
Groups Involved in the Process   417
The Process   420
Findings   423
Outcomes   423
Where Do We Go from Here?   424
Conclusions   424
References   425

Section 6: Future Directors   **427**

**Chapter 26: Next Steps in Rural Health Interprofessional
    Education and Practice**   **429**
Kevin J. Lyons

Introduction   429
Approach to Education   430
Addressing the Needs of Practice in Rural Areas   432
Applying a Leadership Model   435
Conclusions   436
References   436

Chapter 27: Interprofessional Education: Themes and Next Steps   **439**
Charlotte Brasic Royeen, Gail M. Jensen, Robin Ann Harvan

Introduction   439
Gestalt of the Conference   440
Themes   442
Next Steps   444
Final Challenges   445
Conclusions   446
References   446

Appendix A: Content of the Interdisciplinary Education Perception Scale   **449**

**Appendix B: Proposed Cultural Proficiency Elective for Health Care
Professions Schools**   **451**

Course Descriptions   451
Course Goals   451
Learning Objectives   451
Text   452
Evaluative Techniques   452
Student Responsibilities/Clinical Schedules   452
Examples of Questions that will Guide the Student's Inquiry   452
Grading Policy   453

Index   **455**

Contributing Authors

Stephanie W. Adams, MSW
Visiting Assistant Professor
Department of Anthropology, Sociology
  and Social Work
Eastern Kentucky University
Richmond, KY

Joshua J. Alexander, MD
Associate Professor
Department of Physical Medicine and
  Rehabilitation
UNC School of Medicine
University of North Carolina at
  Chapel Hill
Chapel Hill, NC

Marvin Bostic, MS
Manager, Elderly and Disabled Resident
  Initiatives
St. Louis Housing Authority
St. Louis, MO

Barbara F. Brandt, PhD
Assistant Vice President for Education
Academic Health Center
University of Minnesota
Minneapolis, MN

Paul Bray, MA, LMFT
Diabetes Project Coordinator
Bertie Memorial Hospital
Windsor, NC

Patricia Burtner, PhD, OT, FAOTA
Associate Professor, Graduate Program
  in Occupational Therapy
University of New Mexico Health
  Sciences Center
Albuquerque, NM

Deborah E. Bust, BJ
Executive Director
Washington County Community
  Partnership
Potosi, MO

David C. Campbell, MD, MEd
President and CEO
Institute for Family Medicine
St. Louis, MO

Judith H. Carlson, RN, MSN
Associate Professor
School of Nursing
Saint Louis University
St. Louis, MO

Carol W. Cecil, MA, EdD
Executive Director
Kentucky Partnership for Families and
  Children, Inc.
Frankfort, KY

Siobhan Champ-Blackwell, MSLIS
Community Outreach Liaison
National Network of Libraries
  of Medicine
Creighton University
Omaha, NE

Maria C. Clay, PhD
Interim Chair, Department of Medical
  Humanites, Professor of Family Medicine
Director of Clinical Skills Assessment
  and Education
Co-director of the Office of Interdisciplinary
  Health Sciences Education
East Carolina University
Greenville, NC

Keith M. Cochran, MS
Program Manager
Department of Pediatrics
School of Medicine
University of North Carolina at Chapel Hill
Chapel Hill, NC

Teresa M. Cochran, PT, DPT, GCS, MA
Associate Professor and Vice Chair
Department of Physical Therapy
Co-Director, Office of Interprofessional
    Scholarship, Service, and Education
School of Pharmacy and Health Professions
Creighton University
Omaha, NE

Brenda M. Coppard, PhD, OT, FAOTA
Associate Professor and Chair
Department of Occupational Therapy
School of Pharmacy and Health Professions
Creighton University
Omaha, NE

Patrick S. Cross PT, DPT
Assistant Professor
Department of Physical Therapy
School of Health Sciences
The University of South Dakota
Vermillion, SD

Terry K. Crowe, PhD, OT, FAOTA
Professor, Graduate Program in
    Occupational Therapy
University of New Mexico Health Sciences
    Center
Albuquerque, NM

**Doyle M. Cummings, PharmD, BCPS, FCP,
    FCCP**
Clinical Professor, Division of Pharmacy
    Practice and Experiential Education
Eshelman School of Pharmacy
School of Pharmacy
East Carolina University
Greenville, NC

Karen Cuvar, PhD, RN
Assistant Professor
School of Nursing
Saint Louis University
St. Louis, MO

Joy D. Doll, OTD, OT
Assistant Professor of Clinical Education,
Department of Occupational Therapy
School of Pharmacy and Health
    Professions
Creighton University
Omaha, NE

Jeanne Donnelly, PhD, MBA, RHIA
Associate Professor
Department of Health Informatics and
    Information Management
Doisy College of Health Sciences
Saint Louis Univeristy
St. Louis, MO

Brent Garrett, PhD, MPA
Research Scientist
Pacific Institute for Research and
    Evaluation
Louisville, KY

Caroline Goulet, PhD, PT
Associate Professor, Department of
    Physical Therapy
Co-Director, Office of Interprofessional
    Scholarship, Service, and Education
School of Pharmacy and Health
    Professions
Creighton University
Omaha, NE

Ann Ryan Haddad, PharmD
Associate Professor
Department of Pharmacy Practice
School of Pharmacy and Health
    Professions
Creighton University
Omaha, NE

Jane Hamel-Lambert, MBA, PhD
Assistant Professor of Family Medicine
Director, Interdisciplinary Mental Health
   Education
Ohio University College of Osteopathic
   Medicine
Athens, OH

Teresa L. Hartman, MLS
Head of Education/Associate Professor
McGoogan Library of Medicine
University of Nebraska Medical Center
Omaha, NE

Margaret M. Herning, PhD, PT
Associate Professor
Department of Physical Therapy and
   Athletic Training
Doisy College of Health Sciences
Saint Louis University
St. Louis, MO

Claudia List Hilton, PhD, OT, SROT
Post Doctoral Fellow
Social Developmental Studies
Department of Psychiatry
Washington University School of Medicine
St. Louis, MO

Marlene Belew Huff, PhD, LCSW
Associate Professor
College of Medicine
University of Kentucky
Lexington, KY

**Omofolasade "Sade" Kosoko-Lasaki, MD,
   MSPH, MBA**
Professor of Surgery (Ophthalmology),
   Preventive Medicine and
   Public Health
Associate Vice President of Health
   Sciences
School of Medicine
Creighton University
Omaha, NE

Mary Ann Lavin, ScD, RN, ANP, FAAN
Associate Professor
Director, Center for Interprofessional
   Education and Research
School of Nursing
Saint Louis University
St. Louis, MO

Brenda Le, MSN, APRN-BC, RN, FNP
Clinical Programs Manager
Institute for Family Medicine
St. Louis, MO

Kevin J. Lyons, MA, PhD
Associate Dean and Director, Center for
   Collaborative Research
College of Health Professions
Thomas Jefferson University
Philadelphia, PA

Amy Marshall, MS, OT
Research Coordinator of Endowed Chair
Department of Occupational Therapy
Eastern Kentucky University
Richmond, KY

Patricia D. Miller, MS, CCC-SLP
Assistant Professor
Director of the Graduate Program
Department of Communication Sciences
   and Disorders
Saint Louis University
St. Louis, MO

Caroline Murphy, PhD
Clinical Child Psychologist
Nationwide Children's Hospital
Clinical Assistant Professor of Pediatrics
The Ohio State University
Columbus, OH

Doris Pierce, PhD, OT, FAOTA
Endowed Chair in Occupational Therapy
Department of Occupational Therapy
College of Health Science
Eastern Kentucky University
Richmond, KY

Carmilla Ratliff
Assistant Youth Council Coordinator
Kentucky Partnership for Families
    and Children
Frankfort, KY

Pamela J. Reynolds, PT, EdD
Professor
Doctor of Physical Therapy Program
Morosky College of Health Professions
    and Sciences
Gannon University
Erie, PA

Victoria F. Roche, PhD
Senior Associate Dean and Professor of
    Pharmacy Sciences
School of Pharmacy and Health
    Professions
Creighton University
Omaha, NE

Irma Ruebling, MA, PT
Assistant Professor
Department of Physical Therapy
Director of Interprofessional Education
Doisy College of Health Sciences
Saint Louis University
St. Louis, MO

Darlene M. Sekerak, PhD, PT
Professor and Associate Chair
Division of Physical Therapy
Allied Health Sciences
University of North Carolina at
    Chapel Hill
Chapel Hill, NC

K. Jody Smith, PhD, RHIA, FAHIMA
Professor and Chairperson
Health Informatics and Information
    Management
Doisy College of Health Sciences
Saint Louis University
St. Louis, MO

Wehnona Stabler, MPH
Indian Health Service
Oklahoma

Laura Lee (Dolly) Swisher, PT, MDiv, PhD
Associate Professor, School of Physical
    Therapy and Rehabilitation Sciences
Assistant Dean for Interprofessional
    Education, College of Medicine
University of South Florida
Tampa, FL

Elizabeth Terhaar, MS, OT
Graduate Research Assistant
Doisy College of Health Sciences
Saint Louis University
St. Louis, MO

Theresa A. Torres, OT
Graduate Program in Occupational Therapy
University of New Mexico Health Sciences
    Center
Albuquerque, NM

Beth P. Velde, PhD, OT
Professor
Department of Occupational Therapy
Assistant Dean
College of Allied Health Sciences,
East Carolina University,
Greenville, NC

Gwen Wagstrom Halaas, MD, MBA
Director
Center for Interprofessional Education
University of Minnesota Academic Health
    Center
Minneapolis, MN

Linn Wakeford, MS, OT
Assistant Professor
Division of Occupational Science
University of North Carolina at
    Chapel Hill
Chapel Hill, NC

Sarah R. Walsh, MOT, OT
Occupational Therapist
Pate Rehabilitation
Dallas, TX

Shirley A. Wells, MPH, OT, FAOTA
Assistant Professor
Department of Occupational Therapy
The University of Texas–Pan American
Edinburg, TX

Nina Westhus, PhD, MSN, RN
Associate Professor
School of Nursing
Saint Louis University
St. Louis, MO

Elaine Wilder, PhD, PT
Associate Professor
Department of Physical Therapy and
    Athletic Training
Doisy College of Health Sciences
Saint Louis University
St. Louis, MO

Marlene Wilken, RN, PhD
Assistant Professor
School of Nursing
Creighton University
Omaha, NE

Rita Wunderlich, PhD, RN
Assistant Professor
School of Nursing
Saint Louis University
St. Louis, MO

Acknowledgments

This book is an example of collaboration from beginning to end. The contributors to this book are all experienced educators, health professionals, or community members who are part of community–academic partnerships. Forty leaders from across the United States who are involved in rural, interdisciplinary training of health professional students gathered at *Leadership in Rural Health Interprofessional Education: A Working Conference for Leaders in Rural Health Care* in Denver, Colorado.

We are grateful for the support of our institutions: Creighton University, Saint Louis University, and University of Colorado Denver, including the conference coordinated by the Office of Interprofessional Scholarship, Service and Education (OISSE) at Creighton University. The conference would not have taken place without the financial support of the Health Resources and Services Administration (HRSA) Grant #1D36HP03158 for *Circles of Learning: Community and Clinic as Interdisciplinary Classroom*, a Quentin N. Burdick Interdisciplinary Training Project.

We thank David Cella for taking a risk to come to Denver to see what we were up to. His vision for the book and support for the project are much appreciated. We also thank Maro Asadoorian, our task master, who was responsible for keeping the editors organized and on a timeline. This is not an easy task. Julia Waugaman's gentle yet skilled hand in editing has greatly enhanced our book.

Finally, we hope that this book will be the first of many interprofessional contributions to health professions education and practice that will target underserved communities and the elimination of health disparities.

Foreword

Interprofessional Education and Practice in Health Care: International Perspectives

"We have to work together to ensure access to a motivated, skilled, and supported health worker by every person in every village everywhere."

Dr. Lee Jong-wook
Director-General (2003-2006)
World Health Organization (WHO)

UNITED KINGDOM PERSPECTIVE

Few regions of Britain compare with the remote expanses of North America, save perhaps for the highlands and islands of Scotland, nor is the rural health deficit as stark as that portrayed in this book. Yet most of the 90 percent of Britons who live in the cities are blissfully unaware of the privation hidden behind the friendly façade of rural life in seemingly idyllic towns and villages where they may retreat to unwind on weekends.

Rural communities in Britain were protected for many years from the full force of economic and social change. A nation that remembered food rationing in the Second World War subsidized agriculture heavily, assisted later by the European Community, in the mistaken belief that as an island it must be self-sufficient in food. As a result, farming flourished during the post-war years. Productivity soared with the benefit of modern agricultural methods, while "townies" made snide remarks about "featherbedded farmers." If that held a grain of truth for the fertile fens of East Anglia, it was wide of the mark in the uplands of Northern England, Scotland, and Wales, where farming had never been much above subsistence level.

Farmers were not prepared for the harsh winds of economic reality as national and European subsidies were redistributed and withdrawn, exacerbated by the ravages of BSE (mad cow disease) and foot and mouth, which drove some into bankruptcy. Sons of farmers now in their fifties are reluctant to follow them onto the land. Stress masquerades as fortitude, but cannot fool the watchful doctor or nurse. The bedrock of the rural economy has been shaken as the last staple industry has been overtaken by a post-industrial society where wealth comes largely from invisible earnings in the city of London.

City shoppers have grown accustomed to cheap imported food from the prairies of Canada and the pastures of New Zealand, while superstores recently threatened to import milk from Ireland and even Poland to undercut "uncompetitive" local producers. Thankfully, some of the major retailers relented and signed long-term agreements. Mindful of the power of "the big four" supermarket chains, the central government appointed an ombudsman, ostensibly to protect the interests of farmers as much as consumers, yet only to find its good intentions greeted with skepticism.

"Rationalization" and "diversification" are now the catchwords as farms merge in search of economies of scale and bed and breakfast signs go up at the roadside gate. Farming may have always had its "ups and downs," as some country folk may still maintain, while crisis creeps up on unsuspecting rural communities. Long-term trends militate against preservation of traditional rural life. Second-home owners from the cities first bought redundant farmsteads, then competed for housing that local young people desperately needed before long distance commuters to the cities moved in, followed by the successful self-employed who set up their high-tech offices in the outbuildings.

"Off-comers" may contribute to the local economy and help to sustain local services, but property prices escalate beyond the reach of local people. Many village schools and post offices-cum-grocery stores face closure, despite the influx from the cities. Most railway branch lines were "axed" fifty years ago, replaced by bus services later deemed to be uneconomic and withdrawn. Decline in local services hits poor, young, elderly, and disabled people hardest, as they lack private transportation to be able to access services and entertainment in the cities. The Countryside Alliance, a rainbow coalition comprising everyone from Masters of Hounds to the Women's Institute, demonstrates en masse in Hyde Park for or against everything from reinstating fox hunting to saving local hospitals, as a bemused metropolis looks on.

Poverty in the countryside is for the most part hidden, masked by the relative affluence of the incoming population, but wages remain low for many in the indigenous population, and prices remain high, compared with the cities, not only for housing but also for food and transportation. Some 900,000 country dwellers (according to the latest official figures) live below the poverty line. Quality of life suffers, as measured by economists and sociologists, although many locals still count themselves lucky to live in the countryside—a countryside to which others flock. Tourism generates ten times more income than farming and helps rescue the economy in scenic areas, even though many of the jobs created are for seasonal migrant labor. Scarred and rundown mining villages miss out.

Improving education, employment, housing, and transportation tend to be higher priorities than health care in rural communities. The National Health Service is charged with the responsibility of delivering the same range and quality of care everywhere. Primary care is generally well-provided in rural areas, with many new purpose-built premises designed to bring specialist services closer, but proposals for polyclinics are dismissed by general practitioners (family physicians) as London-centric in conception and antipathetic to the doctor–patient relationship.

District hospitals are threatened with closure before alternative community-based provision becomes available, as services are redeployed from towns to cities. Hospitals are no longer owned by the local community, nor are their staff working as closely in partnership with primary care professionals. Hospital appointments entail longer and costlier journeys, save for those patients entitled to use the ambulance, while elderly relatives without cars rely on the goodwill of neighbours to provide transportation for visits. Reaching the Accident and Emergency Unit may entail a long and separate journey, while air ambulance services rely desperately on charitable donations raised at domino drives in village halls.

Responsibility rests with local authorities to sustain and restore the quality of rural life in partnership with NHS Trusts, police authorities, and community groups. Elected representatives, senior managers, and grassroots activists provide the leadership. Collaboration is assumed within community development strategies whose success depends upon wide-ranging participation.

Professional education is being strengthened as the latest wave of new universities is established in rural counties by upgrading or merging institutes of higher and further education. Multi-site universities result, working with feeder colleges to improve access to higher education in regions where take-up has been traditionally low. Priority is invariably given to the development of vocational courses for service industries, in the proven expectation that a significant percentage of graduates will opt to work locally in key occupations such as school teaching, medicine, nursing, and social work. The new generation of universities is strategically placed to promote not only professional but also interprofessional education (IPE) that is responsive to rural needs and priorities.

Hugh Barr, PhD
Joint Editor-in-Chief
The Journal of Interprofessional Care
President
The UK Centre for the Advancement of
    Interprofessional Education (CAIPE)
Emeritus Professor of Interprofessional Education
University of Westminster, UK

CANADA PERSPECTIVE

The Canadian Health Services Research Foundation describes "rural" as: "communities based on geographic isolation, economic and labour force characteristics, and availability of services and amenities."[1(p3)] Canada covers a landmass second only to Russia, yet its population is scarcely larger than 35 million people. Much of that population occupies a band of about 200 miles across its entire border with the United States of America. Canada has a large Aboriginal population that is widely dispersed and whose health needs have been documented in many reports. Providing a range of health and social care services to the rural population presents considerable challenges.

Many of those challenges are related both to the distance between rural and urban communities, and to the scarcity of health and human services in rural areas. The spectrum of health problems is wide and includes low life expectancy at birth, high mortality and suicide rates, and above-average chronic disease rates. These health challenges are compounded by low access to physicians, a relatively small number of health care providers, and inadequate access to specialists in all fields. Providing considerable services to very ill patients over large geographic areas is a feat that is accomplished by a very small number of health care providers whose working life expectancy under such conditions is considerably shorter than that of colleagues in urban areas.

The ability of rural communities, health authorities, post-secondary institutions, and others to provide and support the education of health professionals, particularly at the pre-licensure level, is therefore a highly complex issue. Providing leadership in rural health education and practice is heavily dependent on community capacity; i.e., the ability of a rural community to handle a quantity (number and mix) of students and also to provide a high quality practice education experience.

There is growing recognition of the benefits to rural communities and to students (and ultimately to the health care system) from learning in rural communities as part of their educational experience. In British Columbia, Canada's most westerly province, a number of such programs have been initiated over the past several years. These programs include the Interprofessional Rural Program of BC, the Aboriginal Health Elective, and the Vancouver Island Interprofessional Health Project. In addition, there are long-standing uniprofessional rural placements provided through most education programs. Although significant momentum is underway with similar programs across Canada, it has become clear that there is an urgent need to engage a wide range of stakeholders in order to achieve a number of common goals. All jurisdictions recognize that there is a need to carry forward at least the following actions:

- Promote knowledge exchange about models, activities, successes, and challenges relating to interprofessional placements linked to rural practice and research
- Engage in meaningful dialogue regarding a longer term sustainable model, including principles and components for expanding interprofessional practice education linked to rural practice and research
- Identify an action plan that is endorsed by key stakeholders in both urban and rural communities

In the past four years, through the agency and financial support of Health Canada, many rural interprofessional initiatives have been started that are actively engaged in realizing the actions outlined above. Canada's good fortune in mounting these initiatives was that it was able to learn from the Quentin Burdick program in the United States and profit from much of the learning in that program, whose lessons are amply illustrated in a number of chapters in this volume. Canada and the United States share many commonalities in their rural populations and are presented with many of the same problems in providing access to health care. The fundamental underlying attempts to connect the academic and rural communities are generic to both countries, as are our mutual attempts to provide excellent models of interprofessional care through collaborative teamwork.

The wealth of materials focusing on leadership represented in this volume speak to the long history of successes (and failures) in our efforts to mount a sustained interprofessional culture in both countries. The challenges of rural interprofessional practice are many, yet they hold great promise for realizing the long sought-after goal of systemic change to enhance and improve the quality of care given to all people who enter the health care system in our two countries. These challenges, articulately addressed in the contents of this book, are worth carrying forward.

John H. V. Gilbert, PhD
Project Lead
Canadian Interprofessional Health
  Collaborative
President
International Association for Interprofessional
  Education And Collaborative Practice
  (InterED)

Co-Chair
World Health Organization (WHO)
  Study Group on IPE & Collaborative
  Practice
Principal and Professor Emeritus
College of Health Disciplines
University of British Columbia
Vancouver, BC

UNITED STATES OF AMERICA PERSPECTIVE

The concept of *rural* is first, and foremost, a statement about geography. But defining more specifically what rural means is not straightforward, as geographers have noted. In their survey of the literature, Williams and Cutchin identified seven ways in which rural has been descriptively defined: land use, demographic structure, non-metropolitan area, environmental characteristics, and, less commonly, population density, population characteristics, and commuting patterns. They also identified "universals" that define the overall characteristics of rural areas.[2]

First, there are the poor socioeconomic circumstances of rural areas that contribute to health disparities. Globalization, the shift to service economies, technological change, and resource depletion are economic forces identified by Williams and Cutchin that have generated "restructuring" processes, impoverishing many rural places. Population shifts to more urban areas have left the poorest and most vulnerable behind. Second, rural places exist within a larger political context where an urban bias in the distribution of health care resources has dominated. Third, the cultural character of rural places is tremendously varied, and appropriate provision of health promotion and health care takes this cultural diversity into account. The geographic remoteness of rural places coupled with their universal characteristics underlies problems with provider supply, distribution and availability, recruitment and retention, and accessibility for the provision of health care to meet the needs of rural populations.[2] All of these factors are implicated in the more severe nature of health problems that plague residents of rural areas. Although the traditional approach to addressing rural health problems has been to try to increase access to health services, experts are calling for more emphasis on a public/population health approach to the health needs of rural sub-populations, recognizing the need for geographically and culturally sensitive approaches to modifying health behaviors in combination with the provision of health services.[3]

Paradoxically, in contrast to the universals identified, drawing on Halfacree,[4] Williams and Cutchin argue that the particular health care problems of any specific rural place represent a unique combination of geographic and social variables that generates highly local circumstances, and these circumstances need to be explored with residents and understood holistically for successful care provision.

The nature of rural America and the challenge of providing comprehensive health care to rural Americans follows this more universal pattern. The U.S. Census in 2000 estimated that 20 percent of the U.S. population lives in rural areas;[5] in 2007 the estimate for the rural (non-metropolitan) population was 17 percent, spread across 80 percent of the land area.[6] Although the vast majority of those living in rural areas are classified as White (non-Hispanic), 18 percent of the rural population is minority.[7]

From a cultural perspective, data from 2002 showed that three times as many minorities in rural areas lived in poverty as compared to rural Whites (non-Hispanic).[8] As of 2002, among African-Americans, who represent the largest of the rural minority populations, one-third were poor, compared to 13 percent of Whites.[9] Among Native Americans, the only minority group with a greater presence in non-metro than in metro counties,[7] a percentage similar to that of African-Americans were poor.[9] Although most Hispanics reside in large metropolitan areas, the presence of persons of Hispanic background has doubled in rural areas since 1990,[10] and 25 percent of them are poor when compared to rural (non-Hispanic) Whites. Asians make up the smallest minority in rural areas, and their poor make up a lesser percentage than that of rural Whites (non-Hispanic).[9] Asians are the exception in another way; they are not geographically concentrated in particular regional areas and physical environments of the U.S. as are the other three minority populations. Additionally, according to the United States Department of

Agriculture Economic Research Service, "foreign-born immigrants add a relatively new dynamic to rural population growth: between 2000 and 2005, immigration accounted for almost 30 percent of non-metro population growth."[7]

Rural U.S. residents have poorer health than urban residents on many health indicators. This includes indicators of multiple chronic illnesses and activity limitation rates related to these illnesses, traffic-related injuries, suicide rates, dental problems, and risk factors, such as obesity, that implicate health-related lifestyle behaviors.[11]

Most rural areas in the United States are designated health professions shortage areas (HPSAs) for primary medical care.[12] The physician shortage in rural areas of the United States has been long-standing; presently only about 9 percent of U.S. physicians practice in rural areas, and the majority of these are prepared at a small number of comprehensive medical schools, mostly in the Midwest.[13] Twenty-two percent of nurse practitioners practice in rural areas. Nurses, pharmacists, dentists, and mental and behavioral health professionals also are all in undersupply in rural areas.[14] Although the Association of Schools of Allied Health Professions has proposed expansion of scope of practice for allied health professionals to help address rural shortages, several of these professions, including occupational and physical therapy, clinical laboratory sciences, dental hygiene, and respiratory therapy are experiencing or are expected to experience serious shortages by 2014.[15] Trained emergency medical service personnel are also in serious undersupply in rural areas.[12]

Since the new millennium, key Institute of Medicine (IOM) reports have focused on the issues of health care quality and safety in our health care system and strategies for addressing those concerns.[10,16] Concerns for quality and safety apply as much in rural health care as they do to metropolitan areas. However, the content of reports and the nature of recommendations for change, guidelines, regulations, and initiatives that have grown out of the patient safety movement are a good example of the urban bias that contributes to perpetuating disparities in care available to populations living in isolated rural areas. The emphasis of the patient safety movement has been largely on the nature of care in larger urban and suburban hospitals. There needs to be greater attention to the rural contexts of health care quality and patient safety issues.[17] Such contexts include the distinct nature of rural hospitals and the geographically dispersed and varied nature of rural ambulatory health care services.

Williams and Cutchin note that, increasingly, telemedicine is offered as a technical solution to addressing many of the issues surrounding the provision of health care in rural areas, but this solution creates its own "have-nots."[2] The potential for telemedicine to address rural health disparities through access to specialist services as well as continuing education of local health care providers currently is best exemplified by the Arizona Telemedicine Program, created in 1996 as a partnership between the Arizona State Legislature and the University of Arizona Health Sciences Center in Tucson. It has its own telecommunications network with 65 direct links and 85 links through affiliates throughout the state, which include many remote Native American health services sites as well as State Department of Corrections rural prison health care sites.[18] However, the resources and scope of this program far surpass what is available throughout most of the U.S.

It is often said that the best place for interprofessional team training in the health care professions is in rural areas. [A similar argument has been made that rural settings have certain advantages as test sites for quality improvement efforts.[17]] The prevalence of unmet needs and the scarcity of health care personnel necessitating use of all available resources in a cooperative and coordinated fashion provide ample opportunities for students to both observe and enhance teamwork and to provide some of the needed services in physically and culturally diverse rural settings. In fact, under the Health Resource Service Administration (HRSA), federal programs for interprofessional training in the health professions in the United States since the 1970s have targeted rural areas. This has been done with the hope of recruiting and retaining future health professionals to practice in rural areas and through the training programs, indirectly improving the quality of health care, especially with prevention, health promotion, and screening services. Notably, these programs have included Area Health Education Centers (AHECs), geriatric education centers (GECs), and rural interdisciplinary training, the latter culminating in the Quentin Burdick Rural Training Program. Unfortunately, the Burdick program has completely lost its funding in the current federal administration, while others have been repeatedly threatened or have lost their funding intermittently.

The contents of this book, rooted in the experience of those who deliver health care and interprofessional team training in rural environments in the United States, illustrate the variety of universal rural issues relevant to effective interprofessional care and training identified by Williams and Cutchin and successfully capture how those universal issues play out as they are uniquely mixed in a variety of rural U.S. localities and cultures.

The book begins with a general introduction to the field of rural health IPE and practice. One chapter in the introduction, unusual for this type of book, is focused on IPE and the common good. The authors explore the cognitive and moral framework required to motivate individual faculty, administrators, and, in turn, students, of various health professions, as well as the educational and professional organizations they are a part of, to learn and work together to serve the common good of their patients and society. Although not made specific to the book's rural focus, the chapter seems particularly relevant to inequity issues of rural care provision and health care training to serve rural populations. This chapter effectively frames the moral and ethical context for numerous chapters describing specific experiences of rural health care and training in the book. Another chapter addresses the limitations of current accreditation guidelines for fostering interprofessional learning in health professions curricula. Other issues raised by these introductory chapters focus on theories of IPE, assessing interprofessional competencies, promoting interprofessional practice in rural settings, and engaging faculty in interprofessional scholarship, education, and service.

In a recent article discussing the foci for IPE, Barr adds a fourth focus to three that previously have been identified (preparing individuals for collaborative practice, learning to work in teams, and developing services to improve care). The fourth focus is to improve the quality of life in communities. Barr noted that this focus has much in common with the community–campus partnerships movement and with service learning.[19] The second section in this book places rural IPE squarely in a community context, and various chapters explore the dynamics of relationships between educational institutions and the communities where interprofessional learning takes place, always emphasizing the partnership status and "give back" that rural, underserved communities need and deserve as part of the exchange that transpires around student learning. There has been much pressure on federally funded IPE programs' evaluation to show that these programs make a difference in patient outcomes. The rural model of community-embedded IPE has clear potential to demonstrate these linkages, as many chapters of this book illustrate.

The third section of the book brings attention to the diverse local contexts, including cultural contexts, rural care, and training from a variety of perspectives. One chapter focuses on how federally funded Area Health Education Centers (AHECs) have fostered rural interprofessional training. A chapter in Section Four provides a specific example of how an academic health center has used AHECs statewide to organize rural interprofessional training. In Section Three, one chapter provides important insights into how Wagner's chronic illness model, with a focus on diabetes care, can be adapted to a rural setting to improve outcomes.

Gross under-representation of minorities in the health care workforce is an important issue in rural settings, as it is more broadly, with the greatest disparities for Native American health personnel. One chapter in Section Three calls attention to a successful effort to prepare Hispanic and Native American occupational therapists. Other chapters in Section Three and Section Four illustrate how a particular isolated Native American community has built onsite health services and resources that are sensitive to the unique needs and culture of the community and how a culturally sensitive model of IPE has been integrated into that setting. Other chapters throughout the book, especially others in Section Four on "Better Practice Exemplars," also contain excellent examples of culturally sensitive interprofessional training and care. One chapter each in Section Three and Section Four, respectively, reminds us of the possibilities for extending training into remote areas through the use of telehealth technology and the important role of health literacy in improving health promotion among culturally diverse rural populations.

The timing of this book is an important reminder of the continuing need for leadership in resolving health care disparities in rural communities and the potential for interprofessional care and training to contribute to addressing those health disparities. The contents of the book repeatedly demonstrate what can be accomplished through health care services tailored to unique rural settings and populations as well as university-rural community partnerships for service provision and interprofessional student team training experiences. It keeps attention focused on the values and contributions of rural interprofessional training when the funding of interprofessional team training has mostly shifted to a focus on patient safety in the context of institutional, and usually urban, settings.

A final important reminder of what it takes to prepare health care professionals for a future of greater collaboration and to deliver truly patient-centered, team-oriented care is suggested by the collective authorship of the book. A great deal of the literature on IPE and practice is generated by or focuses on the two dominant health professions of medicine and nursing, whereas the health professions collectively encompass many more discrete fields of expertise, without which the quality of health care individuals and populations receive would be greatly compromised. This is certainly true in rural areas in the United States where the professions are challenged together to meet the health and health-related needs of diverse rural populations. The authors of this book represent the diverse health professions of physical therapy, occupational therapy, pharmacy, social work, physician assistants, library science, and health educators, as well as medicine and nursing. Many of the chapters are written in partnership with representatives of the communities described, as well as leaders in health advocacy groups. Collectively, their contributions capture what rural health care leadership for IPE and practice in the United States is all about.

Madeline H. Schmitt, PhD, RN, FAAN, FNAP
Editor, North American Division
Journal of Interprofessional Care
Professor Emeritus
University of Rochester School of Nursing
Rochester, NY

REFERENCES

1. Canadian Health Services Research Foundation. Rural health research in the Canadian Institutes of Health Research. Available at: http://www.chsrf.ca/final_research/commissioned_research/programs/pdf/hidg/pong.pdf. Accessed August 22, 2008.
2. Williams AM, Cutchin MP. The rural context of health care provision. *J Interprof Care*. 2002;16(2):107-115.
3. Hartley D. Rural health disparities, population health, and rural culture. *Am J Public Health*. 2004;94(10):1675-1678.
4. Halfacree K. Locality and social representation: space, discourse, and alternative definitions of the rural. *J Rural Studies*. 1993;9(1):23-37.
5. U.S. Department of Transportation, Federal Highway Administration. Census 2000 Population Statistics. Available at: http://www.fhwa.dot.gov/planning/census/cps2k.htm. Accessed March 23, 2008.
6. United States Department of Agriculture, Economic Research Service. Briefing room, rural population and migration. October 25, 2007. Available at: http://www.ers.usda.gov/Briefing/Population/. Accessed March 23, 2008.
7. United States Department of Agriculture, Economic Research Service. Amber Waves. April 2007. Available at: http://www.ers.usda.gov/AmberWaves/April07/Features/Population.htm. Accessed March 23, 2008.
8. United States Department of Agriculture, Economic Research Service. Rural poverty at a glance. Available at: http://www.ers.usda.gov/publications/rdrr100/rdrr100.pdf. Accessed March 23, 2008.

9. Probst JC. Minorities in rural America: An overview of population characteristics. South Carolina Rural Health Research Center, University of South Carolina. 2002. Available at: http://rhr.sph.sc.edu/report/MinoritiesInRuralAmerica.pdf. Accessed March 23, 2008.

10. Institute of Medicine. *Crossing the Quality Chasm: A New Health System for the 21st Century.* Washington, DC: National Academy Press; 2001.

11. National Rural Health Association. Health disparities in rural populations: An introduction. May 2006. Available at: http://www.nrharural.org/advocacy/sub/policybriefs/HlthDisparity.pdf. Accessed March 23, 2008.

12. National Organization of State Offices of Rural Health. National rural health issues. September 2006. Available at: http://www.nosorh.org/pdf/Rural_Impact_Study_States_IT.pdf. Accessed March 23, 2008.

13. Rabinowitz HK, Diamond JJ, Markham FW, Wortman JR. Medical school programs to increase the rural physician supply: A systematic review and projected impact of widespread replication. *Acad Med.* 2008;83(3):235-243.

14. Institute of Medicine. *Quality through collaboration: The future of rural health care.* Washington, DC: National Academies Press; 2005.

15. Association of Schools of Allied Health Professions. Health care in America. *Trends.* May 2006. Available at: http://www.asahp.org/trends/2006/May.pdf. Accessed March 28, 2008.

16. Institute of Medicine. *To Err is Human.* National Academies Press; 2000.

17. The National Advisory Committee on Rural Health and Human Services. Health care quality: The rural context. 2003. Available at: http://ruralcommittee.hrsa.gov/QR03.htm#execsum. Accessed March 22, 2008.

18. Arizona State Senate. Issue Brief: Telemedicine in Arizona. October 20, 2006. Available at: http://www.azleg.state.az.us/briefs/Senate/TELEMEDICINE.pdf. Accessed March 22, 2008.

19. Barr H. Interprofessional education: The fourth focus. *J Interprof Care.* 2007;21(S2): 40-50.

SECTION 1

Introduction to Interprofessional Education and Practice

CHAPTER 1

Interprofessional Education: Context, Complexity, and Challenge

Gail M. Jensen, PhD, PT, FAPTA
Robin Ann Harvan, EdD
Charlotte Brasic Royeen, PhD, OT, FAOTA

INTRODUCTION

The changing and challenging landscape of health care provides the environment in which graduates of health professions education will work. Graduates face a more diverse patient population, a growing number of people living with chronic illness, increasing rates of obesity and diabetes among our youth, and escalating health care costs.[1] Once graduates move into clinical practice, they are often asked to work in interprofessional teams, yet these young health professionals often have little or no experience in team-based skills. How do we prepare graduates who have the competencies and skills to work in these challenging times? The response to this question continues to be the need and call for reform in health professions education.

The creation of this book represents a collective response from a group of health professionals (educators, clinicians, and community health center leaders) to create a resource for interprofessional education and practice and a stimulus for continued discussion, debate, and action in the field. Chapter 1 sets the context for the book as we address the following: (a) the key events that are triggering the national conversation in the United States and focus on interprofessional education and (b) the background and structure for this book.

Interprofessional education and interprofessional collaboration have not often found a place in the education and practice of health. . . . Each profession owns a professional jurisdiction or scope of practice, which impacts delivery of services. This silo-like division of professional responsibilities is rarely naturally nor cohesively integrated in a manner which meets the needs of both clients and the professionals (p. 9).[2]

We all know well the "silo culture" of health professions education as different units compete for resources across a campus. The building of a cohesive, shared approach to education and practice is challenging. We hope this book provides both a stimulus and resource for change.

INTERPROFESSIONAL EDUCATION IN THE UNITED STATES: KEY EVENTS

Numerous reports conclude that health professionals are neither adequately prepared in the academic or clinical settings to address shifts in the national's patient population nor educated together or trained in team-based skills that would enhance their ability to work as part of interprofessional teams.[3–7] Furthermore, these reports highlight the critical areas of practice that are in need of transformative educational reform.

The Institute of Medicine (IOM) report on *Health Professions Education: A Bridge to Quality*[6] makes the case that education reform is critical to enhancing the quality of health care in the United States. This report represented the third phase of the IOM's Quality of Health Care in America project that began in 1998. The IOM's Committee on the Quality of Health Care in America focused on the first two phases of the quality initiative and authored the reports *To Err Is Human: Building a Safer Health System*[4] and *Crossing the Quality Chasm: A New Health System for the 21st Century.*[5] These reports documented the nature of the quality problem and laid the foundation for a vision of transforming the health care system. This vision of transformation is recommended to close the chasm that exists between what we know is good quality care and what actually exists in practice. The first two phases of the IOM's quality initiative focused on developing a vision for health care system transformation. The IOM's Committee on the Quality of Health Care in America was charged to

1. Review and synthesize findings in the literature pertaining to the quality of health care in the health care system;
2. Develop a communication strategy for raising the awareness of the general public and key stakeholders of quality of care concerns and opportunities for improvement;

3. Articulate a policy framework that provides positive incentives to improve quality and foster accountability;
4. Identify characteristics and factors that enable or encourage providers, health care organizations, health plans, and communities to continuously improve the quality of care;
5. Develop a research agenda in areas of continued uncertainty.

The first report, *To Err Is Human: Building a Safer Health System*, focused on a specific quality of care concern—patient safety. According to the committee, "to err is human, but errors can be prevented ... safety is a critical first step in improving quality of care." This report sets an agenda and comprehensive approach for reducing medical errors and improving patient safety through the design of a safer health care system.[4]

The recommendations in this first report present a comprehensive approach organized according to the following themes:

1. Establishing a *national focus* to create leadership, research, tools and protocols to enhance the knowledge base about safety;
2. Identifying and learning from errors through immediate and strong *mandatory reporting efforts* and encouragement of voluntary efforts, both with the aim of making sure the system continues to be made safer for patients;
3. *Raising standards and expectations* for improvement in safety through the actions of oversight organizations, group purchasers, and professional groups;
4. *Creating safety systems* inside health care organizations through the implementation of safe practices at the delivery level. This level is the ultimate target of all the recommendations.

The second and final report of the IOM's Quality of Health Care in America Committee, *Crossing the Quality Chasm: a New Health System for the 21st Century,*[5] focused more broadly on quality-related issues and how the health care delivery system can be redesigned to innovate and improve care. The recommendations in this second report, organized according to the following themes, provided a strategic direction for establishing aims and redesigning the health care delivery system of the 21st century to ensure that all Americans receive care that is safe, effective, patient centered, timely, efficient, and equitable:

1. Formulating new rules to redesign and improve care;
2. Taking the first steps to providing evidence-based care that is responsive to individual patient's needs and preferences and focusing greater attention on the development of care processes for the common priority conditions that affect many people;

3. Building organizational supports for change;
4. Establishing a new environment for care in four major areas—the infrastructure that supports the dissemination and application of new clinical knowledge and technologies, the information technology infrastructure, payment policies, and preparation of the health care workforce.

The preparation of the health care workforce and the need to reform clinical education was the focus of the third phase of the IOM's quality initiative. Upon examination and review of the literature on clinical education, particularly medical education, the second report stated that "despite the changes that have been made [in undergraduate medical education], the fundamental approach to clinical education has not changed since the Flexner report of 1910."[5]

The specific recommendation in the second report that prompted the establishment of the IOM's Committee on the Health Professions Education Summit and subsequent recommendations in the third report, *Health Professions Education: A Bridge to Quality*,[6] was as follows:

> *Recommendation 12: A multidisciplinary summit of leaders within the health professions should be held to discuss and develop strategies for (1) restructuring clinical education to be consistent with the principles of the 21st century health system throughout the continuum of undergraduate, graduate, and continuing education for medical, nursing, and other professional training programs; and (2) assessing the implications of these changes for provider credentialing programs, funding, and sponsorship of education programs for health professions.*

Health Professions Education Summit

With this recommendation in mind, the IOM established the Committee on the Health Professions Education Summit that included members with expertise in academic and continuing allied health, medical, nursing, and pharmacy education; multidisciplinary clinical training; health professions licensure and oversight processes; professional credentialing; and health care delivery and quality. In preparation for the summit, the committee reviewed the *Quality Chasm* chapter on "Preparing the Workforce." This chapter examined three specific issues: clinical training and education, regulation of health professions, and legal liability issues.[5]

The *Quality Chasm* report identified patient-centered concepts for the delivery of competent care in a redesigned health care system. In addition, the

Quality Chasm report also addressed key skills such as transparent communication, collaboration among health professionals, and the use of evidence in clinical decision making for all health professionals. The IOM's Committee on the Health Professions Education Summit used these patient-centered concepts and key skills along with review of other seminal reform efforts to generate a set of core competencies applicable to all health professions (Table 1-1).[5]

The Health Professions Education Summit convened over 150 national experts in health professions education, regulation, quality, health policy, and industry to discuss and develop strategies for restructuring health professions education to advance quality and better prepared health care professionals to practice in the 21st century health system. Table 1-2 lists the five

Table 1-1. Core Competencies for Health Professionals[5]

Provide Patient-Centered Care
Identify, respect, and care about patients' differences, values, preferences, and expressed needs; relieve pain and suffering; coordinate continuous care; listen to, clearly inform, communicate with, and education patients; share decision making and management; and continuously advocate disease prevention, wellness, and promotion of healthy lifestyles, including a focus on population health.

Work in Interdisciplinary Teams
Cooperate, collaborate, communicate, and integrate care in teams that is continuous and reliable.

Employ Evidence-Based Practice
Integrate best research with clinical expertise and patient values for optimum care, and participate in learning and research activities to the extent feasible.

Apply Quality Improvement
Identify errors and hazards in care; understand and implement basic safety design principles, such as standardization and simplification; continually understand and measure quality of care in terms of structure, process, and outcomes in relation to patient and community needs; and design and test interventions to change processes and systems of care, with the objective of improving quality.

Utilize Informatics
Communicate, manage knowledge, mitigate error, and support decision making using information technology.

Adapted from Institute of Medicine. *Crossing the Quality Chasm: A New Health System for the 21st Century.* Washington, DC: National Academy Press; 2001.

Table 1-2. Five Cross-Cutting Strategies for the Reform of Health Professions Education[6]

1. Build consensus around a core set of competencies with a shared definition of key terms and language.

2. Integrate core competencies into oversight processes (accreditation, licensing, and certification).

3. Motivate and support education leaders (from academic, continuing education, and practice settings, including consumers and students) and monitor the progress of educational reform efforts.

4. Develop evidence-based curricula and teaching approaches as they relate to the core set of competencies.

5. Develop faculty as teaching/learning experts in the core set of competencies.

Adapted from Institute of Medicine. *Health Professions Education: A Bridge to Quality.* Washington, DC: National Academy Press; 2003.

cross-cutting strategies for the reform of health professions education developed from this summit.[6]

Vision for Health Professions Education Transformation

In the *Bridge to Quality* report,[6] the IOM's Committee on the Health Professions Education Summit developed a comprehensive new vision for clinical education in the health professions that is centered on a commitment to, first and foremost, meeting patients' needs. The committee recommended the following overarching vision for all programs and institutions engaged in the education of health professionals:

All health professionals should be educated to deliver patient-centered care as members of interdisciplinary teams, emphasizing evidence-based practice, quality improvement approaches, and informatics.

The committee proposed the aforementioned set of five core competencies that all health clinicians should possess (Table 1-1),[5,6] regardless of their discipline, to meet the needs of the 21st century health care system. In the report, the committee recognized that these competencies are meant to be core, citing that there are many other competencies health professionals should possess, such as a commitment to lifelong learning, but believed those listed are the most relevant across the clinical disciplines. The committee believed that the overall goal is a competency-based education system that better prepares clinicians to meet the needs of patients and communities and the requirements of a changing health care system.

Although the IOM's reports provide strong recommendations for change,[4-7] the implementation of such changes in health professions education continues to emerge at a rather slow pace. Competition for scarce resources in higher education as well as health care dollars only reinforces the tendency for health professions to focus, promote, and protect their core identity in both higher education and practice settings. In addition, external incentives such as federal funding for interprofessional activities have never been robust but have decreased significantly in recent years, particularly for nonphysician health professions. One critical reform strategy identified at the Health Professions Education Summit is to motivate and support education leaders (from academic, continuing education, and practice settings, including consumers and students) and monitor the progress of educational reform efforts. This book is an example of implementing such a reform strategy where educators, clinicians, and community members came together to discuss and plan what is needed to promote patient-centered, quality care that focuses on interprofessional teamwork.

INTERPROFESSIONAL EDUCATION CONFERENCE AND BOOK CREATION: KEY EVENTS

In the Fall of 2006 a conference was held at the University of Colorado Health Sciences Center in Denver for leaders in rural interprofessional education and practice. This book is the result of this conference funded in part by a Health Resources Services Administration grant (no. 1D36HP03158, Circles of Learning: Community and Clinic as Interdisciplinary Classroom, a Quentin N. Burdick Interdisciplinary Training Project). The conference, entitled Leadership in Rural Health Interprofessional Education & Practice: A Working Conference for Leaders in Rural Health Care, gathered 38 leaders in rural interprofessional education and practice to discuss best practices and to develop strategies for impacting the future of rural health care. The conference focused on the challenges and successful strategies for interprofessional education and practice in rural and underserved communities. The conference was a combined effort for funding; Creighton University's Office of Interprofessional Scholarship, Service and Education, within the School of Pharmacy and Health Professions; and the Center for Health Policy and Ethics; and the University of Colorado's Health Sciences Center. Although the key focus of the conference was on interprofessional work, the other core competencies identified for all health professionals (patient-centered care, evidence-based practice, quality improvement, and the use of informatics) were also considered.

The working conceptual model for the conference focused on the integrative and interactive relationship between the practice environment in medically underserved areas and interprofessional education. The model in Figure 1-1 demonstrates the tightly integrated nature of these key concepts:

- Interprofessional education and practice is the foundation or critical building block for the conference. This includes a focus on the basic elements in health professions education: curriculum design, faculty

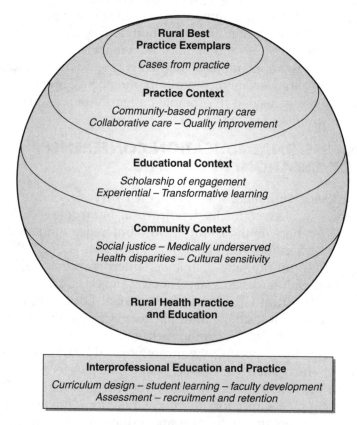

Figure 1-1

Conceptual model demonstrating the integrative and interactive relationships between practice in the medically underserved communities and interprofessional education.

development, assessment of student learning, and recruitment and retention of clinicians in underserved areas.

- Rural health practice and education provide the clinical context for interprofessional work.
- Community context is a critical aspect of education and practice in underserved areas. The issues of health disparities, cultural sensitivity and competence, and social justice are paramount.
- Educational context focuses on the role of faculty and students. The faculty role and reward system needs to embrace the scholarship of engagement that can emerge from study of this community work. Assessment of student learning in this rich experiential setting is critical and requires support of mixed methods to fully understand these transformative learning experiences.
- Practice context is the place where mutual needs of health educators and communities meet. The challenges of interprofessional work and collaborative care must be addressed.
- Rural best practice exemplars provide a structure for sharing the essential practical knowledge that is created from critical reflection on interprofessional work in a rural community setting.

This model was used to assist educators, clinicians, and community members in thinking more deeply about interprofessional education and practice.

BOOK OVERVIEW

The book is divided into six sections focused on (a) introduction to interprofessional education and practice, (b) community context applications, (c) practice context applications, (d) educational context applications, (e) best practice exemplars, and (f) future directions for interprofessional education and practice.

In Section 1, Introduction to Interprofessional Education and Practice, there are seven chapters that explore basic components in interprofessional education from expert commentaries and theoretical concepts to accreditation, assessment issues, and example educational strategies and frameworks. As visible in the model (Figure 1-1), this first section of the book provides the foundational elements for health professions education. This first chapter by the editors provides the grounding for the book as well as an overview of the historical summary of key interprofessional policy statements in the United States. Chapter 2 provides a reflective analysis on the critical importance of social justice and the common good in interprofessional work. Royeen, Terhaar, and Walsh describe the historical context of interprofessional education in accreditation and challenge us with their recommendations for the future in Chapter 3. In Chapter 4, the editors provide examples of how to connect theory to practice in interprofessional education. Coppard and colleagues focus on a critical element in interprofessional education, assessment of student learning, in Chapter 5. Chapter 6, by Roche, and Chapter 7, by Ryan Haddad and Doll, provide examples of successful strategies for implementing interprofessional education (IPE) in rural and underserved communities.

Application of critical educational concepts and foundational elements to an authentic environment is essential for student learning. The next three sections of the book explore three important contextual dimensions for application of the model (Figure 1-1): community, education, and clinical practice. Section 2, Community Context, contains five chapters that highlight different aspects of the academic–community interactions. In Chapter 8, Champ-Blackwell and Hartman outline the critical role of the librarian in rural outreach. Chapter 9 focuses on the cultural foundation that is essential in building interagency health delivery networks. This kind of network building requires skilled leadership. Lavin and colleagues provide a historical perspective of community development models as well as application of those models in practice in Chapter 10. Reynolds, in Chapter 11, explores the opportunities for service learning in interprofessional education and examples of the scholarship of engagement. This section ends with Chapter 12 by Velde on challenges and opportunities for promoting justice in rural communities.

Section 3, Practice Context, contains four chapters highlighting important elements that help build a successful community practice. In Chapter 13, Crowe, Burtner, and Torres-Aragon begin with a strong plea for building a diverse workforce. They provide strategies and recommendations for making this happen. Chapter 14 explores Campus–Community partnerships for rural health education. Swisher, in Chapter 15, gives us a sound rationale for specific focus and pedagogy that enhance student learning and professional formation as they struggle with issues of professional identity and socialization. The final chapter in this section, Chapter 16 by Doll and St. Cyr, is a reflective analysis of an example case from a Native American community where we have lessons learned from both challenging and successful strategies for practice in this community setting.

Section 4, Educational Context, is a cluster of five chapters each sharing a case example from education. Chapter 17, by Cummings, Bray, and Clay, describes a structural process and institutional/community support for building a successful interprofessional model that continues to improve diabetes outcomes. Cross and Doll in Chapter 18 share educational strategies for developing student leaders in IPE. Chapter 19, by Kosoko-Lasaki, is a description of a successful educational model and institutional structure for increasing diversity in health professions education. In Chapter 20, Ruebling and associates provide us with several ideas for building an interprofessional curriculum through collaborative teamwork. Chapter 21, by Sekerek and colleagues, addresses the use of telehealth as a tool for health care delivery in rural areas.

In Section 5, Best Practice, we have selected four innovative cases. In the first case, Chapter 22, Brandt and Halaas provide a macro view of the challenges and opportunities in an academic health center for promoting IPE. Pierce and colleagues in Chapter 23 demonstrate the success of a mental health model in rural Appalachia. In Chapter 24, Wells reflects on lessons learned from working in a rural ethnic community. Wilkin in Chapter 25 shares an innovative application of a health report card in a Native American community-based quality improvement project.

Section 6 revisits our initial question—How do we best prepare graduates to have the skills and competencies to work in a diverse and challenging health care system? In Chapter 26, Lyons challenges us to address critical needs in demonstrating outcomes in IPE and outlines strategies for future progress in interprofessional education and practice. Chapter 27 summarizes our progress in interprofessional education and poses critical issues and potential next steps for continued growth and development.

We challenge the reader to think about what can be done to promote good, interprofessional work in difficult times.

REFERENCES

1. Rubin ER, Schappert SL, eds. *Meeting Health Needs in the 21st Century*. Washington, DC: Association of Academic Health Centers; 2003.
2. D'Amour D, Oandasan I. Interprofessionality as the field of interprofessional practice and interprofessional education: an emerging concept. *J Interprof Care*. 2005; 1S:8–20.
3. O'Neil EH. *Recreating Health Professional Practice for a New Century*. San Francisco, CA: Pew Health Professions Commission; 1998.
4. Institute of Medicine. *To Err is Human: Building a Safer Health System*. Washington, DC: National Academy Press; 2000.

5. Institute of Medicine. *Crossing the Quality Chasm: A New Health System for the 21st Century.* Washington, DC: National Academy Press; 2001.
6. Institute of Medicine. *Health Professions Education: A Bridge to Quality.* Washington, DC: National Academy Press; 2003.
7. Institute of Medicine. *Priority Areas for National Action: Transforming Health Care Quality.* Washington, DC: National Academy Press; 2003.

CHAPTER 2

Interprofessional Education and the Common Good: A Reflective Analysis

Gail M. Jensen, PhD, PT, FAPTA
Teresa M. Cochran, PT, DPT, GCS, MA
Caroline Goulet, PhD, PT
Brenda M. Coppard, PhD, OT, FAOTA

INTRODUCTION

There is a renewed interest and call for professionalism across the health professions. How do we best prepare health professions students for current and future roles in meeting societal needs? Although the traditional focus in health professions education is on promoting good or promoting beneficence with individual patients, we argue that there is a need to expand the concept of beneficence to the role of health professions in working in underserved communities where resources are scarce and health professions must collaborate in the delivery of care. In this chapter we use a framework of organizational ethics based on three realms of ethics—individual, institutional, and societal—to take a critically reflective look at interprofessional education (IPE) in the health professions.

The changing and challenging landscape of health care provides the environment in which graduates of health professions education will work. Graduates face a more diverse patient population, a growing number of people living with chronic illness, increasing rates of obesity and diabetes among our youth, and escalating health care costs. Again, we pose this critical question: How do we prepare graduates who have the competencies and skills to work in these challenging times? The response to this question continues to be the need and call for reform in health professions education. Numerous reports conclude that health professionals are neither adequately prepared in the academic or clinical settings to address shifts in the nation's patient population nor educated together or trained in team-based skills that would enhance their ability to work as part of interprofessional teams.[1–4]

What must our institutions and organizations look like to support IPE? What kind of development activities are necessary for academic and clinical faculty to work in IPE and practice settings? What kind of learning environment and learning experiences are necessary to ensure that graduates can meet these societal needs? As health professionals we are familiar with the concept of promoting good or beneficence with our patients. Professional codes of ethics are grounded in the concept of first, do no harm but promote good or beneficence. In this chapter we argue that there is a need to expand the concept of beneficence by using a systems model to engage in a critical self-reflective look at health professions education across individuals, organizations/institutions, and society. The reflective analysis is done with a focus on the value of beneficence, or doing good, and on the need to "rethink learning" because learning is the essential outcome in health professions education. Green and Luke identify that Dewey argued that the most basic questions about learning include who is learning what, for what purposes, under what conditions, and with what educational, social, cultural outcomes, and consequences for learners, communities, and nations.[5] We begin the chapter with an overview of the organizational ethics framework for the analysis of interprofessional health professions education. This is followed by a critical self-reflective look at each of the levels: individuals (students, academic and clinical faculty, and administrators), organizations, and society.

ORGANIZATIONAL ETHICS FRAMEWORK FOR ANALYSIS

Why use an ethics framework to take a critical look at IPE? Health professionals have a long history of having a social contract of both responsibility and accountability to meet societal needs. In the health professions, practitioners frequently work with patients who are vulnerable and, in need of help. The health professional possesses knowledge and skill that the patient needs. Patients trust professionals to be competent and to do good work for them as a part of a special fiduciary relationship.[6] Professionals have also been the target of scandals and cited for highly unethical behavior that has led to public mistrust.[7] Professional schools are the "portals to professional life" and as such have responsibility for the "reliable formation" of students. Although there is increased awareness and interest in the importance of ethics and human values in professional preparation, there is also a dramatic loss of public confidence in the authority of health professionals, their ability to self-police, and their authenticity as collaborators in societal efforts to improve the health and well-being of all people.[7] Health professionals, particularly nonphysician health professionals, practice in a range of health care settings from institutions to home care and communities. The interdependence of patients, professionals, institutions, communities, policymakers, and other stakeholders in this larger organizational and societal context has an effect on health professions education and practice.

The organizational ethics model is based on three realms or levels: individual, organizational, and societal (Figure 2-1).[8,9] At the level of the individual, the focus is on doing good or beneficence of individuals. One may be weighing the relative importance of various values and needs (e.g., physical, emotional, mental). The level also deals with weighing and balancing values/goods between individuals. In our case we use the individual level to explore individual stakeholders in IPE (students, faculty, administrators, and clinicians). At the organizational level we focus on the organizations in which IPE takes place, such as academic and health care institutions. The primary aim of organizational beneficence is addressing the question, what is the organizational good? How does the organization have systems and structures that respect and promote human dignity and how does the organization attend to

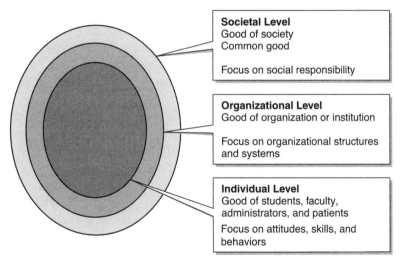

Figure 2-1
The three realms of an organizational framework for ethics.[8,9] Adapted from Glaser J. *Three Realms of Ethics*. Kansas City, MO: Sheed and Ward; 1994 and Glaser J. Three realms of ethics: an integrating map for the future. In: Purtilo R, Jensen G, Royeen C, eds. *Educating for Moral Action: A Sourcebook in Health and Rehabilitation Ethics*. Philadelphia: FA Davis; 2005.

and promote the common good of the society? Organizational goods must also attend to the organization as well as using the individual to represent the individual health profession. The third dimension is the societal level. Here the central focus is on the common good of society. The common good is what we would see as promoting the well-being of a community. This would include community safety, the integrity of its basic institutions and practices, and the preservation of respect for human dignity.[8] At this level we look at the profession's role in promoting the common good.

IPE AND INDIVIDUALS

At the individual level where students enter professional preparation, they are quickly introduced to the culture of their chosen profession. The social-ization process of students begins immediately as they interact with faculty and fellow students in the professions education environment. Here the atti-tudes, beliefs, and behaviors begin to take shape in the professional culture. Students in academic health science campuses quickly learn that there are of-ten differences across health professions for resource allocation of space, number of faculty, and staff support. The emphasis in the types of profes-sional knowledge, whether you have more of a social science background or a physical science background, can also contribute to a perception that your professional knowledge is not as rigorous. For example, students may per-form differently in foundation science courses depending on the depth and breadth of their prerequisite coursework and how that coursework is inte-grated into the professional curriculum.[10,11] This can lead to an early percep-tion among students that some disciplines are "smarter" than others or have more important or prestigious knowledge.

Both academic and clinical faculty are critical players in the early social-ization of health professions students. Faculty are powerful role models, and the extent to which they value or devalue their colleagues through attitudes, beliefs, behaviors, and actions has a profound effect on students.[7,12] Many faculty may see knowledge transmission as paramount and not realize that it is the implicit aspects of what they do in classroom and laboratories that has a long-lasting effect on student learning.[13] For example, physical therapy fac-ulty members who express to students that occupational therapists are not qualified to work with patients with upper extremity musculoskeletal prob-lems have just planted seeds for potentially noncollaborative attitudes within their students. Clinical faculty are also powerful role models as they interact with students in patient care settings. How clinicians interact with their colleagues in the delivery of patient-centered care can have a lasting impression with students.

Health professions educational administrators as individuals can have a profound influence on the behaviors and actions of their faculty and students. Do their words and actions support an educational culture of collaboration or competition? Do their administrative structures provide opportunities for department heads to work together to solve problems? Is there a culture that supports respect for the values and needs of individuals and the individual health disciplines?

Rethinking Learning for Individuals in IPE

Professional socialization is a critical component of professional education that begins with the admissions process. If we are serious about the importance and the "good" that will come from integrating the concept of IPE as part of the professional socialization of students, then we must ensure that individual faculty and administrators have the appropriate knowledge, skills, and attitudes to teach and lead.

We propose that development activities are necessary and needed for both health professions faculty and administrators. Steinert[14] in her article on IPE and faculty development argues that faculty development initiatives must bring about change at both the individual and organizational level. "Clearly, faculty members play a critical role in the teaching and learning of IPE and they must be prepared to meet this challenge."[14] She proposes seven development approaches for promoting IPE (Table 2-1). The three core areas of content for these development initiatives include IPE, teaching and learning, and leadership and organizational change.

In addition to engaging in IPE faculty development, administrators also need leadership competencies that facilitate the growth and development of IPE. These competencies include the ability to (a) develop a shared vision and focused attention to a shared goal, (b) communicate a sense of purpose and meaning, (c) foster collaboration and cooperation, and, perhaps most importantly, (d) build trust within the organization.[14,15]

Students follow the lead of their leaders. Students also need structure or a blueprint for their interprofessional learning. Two core competencies from the document *Health Professions Education: A Bridge to Quality*[2] are central for grounding the learning outcomes for students:

1. Provide patient-centered care: Identify, respect, and care about patients' differences, values and preferences, and expressed needs; relieve pain

Table 2-1. Seven Approaches for Faculty Development in IPE[14]

1. Aim to facilitate change at the individual and organizational levels.

2. Target diverse stakeholders.

3. Address major content areas:

   a. IPE and collaborative patient-centered care;

   b. Teaching and learning challenges and opportunities in IPE;

   c. Leadership and organizational change.

4. Use a variety of settings, including both informal and formal settings, and strategies.

5. Model the principles and practices of IPE and collaborative practice in development activities.

6. Integrate principles of effective teaching and educational design.

7. Consider use of a dissemination model for implementation.

Source: Steinert Y. Learning together to teach together: interprofessional education and faculty development. *J Interprof Care.* 2005;15:60–75; 2005.

and suffering; coordinate continuous care; listen to, clearly inform, communicate with, and educate patients; share decision making and management; and continuously advocate disease prevention, wellness, and promotion of healthy lifestyles, including a focus on population health.

2. Work in interdisciplinary teams: Cooperate, collaborate, communicate, and integrate care in teams to ensure that care is continuous and reliable. This means students should be able to describe one's role and responsibilities to other professions; recognize the limitations of their role and competence, recognize and respect the roles, and responsibilities of other professions; work together with other professions to effect change and resolve conflict in the delivery of care; and enter into interdependent relationships with other professions.[15]

Finally, perhaps the most important learning outcome for students is the ability to engage in critical self-reflection. Students need to develop metacognitive strategies to be aware of their thinking or habits of mind. This is a critical skill for all health professionals. Critical self-reflection on one's practice can lead students to engage in higher order thinking and the ability to exercise judgment in uncertain situations.[16] Learners who are challenged by their peers in collaborative team settings as found in IPE need these reflective skills. Also, reflection done in an interprofessional group provides an opportunity to make the reflections public across peers. This public sharing becomes an opportunity for a "reflection on the reflection" and can lead to growth of the individual as well as growth of the team.

IPE AND ORGANIZATIONS

Although most often individuals are held responsible for promoting good or allowing harm to occur, organizations are the places in which we do most of our work. Organizations have commitments, claims, relationships, and responsibilities for promoting good. The future growth and success of IPE depend to a large extent on how successful individuals are working within educational, health, and professional organizations.

We start with an examination of the structure of the educational organization. In much of health professions education, individual programs are often physically housed in different buildings on a campus or different floors. The organizational structure of the university usually allows the larger health professions to have their own school (e.g., school of medicine, dentistry, pharmacy, or nursing), whereas the other smaller health professions may be together in a school of health professions. The health professions across schools may indirectly or directly compete for resources. The reporting structure of administrators in the school is usually divided across health disciplines where faculty hold primary appointments in their discipline. Budgets are generally structured around single disciplines and core activities of those disciplines. The role and reward structure of the department, school, and educational institution (university or college) is generally based on individual competence and productivity within a discipline, not interdisciplinary work.

Although the accrediting agencies for the health professions have some criteria that address the importance of interprofessional teams, these criteria generally are more about providing students with opportunities to participate in interprofessional teams than about focusing on core competencies and robust learning outcomes. Part of the challenge with accreditation and IPE is that IPE is often poorly understood.[17]

Within the department, curriculum is the organizational structure that provides the guiding map for the courses, learning experiences, and learning outcomes. Curriculum design reflects the input from many difference sources, from accreditation agencies to licensure standards, clinicians, professional associations, faculty, and students.[18] Perhaps the most critical element of curriculum design and continued evolution of the curriculum is understanding the critical importance of the presence or absence of faculty-shared beliefs and values as a basis for deliberation and design decisions.[19] One of the core goals in IPE is collaborative practice, yet if faculty and administrators do not share that belief, moving forward with IPE will be difficult. Often, we have a few champion faculty within disciplines who value collaboration and are not threatened by the notion of sharing resources, including time with other professions. Although these champion faculty cannot transform an organization, they are critical resources in the curriculum deliberative process because they challenge strong traditions in health professions curricula that maintain our "silo" mentality. A silo mentality keeps us working only within our own disciplinary perspective, i.e., disciplinary silos.

Rethinking Learning for Organizations in IPE

Organizations are the structure in which most of our work occurs in health professions education. If we believe that IPE is an important "organizational good," then what must we do to promote change? We suggest that educational organizations in the health professions should aspire to become "learning organizations." Learning organizations are defined as

> *Organizations where people continually expand their capacity to create results they truly desire, where new and expansive patterns of thinking are nutured, where collective aspiration is set free, and where people are continually learning to see the whole together* (p. 3).[20]

Learning organizations need to have a high capacity for learning and for implementing change. Innovative learning organizations engage in systems thinking in that they see how the key elements of the system connect and work interdependently. Problems are not caused by someone else but need to be recognized through feedback and analysis systems. In trying to implement IPE, seeing the health professions as an interdependent system within the educational organization versus disciplinary silos would be an important first step.[20,21]

Organizations depend on the learning of individuals, but that does not ensure organizational learning.[20] Organizations need to build a shared vision and engage in team learning. How is this done? Leaders in learning organizations are responsible for building organizations where people expand their ability to learn, clarify, and contribute to the vision. Leaders are seen as designers of a shared vision, stewards of the collective vision, and teachers who are fostering learning within the organization to develop this systematic understanding of the organization.[20] If we see the role of educational organizations in the health professions to work toward a more collaborative, interdependent model of care delivery, then we need educational leaders at all levels from curriculum chairs, to directors of clinical education, department heads, and academic administrators to aspire to becoming learning organizations.

IPE AND SOCIETY

This third level of analysis, the societal level, deals with the common good of society. Remember, as defined earlier, the common good represents the good life, how we would all like to live in safety and well-being.[9] Glaser citing Hardin shares a simple story of how the common good can conflict with the good of individuals.[22] Think of a group of herdsmen who share a grazing pasture. As long as there is enough pasture to feed the cattle, each herder is satisfied without jeopardizing the common good. If at some point there is overgrazing from individuals increasing the size of their herds but only looking at the impact the increase has on his individual herd, it will be difficult to identify and resolve the problem. Eventually, the pasture will be ruined and not meet anyone's needs.

What does society need from the health professions? Are we able to meet the common good health care needs of our citizens? Patients in the United States are becoming more diverse, are aging with increasing numbers of chronic diseases, and at the same are more likely to seek health information. The number of uninsured adults continues to grow. Uninsured adults have less access to care, are less likely to get needed care or preventive care, are less likely to manage chronic conditions, and are more likely to have poor health outcomes.[23] Once in practice, health professionals are asked to work in interdisciplinary teams often in the area of chronic disease, but the depth and breadth of health professions education in IPE varies across institutions.[2]

What is the interdependence of health professions when it comes to health care goods? Are we more likely to focus on our internal professional needs and defend our turf when it comes to societal needs in health care, or do we work to form coalitions that bring about the most good for patients? Are we individual herders on the common pasture who are only interested in increasing the size of our own herd regardless of what may happen to that resource?

Rethinking Learning for IPE and the Common Good

All health professions share the responsibility for promoting good for their individual patients as well as for promoting "good" or the health of society. Sullivan[7] argues that "professional schools have too long held out to their students a notion of expert knowledge that remains abstracted from context." He challenges professional education to promote the professional life where the professional is working toward improving the quality of life, particularly for those in most need. To that end, he encourages professional schools to focus on developing habits of mind:

> Since professional schools are the portals to professional life, they bear much of the responsibility for the reliable formation in their students of integrity of professional purpose and identity. In addition to enabling students to become competent practitioners, professional schools always must provide ways to induct student into the distinctive habits of mind . . . basic knowledge must be expanded to include an understanding of the moral and social ecology within which students will practice.[24]

The context that is critical for all health professions students is understanding the meaning of social responsibility and concern for the common good in health care. Promoting the common good in health care requires health professionals to work together as stewards of scarce resources to deliver quality care, to take responsibility for shaping health policy that ensures access to care and promotes health. A central challenge for health professionals in understanding the common good is the ability to see the multiple dimensions of common good, particularly in underserved communities. Although health care may be the focus for the health professions student or IPE team, in underserved communities it is only one of several needs, including basic needs such as housing, safety, and education (Figure 2-2). Furthermore, the health care team needs to realize that resources in health care are scarce and the ability to promote good or beneficence is a distributive justice dilemma. Members of the health care team in IPE must be adaptive and flexible in meeting diverse needs. Ideally, health professionals must see their role as moral agents in assuming the responsibility and authority for taking action in promoting the common good in health care.

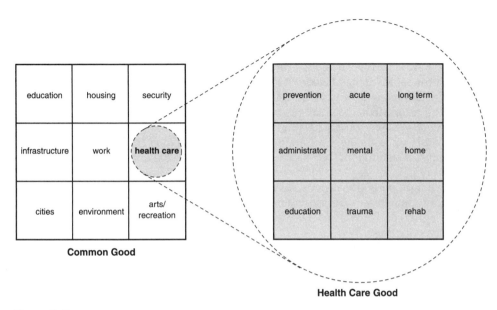

Figure 2-2
A description of the possible "competing" elements that underlie the concept of common good in communities and health care.[8,9] Adapted from Glaser J. *Three Realms of Ethics.* Kansas City, MO: Sheed and Ward; 1994 and Glaser J. Three realms of ethics: an integrating map for the future. In: Purtilo R, Jensen G, Royeen C, eds. *Educating for Moral Action: A Sourcebook in Health and Rehabilitation Ethics.* Philadelphia: FA Davis; 2005.

CONCLUSION

IPE is an essential pedagogical strategy for preparing health professionals for present and future practice. Reform in health professions education in the United States is a complicated and challenging process. We believe that IPE is the key to changing what is to what could be. Working together as a community of health professionals to create a healthier society requires that we also begin learning together. IPE is a tool for addressing those basic questions about learning raised by John Dewey—who is learning what, for what purposes, under what conditions, and with what educational, social, cultural outcomes, and consequences for learners, communities, and nations?[5] We must work at all three levels; societal, organizational, and individual, to promote and support meaningful change that will promote good or beneficence for the patients and communities we serve.

REFERENCES

1. O'Neil EH. *Recreating Health Professional Practice for a New Century.* San Francisco, CA: Pew Health Professions Commission; 1998.
2. Institute of Medicine. *Health Professions Education: A Bridge to Quality.* Washington, DC: National Academy Press; 2003.
3. Institute of Medicine. *Priority Areas for National Action: Transforming Health Care Quality.* Washington, DC: National Academy Press; 2003.
4. Institute of Medicine. *Crossing the Quality Chasm:A New Health System for the 21st Century.* Washington, DC: National Academy Press; 2001.
5. Green J, Luke A, eds. *Rethinking Learning: What Counts as Learning and What Learning Counts.* Review of Research in Education. Washington, DC: American Educational Research Association; 2006.
6. Pellegrino E, Thomasma D. *The Virtues in Medical Practice.* New York: Oxford University Press; 1993.
7. Sullivan W. *Work and Integrity: The Crisis and Promise of Professionalism in America,* 2nd ed. San Francisco: Jossey-Bass; 2005.
8. Glaser J. *Three Realms of Ethics.* Kansas City, MO: Sheed and Ward; 1994.
9. Glaser J. Three realms of ethics: an integrating map for the future. In: Purtilo R, Jensen G, Royeen C, eds. *Educating for Moral Action: A Sourcebook in Health and Rehabilitation Ethics.* Philadelphia: FA Davis; 2005.
10. Oandasa I, Reeves S. Key elements for interprofessional education. Part 1: The learner, the educator and the learning context. *J Interprof Care.* 2005;1S:21–38.
11. Oandasa I, Reeves S. Key elements for interprofessional education. Part 2: Factors, processes and outcomes. *J Interprof Care.* 2005;1S:39–48.
12. Weidman J, Twale D, Stein E. *Socialization of Graduate and Professional Students in Higher Education.* ASHE-ERIC Higher Education Report. San Francisco: Jossey-Bass; 2001.
13. Eisner E. *The Educational Imagination: On Design and Evaluation of School Programs,* 3rd ed. New York: Macmillan; 1994.
14. Steinert Y. Learning together to teach together: interprofessional education and faculty development. *J Interprof Care.* 2005;1S:60–75; 2005.
15. Barr H, Koppel I, Reeves S, Hammick M, Freeth D. *Effective Interprofessional Education: Argument, Assumption and Evidence.* London: Blackwell; 2005.
16. Purtilo R, Jensen G, Royeen C, eds. *Educating for Moral Action: A Sourcebook in Health and Rehabilitation Ethics.* Philadelphia: FA Davis; 2005.
17. Gilbert J. Interprofessional learning and higher education structural barriers. *J Interprof Care.* 2005;1S:87–106.
18. Shepard K, Jensen G. *Handbook of Teaching for Physical Therapists,* 2nd ed. Boston: Butterworth-Heinemann/Reed Elsevier; 2002.
19. Walker D. The process of curriculum development: a naturalistic model. *School Rev.* 1971;80:51–60.
20. Senge P. *The Fifth Discipline: The Art and Practice of the Learning Organization.* New York: Doubleday; 1990.

21. Argyris C, Schon D. *Theory in Practice: Increasing Professional Effectiveness.* San Francisco: Jossey-Bass; 1992.

22. Hardin G. The tragedy of the commons. *Science.* 1969;162:1243–1248.

23. Rubin E, Schappert S. *Meeting Health Needs in the 21st Century.* Washington, DC: Association of Academic Health Centers; 2003.

24. Sullivan W. Preparing professionals as moral agents. Carnegie Perspectives. Available at: http://www.carnegiefoundation.org/perspectives/sub.asp?key=245 &subkey=572. Accessed May 6, 2008.

Interprofessional Education: History, Review, and Recommendations for Professional Accreditation Agencies

Charlotte Brasic Royeen, PhD, OT, FAOTA
Sarah R. Walsh, MOT, OT
Elizabeth Terhaar, MS, OT

INTRODUCTION

Fifteen years ago the Pew Health Professions Commission released a document that identified the need for reform in education of health care professionals and outlined basic competencies expected of those entering the health care field.[1,2] One of the competencies defined by the Pew Health Professions Commission was an ability to work in interdisciplinary teams. In the commission's fourth and final major report, it was suggested that institutions of higher education "require interdisciplinary competence in all health professionals."[3]

Although fostering the development of interprofessional skills through education is increasingly becoming a focal point of the training of health professionals, it is not a new development. Interprofessional education is a topic that has been discussed in the United States and abroad for over 40 years.[4] In fact, one could argue that the United Kingdom and Canada are much more advanced than the United States in development of interprofessional education.

In the 1960s documents addressing the need for interprofessional practice were published. In 1968 Magraw, Deputy Secretary for Health Manpower in the Department of Health, Education, and Welfare, called for the use of interdisciplinary teams in "comprehensive, community-wide, program-oriented approaches to primary care" to decrease the division of labor within the health care field.[5] Additionally, interprofessional training initiatives were developed. Sifneos studied an interdisciplinary education program for public health and social science students with a focus on assessing hazards in mental health settings. Early programs such as this were fraught with high levels of "student dissatisfaction, interdisciplinary absenteeism, and attempts to discourage others from applying to the program."[5,6] Through experience it was learned that student satisfaction increased when they were allowed to maintain their professional identity while participating in interprofessional education opportunities. Early revelations, such as this, were used to guide the development of future interprofessional education programs.

The 1970s saw an increase in the development and expansion of interprofessional programs for health professions students at institutions of higher education.[7] In response to a World Health Organization paper promoting the implementation of interprofessional education programs, the federal government began to provide funding in hopes of preparing students to effectively engage in interprofessional collaboration.[8,9] An array of classes were established,[5] and committees and conferences were devoted to the discussion and further development of interprofessional education initiatives.[10] In 1972 a conference on "Education for the Health Team" was held by the Institute of Medicine during which the concept of interdisciplinary education was supported.[9] Edmund Pellegrino, the chairman of the conference, stated that "A major deterrent to our efforts to fashion health care that is efficient, effective, comprehensive, and personalized is our lack of design for the synergistic interrelationship of all who can contribute to the patient's well-being. We face . . . a national challenge to redeploy the functions of health professionals in new ways, extending the roles of some, perhaps eliminating others, but more closely meshing the functions of each than ever before."[10] Pellegrino suggested the development of educational programs aimed at preparing future professionals for interprofessional collaboration, and offered definitions of interdisciplinary teaching and learning as presented in Table 3-1.

To streamline education of students, conserve funds, and eliminate duplication of courses within colleges, basic science colleges were formed and were seen as early preparation for health care professionals to collaborate as team members.[5]

In the United States the 1980s brought about large changes in interprofessional education, including clarification of concepts and a growing separation

Table 3-1. Definitions for Interdisciplinary Teaching and Learning by Pellegrino[10]

An educational experience can be interdisciplinary at the level of students, at the level of faculty, or at both levels. Thus each of the following combinations is properly interdisciplinary:

1. Students from more than one health profession taught by faculty from one health profession;

2. Students in one health profession taught by faculty from more than one profession;

3. Students from more than one health profession taught by faculty from more than one profession.

Source: Pellegrino ED. Interdisciplinary education in the health professions: assumptions, definitions, and some notes on teams. In: *Education for the Health Care Team.* Washington, DC: National Academy of Sciences; 1972.

between the United States and the rest of the world.[5] Whereas internationally interprofessional education broadly covered a variety of practice areas, in the United States it became primarily focused on the field of gerontology—the only area where funding for the development of programs remained prevalent. As federal funding for the development of interprofessional programs decreased, so did the development of new programs—collaborative education programs were seen as "an expensive luxury."[9]

Research in the 1980s focused on characteristics of successful interprofessional programs. Among the characteristics found to be important to successful interprofessional education programs were support from institutional authorities; leadership from autonomous, cooperative teams, based on honesty, trust, and respect; and an understanding that benefits to the students are more important than financial or political gain.[5,11] In 1988 in *Learning Together to Work Together,* the World Health Organization recommended the development of interprofessional education programs for the purpose of fostering a "type of educational program for health personnel that will enable them to respond to the needs of the populations they serve as part of efforts to achieve the goal of health for all through primary health care. Multiprofessional education oriented to the priority health needs of populations is one such program."[12]

It was in the 1990s that the number of medically uninsured citizens in the United States increased,[5] as did awareness that the U.S. health care system was not meeting the needs of its citizens.[9] Rising health care costs regenerated the need for research into the value of interprofessional education and practice and became more prevalent. Investigation of a variety of interprofessional education models was seen. Innovative interdisciplinary courses addressed topics of current interest, such as acquired immunodeficiency syndrome. In 1998, based on a review of literature, Parsell, Spalding, and Bligh[13] defined criteria for effective interprofessional education programs, which are presented in Table 3-2.

Since the late 1990s, research has become focused on students' perception of the effectiveness of interprofessional education initiatives. Information gathered from qualitative and quantitative studies has been used to create models for educational interprofessional programs. For example, Turnstall, Rink, and Hilton, after studying student attitudes toward undergraduate interprofessional education, assert that problem-based learning groups involving discussion of clinical problems provide an ideal environment for interprofessional education[14]; Ker, Mole, and Bradley advocated for interprofessional learning in a simulated clinical environment[15]; and Hope and colleagues advocated for an extracurricular multicultural, interdisciplinary experience to promote development of interdisciplinary understanding and attitudes, interprofessional teamwork skills, and multicultural skills.[16] Although a variety of methods of interprofessional education models have

Table 3-2. Criteria for Effective Interprofessional Education Programs Based on Parsell, Spalding, and Bligh[13]

1. Detailed planning and organization involving all stakeholders (steering group timing, program location, and student selection)

2. Integration of theory with practice and relevance to work (content—task based and problem oriented)

3. Interactive student-centered learning activities (process—small groups, discussion and debate)

4. Teachers as role models for multiprofessional working (experience, status, and prestige)

5. Establishment of a comfortable learning climate (both physical and emotional)

6. Thorough evaluation for research and further development (before, during, and after the course)

Source: Parsell G, Spalding R, Bligh J. Shared goals, shared learning: evaluation of a multi-professional cause for undergraduate students. Medical Education, 32:304-311; 1998.

been investigated, development and implementation of interprofessional education programs continues to be plagued by inadequate funding.[17]

Inadequate funding for interprofessional education is but one of the many barriers that exist when trying to conceptualize, implement, and assess effectiveness of interprofessional education in the health professions. Five other barriers are of concern when thinking about interprofessional education: attitudes of faculty, sense of tradition/change, time, administration, and resources. Two additional barriers are of major concern regarding barriers to interprofessional education: language used (terminology) and accreditation standards of the health care professions. The next section addresses the five barriers. Subsequently, language and accreditation—two major barriers—are considered.

Five Barriers to Interprofessional Education

In addition to the loss of federal funding sources for implementation of interprofessional education and other related financial issues, five common barriers to interprofessional education are discussed: attitudes of faculty, sense of tradition/change, time, administration, and resources. Faculties in the academy often have primary identity with their profession such that any curricular content not directly addressing their profession may be viewed askance. Most faculty were not educated in an interprofesional model, and it is therefore a challenge for them to see the importance of doing so with new generations of students. In the academy, sense of tradition is very strong and change is a challenge. Without clear and compelling reasons for immediate change, the academy persists in doing things the way they have always been done. To introduce change in terms of how students are educated in a uniprofessional view is a threat to the status quo and requires change in long-standing systems such as schedules, transportation, student group organizations, and celebratory rituals.

In every professional curriculum for every health profession, there never seems to be enough time to teach a student everything they need to know. Thus it is a great challenge to ask for time to be taken away from a uniprofessional curriculum to add interprofessional activity and still cover all that is deemed essential in education of that professional student. Many in administration have little understanding of professional education in the health care area overall, let alone a deep and meaningful understanding of the importance of interprofessional education integrated with professional education.

One final barrier to interprofessional education is resources. Something as simple as space can be a major determinant in offering students opportunities to participate in education in an interprofessional manner. For example, one has to consider whether there are sufficient large lecture rooms to house a class with nutrition and dietetics, physical therapy, and occupational therapy students. Or, one must consider whether there are sufficient small conference rooms to allow for break-out discussion groups of small cases across interprofessional teams of students. Without these very necessary physical resources, alternative methods of promoting interprofessional educational experiences must be constructed.

Language of Interprofessional Education

Language shapes our thoughts and actions. Accordingly, the following definitions from Clark[18] are put forth as supplements to the previous ones supplied by Pellegrino and are presented in Table 3-3.

Table 3-3. Basic Interprofessional Definitions by Clark[18]

Uniprofessional education (UPE): Students are all from the same discipline or profession. The mastery of a specific body of knowledge, types of skills, and modes of conduct are emphasized.

Multiprofessional education (MPE): Various disciplines are brought together to understand a particular problem or experience. They afford different perspectives on the issue at hand. For example, aging may be conceptualized as a physical or biological process, a psychological process, or a set of characteristics. The World Health Organization[12] defines MPE as the process by which a group of students from the health-related occupations with different education backgrounds learn together during certain periods of their education with interaction as an important goal. Its key objectives are the specific team competencies needed to ensure effective team functioning.

Interprofessional education (IPE): Students from various professions learn together as a team. Their collaborative interaction is characterized by the integration and modification of different professions' contributions in light of input from other professions. The hallmark of interprofessional education is the type of cognitive and behavioral change that occurs: Participants understand the core principles and concepts of each contributing discipline and are familiar with the basic language and mindsets of the various disciplines. Before participating in interprofessional education, students must have basic knowledge and skills related to their own profession.

Source: Clark PG. A typology of interdisciplinary education in gerontology and geriatrics: Are we really doing what we say we are? *J Interprof Care.* 1993;7:219–220. Available from: http://www.ipe.utoronto.ca/aboutipe.html. Accessed March 9, 2008.

In addition to these three basic definitions, we share current definitions of many words found in recent literature pertaining to interprofessional education.[19] These or similar words are the key words or phrases that we look for in the accreditation standards of the various professions. They are presented in Table 3-4.

Table 3-4. Glossary of Current Terms in Interprofessional Education Literature

Autonomy: The ability and support to make independent decisions and take independent action

Collaboration: Working together; thinking together; doing together

Communication: Two entities enhancing information that is in some way meaningful to them.

Community or practice: A group of like-minded individuals who join together around a theory, framework, conceptual model idea, or action

Coordination: Assisting operations, people, or systems to work together

Independent: Standing alone

Interdisciplinary: Across the disciplines

Interprofessional: Across the professions

Interprofessionality:[20] Having the character or nature of across the professions

Interprofessional education: Education that is developed and executed through collaboration across the professions

Interprofessional practice: Practice that is developed and executed through collaboration across the professions

Multidisciplinary: Including many disciplines

Parity: Equality

Shared leadership:[21] Taking action to move format in a collaborative manner

Team treatment:[22] Providing services in a group

Source: D'Amour D, Oandasan I. Interprofessionality as the field of interprofessional practice and interprofessional education: an emerging concept. *J Interprof Care.* 2005;(Suppl 1): 8–20, Steinert Y. Learning together to teach together: interprofessional education and faculty development. *J Interprof Care.* 2005;(Suppl1):60–75; Tamura Y, Bontje P, Nakata Y, Ishikawa Y, Noriko T. Can one eat collaboration? Menus as metaphors of interprofessional collaboration. *J Interprof Care.* 2005;19:215–222.

Accreditation of Health Professions and Interprofessional Education

Educational institutions such as colleges and universities have regional accreditation to which they must apply and be accredited for to ensure educational quality, student access to federal and state funds, and fostering transferability of educational credits.[23] Regional accreditation agencies accredit public and private, nonprofit 2- and 4-year institutions. Two examples of these are the Higher Learning Commission of the North Central Association of Schools and Colleges and Southern Association of Colleges and Schools. If a college or university, however, is to offer professional education in addition to traditional arts and sciences types of curriculum, there is typically at least one specialty accreditation agency from which they must also be accredited. For example, in law education it is the American Bar Association and in medicine it is the Liaison Committee on Medical Education. In nursing it is the National League for Nursing Accrediting Commission depending on the level of educational program offered. In what has been typically referred to as the allied health professions or health sciences professions, there is similarly a professional accreditation agency for each and every profession in this arena. To illustrate, for clinical laboratory sciences there is National Accrediting for Clinical Laboratory Science, for health informatics there is the Commission on Accreditation for Health Informatics and Information Management Education, for nuclear medicine technology there is Joint Review Committee on Educational Programs in Nuclear Medicine Technology, and so on. These regional accreditation agencies and agencies in health professions are under the auspices of the Council for Higher Education Accreditation, a not-for-profit, private, national organization responsible for coordination of accreditation in the United States. The mission of CHEA is to

> . . . serve students and their families, colleges and universities, sponsoring bodies, governments, employers by promoting academic quality through formal recognition of higher education accrediting bodies and will coordinate and work to advance self-regulation through accreditation (1996).

The accreditation standards issued by each of the respective organizations of accreditation related to a particular profession typically has lengthy, detailed, and prescriptive standards of education that must be met by a college or university to offer a degree in that profession and that will allow the graduate to take an eligible registration or licensure examination. Thus access into the respective profession is linked to graduating from an "accredited" program, after which one is able to take the test for entry into the profession as a "publicly recognized" and properly credentialed professional.

We believe that more variables are at play than just lack of funding for interprofessional education, though that is true. Accountability of the professions for interprofessional education should be reflected in standards for practice of the professions and for accreditation of the programs educating professionals in those programs. Thus here we review the accreditation standards of the various health professions so identified and determine to what extent, if any, interprofessional education is a standard in accreditation of their respective educational programs.

Table 3-5 reviews the accreditation standards, or summaries thereof, of the various accreditation agencies for the professions reviewed in this chapter: clinical laboratory science, health information management, nuclear medicine technology, nutrition and dietetics, occupational therapy, pharmacy, physical assistant, and physical therapy. Physician and nursing education are not covered in this chapter, and for more information on education and accreditation in these professions the reader is referred to The Carnegie Foundation for the Advancement of Teaching and their respective studies on Professional Preparation of Physicians and Study of Nursing Education.

Cross-Professions Analysis

If one agrees that language shapes our thoughts and action, then the language of interprofessional education found in accreditation standards of these nine health-related professions is lacking. The words used pertaining to interprofessional education were as follows: consultative, responsiveness, instruct, assist, consultation, interact, refer, educating, effective information exchange, and communicate. These do not match or barely begin to address the language of interprofessional education from current literature as presented in Table 3-4. The language of current interprofessional terminology is inadequately reflected. Two of the professions, nutrition and dietetics and physical therapy, came the closest to some sort of reference to interprofessional education with "collaborate and team building" (nutrition and dietetics) and "interdisciplinary team conference" (physical therapy).

Table 3-5. Review Summaries of Accreditation Standards Across Nine Health-related Professions Related to Interprofessional Education

Profession Accreditation	Accreditation Agency	Source and Year	Competencies/Requirements Judged to Pertain to IPE
Clinical laboratory science	National Accrediting Agency for Clinical Laboratory Science	Accessed August 25, 2006 from http://www.naacls.org/accreditation/cls-mt/ 2006 National Accrediting Agency for CLS	Under Description of Career Entry of the Clinical Laboratory Scientist/Medical Technologist—A: The clinical laboratory scientist/medical technologist will also possess basic knowledge, skills, and relevant experiences in communications to enable consultative interactions with members of the health care team, external relations, customer service, and patient education (p. 3).
Health informatics	Commission on Accreditation for Health Informatics and Information Management Education	Accessed August 25, 2006 from http://library.ahima.org/xpedio/groups/public/documents/accreditation/bok1_026307.pdf CAHIIM 2005 Standards	Under Program Goals, Assessment, and Outcomes—II.A.4: Communities of Interest. Demonstrate monitoring and responsiveness to the substantiated needs of the various communities of interest including healthcare providers and employers (p. 2).

Nuclear medicine technology	Joint Review Committee on Educational Programs in Nuclear Medicine Technology	Accessed August 25, 2006 from http://www.jrcnmt.org/pd/2003 %20Essentials.pdf JRCNMT Essentials, revised 2003	Under Radiation Safety—F: A nuclear medicine technologist participates in a hospital's in-service education program to instruct other personnel regarding radiation and principles of radiation protection (p. 10). Under Diagnostic Procedures—A.4: A nuclear medicine technologist performs imaging procedures by assisting the physician or practitioner in cardiac stress testing when performed in conjunction with nuclear medicine procedures (p. 14).
Nutrition and dietetics	Commission on Accreditation for Dietetics Education	Accessed on August 25, 2006 from http://www.eatright.org/cps/rd/e/xchg/ada/hs.xsl/CADE 812 E NU HTML.htm 2006 CADE	Under Examples of Evidence in the Self-study—Planned learning experiences may include collaborating and team building with individuals from other disciplines in such activities as team meetings, case management, discharge planning, quality improvement, product/menu development and marketing, public affairs, communications, entrepreneurship, and so on (p. 23). Under Core Competencies for Dietitians—CD38: Conduct nutrition care component of interdisciplinary team conferences to discuss patient/client treatment and discharge planning (p. 33).

(Continues)

Table 3-5. Review Summaries of Accreditation Standards Across Nine Health-related Professions Related to Interprofessional Education *(Continued)*

Profession Accreditation	Accreditation Agency	Source and Year	Competencies/Requirements Judged to Pertain to IPE
Occupational therapy	Accreditation Council for Occupational Therapy Education	Accessed on August 26, 2006 from http://www.aota.org/nonmembers/area13/docs/draftstandards 106.pdf January 2006 Final Draft of Standards for an Accredited Master's Level Educational Program for the Occupational Therapist and Standards for an Accredited Educational Program for the Occupational Therapy Assistant	Under Intervention Plan. Formulation and Implementation—B5.17: The student will be able to apply the principles of the teaching-learning process using educational methods to design educational experiences to address the needs of the client, family, significant others, colleagues, other health providers, and the public. B5.18: The student will be able to effectively interact through written, oral, and nonverbal communication with the client, family, significant others, colleagues, other health providers, and the public in a professionally acceptable manner. B5.23: The student will be able to refer to specialists, both internal and external to the profession for consultation and intervention (p. 17) Under Professional Ethics, Values, and Responsibilities—B9.3: The student will be able to promote occupational therapy by educating other professionals, service providers consumers, third-party payers, regulatory bodies, and the public (p. 20).

Pharmacy	Accreditation Council for Pharmacy Education	Accessed on August 25, 2006 from http://www.acpe-accredit.org/pdf/ACPE Revised PharmD Standards Adopted Jan 152006.pdf Revised and adopted, January 2006	Guideline 13.4: When content is integrated across disciplines, the core knowledge base and outcomes for each discipline should be provided in adequate depth, scope, and emphasis to ensure attainment of the desired competencies (p. 20).
Physician assistant	Accreditation Review Commission on Education for the Physician Assistant, Inc.	Accessed on August 25, 2006 from http://www.arc-pa.org/Standards/finalcopy926 05.pdf Revised September 26, 2005	Under Clinical Preparatory Sciences—B3.01: The Program must provide instruction in interpersonal and communication skills that result in the effective exchange of information and collaboration with patients, their families, and other health professionals (p. 12).
Physical therapy	Commission on Accreditation in Physical Therapy Education	Accessed on August 25 2006 from http://www.apta.org/AM/Template.cfm?Section-CAPTE1&TEMPLATE=/CM/Content Displaycfm&CONTENTID=32651	Under Curriculum Content: Professional Practice Expectation: Communication—CC-5.17: Expressively and receptively communicate in a culturally competent manner with patients/clients, family members, caregivers, practitioners, interdisciplinary team members, consumers, payers, and policymakers (p. B-29). Patient/Client Management Expectation—CC-5.34: Collaborate with patients/clients, family members, payer, other professionals, and other individuals to determine a plan of care that is acceptable, realistic, culturally competent, and patient-centered (p. B-31).

They are to be commended for having a start but still fall short of fully embracing interprofessional education. Given that in 1998 the Pew Health Professions Commission[24] and in 2001 the Institute of Medicine[25] called for interprofessional outcome competencies, it is a sad state of affairs that no single education accreditation agency that we could find has fully responded to this charge. It may be said that we have come so far only to be so far behind.

RECOMMENDATIONS FOR INTERPROFESSIONAL EDUCATION

Based on this analysis across health care professions, the professional accreditation agencies are contributors to perpetuation of the silo approach. In response to true societal need to focus on the patient or client first and not primarily on professional roles and autonomy, a charge is put forth for accreditation agencies to respond to the Pew Health Professions Commission[24] and the Institute of Medicine's[25] interprofessional outcome competencies and include interprofessional standards in their educational essentials for education of a health care professional.

CONCLUSION

We strongly urge every professional health care education accreditation agency to carefully review their current standards for relevance, support, and integration of interprofessional education. At a minimum, each accreditation agency should include some version of the Institute of Medicine and Pew Health Professions Commission outcome competency related to ability to work in interdisciplinary teams by being educated in interprofessional teams. For better practice, acknowledgment of the important role interprofessional education could play at every year of preprofessional and professional education should be included in the professional educational standards in a meaningful way.

We believe that two ways to change the health care delivery system in the United States to reduce patient error, promote cost-effective practice, and increase humanistic care (i.e., to better serve societal need) are

1. Through incorporation of the identified interprofessional education competencies,
2. Through thorough assessment and accountability measure for those educational competencies.

Thus this chapter ends with a call to action for change in accreditation review standards for health professions education accreditors to include outcome competencies for interprofessional education.

REFERENCES

1. Shugars DA, O'Neill EH, Bader JD. *Healthy America: Practitioners for 2005. An Agenda for Action for US Health Professional Schools.* Durham, NC: The Pew Health Professions Commission; 1991.
2. Herrick CA, Arbuckle MB, Claes JA. Teaching interprofessional practice: a course on a system of care for children with severe emotional disturbance and their families. *J Fam Nurs.* 2002;8:264–281.
3. *Recreating Health Professional Practice for a New Century.* The Fourth Report of the Pew Health Professions Commission. The Center for the Health Professions, University of California, San Francisco; December 1998.
4. Kilminister S, Hale C, Lascelles M, et al. Learning for real life: patient-focused interprofessional workshops offer added value. *Med Educ.* 2004;38:717–726.
5. Lavin MA, Ruebling I, Banks R, et al. Interdisciplinary health professional education: a historical review. *Adv Health Sci Educ.* 2001;6:25–47.
6. Sifneos PE. The interdisciplinary team: an educational experience for mental health professionals. *Psych Quart.* 1969;43:123–130.
7. Walker PH, Baldwin DW, Fitzpatrick JJ, Ryan SS. Building community: developing skills for interprofessional health professions education and relationship-centered care. National League for Nursing Appointed Interdisciplinary Health Education Panel. *J Allied Health.* 1998;27:173–178.
8. Hale C. Interprofessional education: the way to a successful workforce? *Br J Ther Rehabil.* 2003;10:122–127.
9. Baldwin DC. Some historical notes on interdisciplinary and interprofessional education and practice in the USA. *J Interprof Care.* 1996;10:173–187.
10. Pellegrino ED. Interdisciplinary education in the health professions: assumptions, definitions, and some notes on teams. In: *Education for the Health Care Team.* Washington, DC: National Academy of Sciences; 1972.
11. Satin DG. The difficulties in interdisciplinary education: lessons from three failures and a success. *Educ Gerontol.* 1987;13:53–69.
12. World Health Organization. *Learning Together to Work Together.* Switzerland: World Health Organization; 1988.
13. Parsell G, Spalding R, Bligh J. Shared goals, shared learning: evaluation of a multiprofessional course for undergraduate students. *Med Educ.* 1998;32:304–311.
14. Turnstall S, Rink E, Hilton S. Student attitudes to undergraduate interprofessional education. *J Interprof Care.* 2003;17:161–172.
15. Ker J, Mole L, Bradley P. Early introduction to interprofessional learning: a simulated ward environment. *Med Educ.* 2003;37:248–255.

16. Hope JM, Lugassy D, Meyer R, et al. Bringing interdisciplinary and multicultural team building to health care education: the Downstate Team Building Initiative. *Acad Med.* 2005;80:74–83.

17. Brashers VL, Curry CE, Harper DC, McDaniel SH, Pawlson G, Ball JW. Interprofessional health care education: recommendations of the National Academies of Practice Expert Panel on Health Care in the 21st Century. *Issues Interdisc Care Natl Acad Pract Forum.* 2001;3:21–31.

18. Clark PG. A typology of interdisciplinary education in gerontology and geriatrics: Are we really doing what we say we are? *J Interprof Care.* 1993;7:219–220. Available from: http://www.ipe.utoronto.ca/aboutipe.html. Accessed March 9, 2008.

19. Royeen CB, Lavin MA. Framing interprofessional education, practice and research: words as determinants of ideas in interprofessional education. Presentation at the American Association of Schools of Allied Health Professional Annual Conference, December 18–20, 1996, Chicago, Ill.

20. D'Amour D, Oandasan I. Interprofessionality as the field of interprofessional practice and interprofessional education: an emerging concept. *J Interprof Care.* 2005;(Suppl 1):8–20.

21. Steinert Y. Learning together to teach together: interprofessional education and faculty development. *J Interprof Care.* 2005;(Suppl 1):60–75.

22. Tamura Y, Bontje P, Nakata Y, Ishikawa Y, Noriko T. Can one eat collaboration? Menus as metaphors of interprofessional collaboration. *J Interprof Care.* 2005;19:215–222.

23. Eaton JS. *An Overview of U.S. Accreditation.* Council for Higher Education Accreditation (CHEA) Author. One Dupont Circle NW, Suite 510, Washington, DC 20036.

24. O'Neill EH, Pew Health Professions Commission. *Recreating Health Professional Practice for a New Century: The Fourth Report of the Pew Health Professions Commission.* San Francisco: Pew Health Professions Commission; 1998.

25. Institute of Medicine. *Crossing the Quality Chasm: A New Health System for the 21st Century.* Washington, DC: National Academy Press; 2001.

CHAPTER 4

Grounding Interprofessional Education and Practice in Theory

Robin Ann Harvan, EdD
Charlotte Brasic Royeen, PhD, OT, FAOTA
Gail M. Jensen, PhD, PT, FAPTA

INTRODUCTION

Theories are constructed to explain, predict, and master phenomena (e.g., inanimate things, events, or the behavior of humans and animals). A phenomenon is any occurrence that is observable. In many instances we are constructing models of reality or theories-in-action. A theory makes generalizations about observations and consists of an interrelated, coherent set of ideas and models.[1] A conceptual model is a theoretical construct that represents something, with a set of variables and a set of logical relationships between them. Models in this sense are constructed to enable reasoning within an idealized logical framework about these processes and are an important component of theories.[2] The traditional process of theorizing rests on the scientific method. This is summarized in the model presented in Figure 4-1.

The first two phases of theorizing in this case rests on (a) what do we know about interprofessional education and practice in health care and (b) what can we assume about interprofessional education and practice in health care based on what we know. These assumptions are then tested, refined, and revised to form new knowledge. The process of theorizing is continuous. New knowledge, new ideas and assumptions, new guiding principles, new methods of testing, and new ways of interpretation all work to form and reform theories-in-action about interprofessional education and practice.[1]

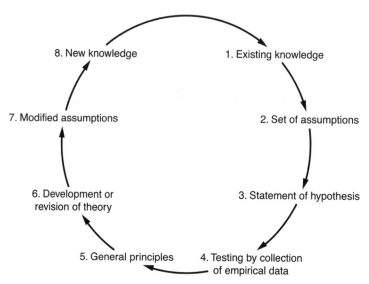

Figure 4-1
The process of theorizing.

There are two purposes of this chapter: (a) to explore theoretical constructs and emerging conceptual models of interprofessional education and practice in health care and (b) to propose the application of theoretically grounded, evidence-based, translational research methods for investigating health care team education and practice. To explore organizational theoretical models of health care team practice we must ask if we were to observe the effective and efficient functioning of interprofessional health care teams, then how would we be able to explain, construct, model, or predict these phenomena? To explore educational theoretical models for interprofessional education we must ask if we were to observe effective and efficient instruction and training for achieving the outcomes of effective and efficient functioning of health care teams, then how would we be able to explain, construct, model, or predict these phenomena? Finally, to contribute to the science and art of interprofessional health care education and practice, translational research is required. Translational research is applying ideas, insights, and discoveries generated through basic scientific inquiry using a variety of research methods from quantitative to qualitative.[3] The creation of knowledge in interprofessional health care education and practice depends on good conceptual thinking and theory development.

KEY DEFINITIONS

Over the years a plethora of terms have been used to describe and define health care team concepts. Since the 1970s key definitions for interdisciplinary practice and education have been offered.

According to Pelligrino, "society and health care would be better served if students in the health professions have opportunities to experience working together" ... in models of cooperative health care delivery.[4] In 1972, Pelligrino and the National Academy of Sciences convened a national meeting that produced this definition of interdisciplinary education: "an educational experience can be interdisciplinary at the level of students, at the level of faculty or at both levels ... (1) students from more than one health profession taught by faculty from one health profession, (2) students in one health profession taught by faculty from more than one profession, and (3) students from more than one health profession taught by faculty from more than one health profession."[5]

In 1979, Ducanis and Golin defined the interdisciplinary health care team as a "functioning unit composed of individuals with varied and specialized training who coordinate their activities to provide services to a client or group of clients." It has been assumed that if coordinated health care team practice is the ultimate goal, then interdisciplinary education and training is the preferred process to prepare practitioners to work together.[6]

In 1988, the World Health Organization defined interdisciplinary education as "the process by which a group of students from the health related occupations with different educational backgrounds *learn together* during certain periods of their education, with *interaction* as an important goal, to *collaborate* in providing promotive, preventive, curative, rehabilitative, and other health related services."[7]

In 1997, Freeth and colleagues at the Centre for the Advancement of Interprofessional Education (CAIPE) in the United Kingdom provided the following definitions:[8]

- *"Interprofessional education:* Members (or students) of two or more professions associated with health or social care, engaged in learning with, from, and about each other. It is an initiative to secure interprofessional learning and promote gains through interprofessional collaboration in professional practice."[8]
- *"Multiprofessional education:* Members (or students) of two or more professions learning alongside one another: parallel learning rather than interactive learning"[8]

- *"Uniprofessional education:* Members (or students) of a single profession learning together: interactively or in parallel"[8]

In 2000, Drinka and Clark defined the interdisciplinary health care team as a group of individuals with diverse training/backgrounds who work together as a unit, consistently collaborate to solve patient problems, share mutual goals, work interdependently to define and treat patient problems, accept and capitalize on disciplinary differences, and share leadership, with effective communication being key to success.[9]

As illustrated, an exploration of defining concepts for interprofessional health care education and practice have included multidisciplinary, multiprofessional, interdisciplinary, interprofessional, transdisciplinary, and cross-professional. "Multi-" refers to "more than one" discipline or profession, "inter-" implies "between or among," and "trans-" and "cross" imply "across" professions and disciplines. It is important to distinguish health care team education and practice that is multidisciplinary (includes more than one) from inter-, trans-, or cross-disciplinary (implying interaction between, among, or across disciplines).[10,11]

- *(Uni)disciplinary:* One provider working independently to care for a patient; little awareness or acknowledgment of practice outside of one's own discipline; may consult with other providers but retains independence.
- *Multidisciplinary:* Different aspects of a patient's case are handled independently by appropriate experts from different professions.[12] Rather than integrated, the patient's problems are subdivided and treated separately, with each provider responsible for his or her own area.
- *Interdisciplinary:* Denotes the provision of health care by providers from different professions in a coordinated manner that addresses the needs of patients. Providers share mutual goals, resources, and responsibility for patient care.[13]
- *Interprofessional:* The term *interprofessional* is used to describe clinical practice, whereas the term *interdisciplinary* is often used to describe the educational process.[13] Either term may be used when referring to health professions education and practice.
- *Interprofessional education:* An educational approach in which two or more disciplines collaborate in the teaching–learning process with the goal of fostering interprofessional interactions.[14]
- *Transdisciplinary:* Requires each team member to become sufficiently familiar with the concepts and approaches of his or her colleagues as to "blur the lines" and enable the team to focus on the problem with

collaborative analysis and decision making that enhance the practice of each discipline[15]

- *Cross-professional education, practice, and research:* An organizational approach that requires each team member to become sufficiently familiar with the concepts and approaches of his or her colleagues as to "blur the lines" and enable the team to focus on the problem with collaborative analysis and decision making.[15]

In 1999, the Association of Academic Health Centers published proceedings from a conference on core issues that must be addressed in redefining education in primary care for the 21st century. In this volume Hirokawa examined the differences between multidisciplinary and interdisciplinary health care teams.[16] He noted a key distinction in the definition of these concepts according to Klein[17] that multidisciplinary is essentially additive and not integrative, whereas the presence of interaction among and between disciplines is a key feature of interdisciplinarity.

A multidisciplinary group becomes interdisciplinary when its members transcend their separate disciplinary perspectives and attempt to weave together their unique perspectives and methods of practice to overcome common problems or concerns. In contrast, "members of the interdisciplinary team perform their work in a collaborative fashion. Each member of the team, while providing the group with the knowledge and skills of his or her disciplinary perspective, also strives to incorporate that perspective with those of others to create solutions to health care problems that transcend conventional, discipline-specific methods, procedures, and techniques."[4] Communication is the key component to this collaboration and interaction.

Senge associates multidisciplinarity with discussion and interdisciplinarity with dialogue.[18] According to Senge, the goal of dialogue is not persuasion but rather the establishment of understanding to "gain insights that simply could not be achieved individually" (p. 241). Given these distinctions in definitions, Hirokawa concludes that interdisciplinary health care teams are not defined by the nature or diversity of their professional membership but by the quality of their communication and the degree of collaboration evident in the interaction of team members.[16]

According to the Pew-Fetzer Task Force, the multidisciplinary approach handles different aspects of a patient's case independently by appropriate experts from different professions.[19] They defined interdisciplinary team care as the provision of health care by providers from different professions in a coordinated manner that addresses the needs of patients, where providers share mutual goals, resources, and responsibility for patient care. Rather than integrated, the patient's problems are subdivided and treated separately, with each provider responsible for his or her own area.

Most recently, D'Amour and Oandasan proposed a distinction of interdisciplinarity from interprofessionality.[20] They argue that interdisciplinarity is a response to the fragmented knowledge of numerous disciplines, whereas interprofessionality is a response to the realities of fragmented health care practices. They define interprofessionality as the development of a cohesive practice between professionals from different disciplines. This concept is similar to the concepts of transdisciplinary and cross-professional approaches previously defined in this chapter. Interprofessionality, transdisciplinary, and cross-professional each implies cohesive, collaborative decision making and team-oriented health care delivery. According to D'Amour and Oandasan, if interprofessionality is to be studied, it is necessary to make a distinction between educational initiatives to enhance learner outcomes and collaborative practice to enhance patient outcomes, yet they acknowledge their interdependency.[20]

ESTABLISHING THE EVIDENCE

Since the dawning of the 21st century, there has been an enormous resurgence of interest, globally, regarding health care teamwork in relation to improving health care quality, cost, and access. For those who have been working in this arena, through various historical cycles of focus and interest in interprofessional education and practice, this is, indeed, good news. In today's global communication networks, information sharing can be more timely and efficient. Together, we can learn with each other and from each other. We can practice what we teach about collaboration.

There is also good news regarding the evidence base and rationale for interprofessional health care teamwork. Several seminal systematic reviews of empirical evidence pertaining to interprofessional education and practice in health care have been conducted in recent years. These systematic reviews regarding the evidence base for interprofessional education and practice include·

- Agency for Healthcare Research and Quality (AHRQ)[21]
- Australian Capital Territory (ACT) Department of Health[22]
- Best Evidence in Medical Education[23]
- Cochrane Collaboration[24]
- Health Canada[25]

Conclusions, although promising, call for more rigorous research, hence the continuation of theorizing conceptual models and theoretical constructs regarding interprofessional education and practice.

The most promising conclusions relate to improving patient safety outcomes. Key conclusions from the AHRQ literature review on medical teamwork and patient safety are summarized in Box 4-1.

Box 4-1: Key Conclusions from the AHRQ Literature Review on Teamwork and Patient Safety[21]

1. **The science of team performance and training can help the medical community improve patient safety.** A general science of team performance and training has evolved and matured over the last 20 years. This science has produced a number of principles, lessons learned, tools, and guidelines that will serve the patient safety movement.

2. **Research has already identified many of the competencies that are necessary for effective teamwork in medical environments.** The science of team performance and training has identified the competencies that are required for effective team functioning in a number of complex settings. Many, if not most, of these competencies apply to the medical community.

3. **A number of proven instructional strategies are available for promoting effective teamwork.** The science of team performance and training has also developed and validated numerous training strategies that can provide requisite competencies to teams who perform in complex environments.

4. **The medical community has made considerable progress in designing and implementing team training across a number of settings.** The review of existing medical team training programs clearly shows that the health care community is striving to implement crew resource management (CRM) training across a number of medical domains. The AHRQ report recommends that this trend be continued. However, the extent to which these programs are being implemented with the help of what is known from the science of learning, of team performance, and of training is less clear. Thus the report recommends strengthening the link between scientific knowledge and medical-team training.

5. **The institutionalization of medical-team training across different medical settings has not been addressed.** To make teamwork a common, effective practice throughout the delivery of health care, there is an imperative need to embed team training in professional development. "Embedding" means implementing and regulating team training throughout a health care provider's career.

Source: Baker D, Gustafson S, Beaubien J, Salas E, Barach P. *Medical Teamwork and Patient Safety: The Evidence-Based Relation.* Literature Review. AHRQ Publication No. 05-0053. Rockville, MD: Agency for Healthcare Research and Quality; 2005.

One of AHRQ's first efforts following the Institute of Medicine report, *To Err Is Human: Building a Safer Health System*,[26] was to commission Evidence Report 43, entitled *Making Health Care Safer: A Critical Analysis of Patient Safety Practices.*[27] This report reviewed "existing data on practices within and outside health care that are regarded as having potential to improve patient safety." Interestingly, "the report reviewed evidence for CRM training, based on its success in the aviation industry, and concluded that CRM has tremendous potential for health care team training."[21] The subsequent AHRQ report on medical teamwork and patient safety extends and updates the previous review and contends that "the training of health care providers as teams constitutes a pragmatic, effective strategy for enhancing patient safety and reducing medical errors."[21]

As previously explored, one widely cited definition of interprofessional education offered by Barr and colleagues at CAIPE is "occasions when two or more professions learn with, from and about each other to improve collaboration and the quality of care."[10] Pairing the conclusion offered by AHRQ with the definition offered by CAIPE captures several dimensions relevant to exploring theoretical models applicable to interprofessional health care education and practice.

EXPLORING THEORETICAL MODELS

Numerous theoretical constructs on interprofessional collaborative learning and interprofessional collaborative practice in health care have been introduced and explored. The theoretical base differs depending on the focus of investigation. A focus on team learning related to learning outcomes may offer a different set of assumptions worth testing than a focus on team functioning related to patient safety outcomes. In general, interprofessional health care education is grounded in educational theory, whereas interprofessional health care practice is grounded in organizational systems theory.

Theoretical Models for Interprofessional Health Care Education

Educational theories generally fall within three broad psychological categories:[28,29]

1. *Behaviorism:* This theory is based on observable changes in behavior. Like animals, humans are assumed to be wired so that any behavior

that is reinforced will be more likely to become automatic. Learning is the acquisition of new behavior.

2. *Cognitivism:* This theory is based on the thought process behind the behavior and that there is a meaningful pattern or structure. Changes in behavior are observed and used as indicators as to what is happening inside the learner's mind.

3. *Constructivism:* This is based on the premise that we all construct our own perspective or meaning of the world, through individual experiences and schema. Constructivism focuses on preparing the learner to problem solve in ambiguous situations.

An excellent resource regarding constructionist and adult learning theories related to interprofessional health care education can be found in *Effective Interprofessional Education: Argument, Assumption, & Evidence.*[10]

In an attempt to explore the development of a theoretical model for interprofessional education, Clark considers five different theoretical approaches from the fields of educational philosophy and psychology:

1. *Cooperative, collaborative, or social learning:* Learning with and from each other in interdependent social groups builds the knowledge and the essential teamwork skills required to work together effectively.

2. *Experiential learning:* Learning as a continuous process grounded in experience.

3. *Epistemology and ontology of interdisciplinary inquiry:* Learning as the philosophical and metaphysical study of professional socialization and the use of cognitive and normative maps that represents professional disciplinary thinking and action.

4. *Cognitive and ethical development:* Learning through transformative stages of intellectual and ethical development.

5. *Educating the reflective practitioner:* Learning from reflecting on the technical (cognitive) and artistic (normative) aspects of professional practice.[30]

Interprofessional socialization has its merits, along with professional socialization. Socializing health professionals is critical to professionalization and induction into the profession. Students learn the knowledge, skills, and mores (values, norms, and behaviors) during the professional socialization process. This process of socialization can contribute to improved quality of care, patient safety, or patient outcomes. Likewise, it can be argued that interprofessional socialization can contribute to the same quality outcomes.

Interprofessionality, therefore, could be considered a conceptual model for interprofessional socialization for cohesive and collaborative team decision making and delivery of health care.

A multitude of educational theories could be explored in relation to interprofessional health care education. There is an excellent resource on the Internet for exploring educational theories and instructional design models developed by a colleague at the University of Colorado Denver, School of Education.[31] Grounding instructional design models in theory allows for systematic and scientific testing and evaluation of guiding principles, general assumptions, and instructional methods for health care team training.

Theoretical Models for Interprofessional Health Care Practice

Focusing on the context of health care team performance, health care delivery, quality, and patient safety requires consideration of organizational theory and systems theory perspectives. An organization is a structured social system consisting of groups of individuals working together to meet some agreed-on objectives. Organizational theory is the study of organizations for the benefit of identifying common themes for the purpose of solving problems, maximizing efficiency and productivity, and meeting the needs of stakeholders.[32]

Organizational theories are interdisciplinary, based on knowledge from the fields of psychology, political science, economics, anthropology, and sociology. They seek to explain behavior and dynamics in individual, group, and organizational contexts. Organizational theories are related to the following processes:

- *Individual processes:* motivation theory, personality theory, and role theory
- *Group processes:* group dynamics and communication, leadership, and power and influence theories
- *Organizational processes:* organizational design, organizational systems, and organizational culture theories

Organizational behavior is widely defined as the study of individual-, group-, and organizational-level behavior, yet organizational researchers often focus on only one of these levels. Individual behavior, however, is likely to be affected by the work group and organization, just as the work group and organization are influenced by the individual.

Systems theory is an interdisciplinary field of study of the nature of complex systems, and it is a framework by which one can analyze and/or describe any group of objects that work in concert to produce some result. A system can be defined as a collection of interrelated parts that work together by way of some driving process.[32] Systems are generalizations of reality. The various parts of a system have functional as well as structural relationships between each other.[32] Functional relationships can only occur because of the presence of a driving force. The parts that make up a system show some degree of integration whereby the parts work well together.

Health care organizations are considered macrosystems and health care teams are microsystems. A plausible argument could be made for grounding organizational and systems theories in the study of the effective and efficient functioning of health care teams in health care organizations.

HEALTH CARE TEAM TRAINING ASSUMPTIONS

According to the AHRQ report on health care teamwork,

- Teamwork is traditionally described using systems theory, which posits that team inputs, team processes, and team outputs are arrayed over time.
- Team inputs include the characteristics of the task to be performed, the elements of the context in which work occurs, and the attitudes brought forth by its members to a team situation.
- Team processes are the interactions and coordination necessary on the part of team members to achieve specific goals.
- Team outputs consist of the products derived from the team's collective efforts.
- Teamwork occurs in the process phase, during which designated members interact and collaborate to achieve the desired outcomes.[21]

Effective team training reflects general learning theory principles, presents information about requisite team behaviors, affords team members the necessary skills practice, and provides them with remedial feedback.[21] Team training can be described as the application of instructional design principles and models based on well-tested teaching–learning methods to a specific set of competencies. Competency-based educational models are widely applied in health professions education.

The team competencies presented in Table 4-1 are a useful supplement to the team training research and practical guidance, in the design of team training programs.

Table 4-1. Primary Teamwork Competencies[21]

Competency	Definition
Knowledge competencies	
Cue/strategy associations	The linking of cues in the environment with with appropriate coordination strategies
Shared task models/ situation assessment	A shared understanding of the situation and appropriate strategies for coping with task demands
Teammate characteristics familiarity	An awareness of each teammate's task-related competencies, preferences, tendencies, strengths, and weaknesses
Knowledge of team mission, objectives, norms, and resources	A shared understanding of a specific goal(s) or objective(s) of the team as well as the human and material resources required and available to achieve the objective. When change occurs, team members' knowledge must change to account for new task demands
Task-specific responsibilities	The distribution of labor, according to team members' individual strengths and task demands
Skill competencies	
Mutual performance monitoring	The tracking of fellow team members' efforts to ensure that the work is being accomplished as expected and that proper procedures are followed
Flexibility/adaptability	The ability to recognize and respond to deviations in the expected course of events, or to the needs of other team members
Supporting/back-up behavior	The coaching and constructive criticism provided to a teammate, as a means of improving performance, when a lapse is detected or a team member is overloaded
Team leadership	The ability to direct/coordinate team members, assess team performance, allocate tasks, motivate subordinates, plan/organize, and maintain a positive team environment

(Continues)

Table 4-1. Primary Teamwork Competencies[21] *(Continued)*

Competency	Definition
Conflict resolution	The facility for resolving differences/disputes among teammates, without creating hostility or defensiveness
Feedback	Observations, concerns, suggestions, and requests communicated by team members in a clear and direct manner, without hostility or defensiveness
Closed-loop communication/ information exchange	The initiation of a message by a sender, the receipt and acknowledgment of the message by the receiver, and the verification of the message by the initial sender
Attitude competencies	
Team orientation (morale)	The use of coordination, evaluation, support, and task inputs from other team members to enhance individual performance and promote group unity
Collective efficacy	The belief that the team can perform effectively as a unit, when each member is assigned specific task demands
Shared vision	The mutually accepted and embraced attitude regarding the team's direction, goals, and mission
Team cohesion	The collective forces that influence members to remain part of a group; an attraction to the team concept as a strategy for improved efficiency
Mutual trust	The positive attitude that team members have for one another; the feeling, mood, or climate of the team's internal environment
Collective orientation	The common belief that a team approach is more conducive to problem solving than an individual approach
Importance of teamwork	The positive attitude that team members exhibit with reference to their work as a team

Source: Baker D, Gustafson S, Beaubien J, Salas E, Barach P. *Medical Teamwork and Patient Safety: The Evidence-Based Relation.* Literature Review. AHRQ Publication No. 05-0053. Rockville, MD: Agency for Healthcare Research and Quality; 2005.

Cannon-Bowers and colleagues contend that team knowledge, skill, and attitude competencies should serve as the starting point for training needs analyses.[33] Trainers then must specify appropriate instructional strategies. Team training should include a feedback component that encourages team members to share their task-performance expectations. Team members also should be encouraged to explain the rationale behind their behaviors as they perform specific tasks. Such strategies provide useful insight into the way each team member processes information, while enabling their peers to better predict one another's behavior and information needs. Finally, the influence of organizational factors above and beyond a training program mandates a needs analysis be conducted to determine the best delivery method or instructional strategy for a given educational intervention.[21]

CONCLUSION

Theory informs practice, the practice of interprofessional team teaching and learning and the practice of collaborative health care teamwork. In the AHRQ review and report regarding teamwork and patient safety, the authors outline a number of conclusions drawn from review and provide specific recommendations for ensuring the design and delivery integrity of medical team training programs with respect to desirable patient safety outcomes. First and foremost, they conclude the following:

> *The medical field lacks a theoretical model of team performance. To date, research has not developed a comprehensive model of team training performance in medical settings. As a result, medical team training programs have not been grounded in a scientific understanding of those human factors that directly influence effective teamwork in medical treatment settings. Given this gap in knowledge, the first research effort we advocate is the development of a theoretical medical team performance model that hypothesizes (1) the interrelationships among predictors of performance, and (2) the interdependencies of predictors and outcome criteria. Despite the absence of a team-performance model uniquely suited to medical treatment scenarios, however, previous research has revealed a considerable volume of relevant knowledge* (p. 39).[21]

D'Amour and colleagues at the University of Montreal conducted a literature review regarding interprofessional collaboration that they identified as a key factor in initiatives designed to increase the effectiveness of health services currently offered to the public.[34] They argue that "the concept of collaboration be well understood, because although the increasingly complex health problems faced by health professionals are creating more interdependencies among them, we still have limited knowledge of the complexity of interprofessional relationships." The review of the literature on interprofessional collaboration was conducted to identify conceptual frameworks that could improve an understanding of this important aspect of health organizations. To that end, they identified and took into consideration "various definitions proposed in the literature and the "various concepts associated with collaboration" and "theoretical frameworks of collaboration."[34] Their results demonstrated the following:

- "The concept of collaboration is commonly defined through five underlying concepts: sharing, partnership, power, interdependency, and process."
- "The most complete models of collaboration seem to be those based on a strong theoretical background, either in organizational theory or in organizational sociology and on empirical data."
- "There is a significant amount of diversity in the way the various authors conceptualized collaboration and in the factors influencing collaboration."
- "These frameworks do not establish clear links between the elements in the models and the outputs."
- "The literature does not provide a serious attempt to determine how patients could be integrated into the health care team, despite the fact that patients are recognized as the ultimate justification for providing collaborative care."[34]

Clearly, more research is needed in this area, yet much has been learned. As we continue to review the literature across multiple disciplines of inquiry, we will continue to add to this knowledge base on interprofessional health care education and practice. As stated in the introduction of this chapter, the first two phases of theorizing in this case rest on (a) what do we know about interprofessional education and practice in health care and (b) what can we assume about interprofessional education and practice in health care based on what we know. These assumptions are then tested, refined, and revised to form new knowledge. The process of theorizing is continuous. New knowledge, new ideas and assumptions, new guiding principles, new methods of testing, and new ways of interpretation all work to form and reform theories about interprofessional education and practice.

One guiding practical principle for continued research in this area can be learned from health sciences colleagues in the basic science and clinical science arenas. Following the National Institutes of Health Roadmap for Medical Research, research teams are being formed that are interdisciplinary and include public–private partnerships, and the clinical research enterprise is being reengineered with a fundamental focus on translational research. According to the National Institutes of Health,

> [T]o improve human health, scientific discoveries must be translated into practical applications. Such discoveries typically begin at "the bench" with basic research—in which scientists study disease at a molecular or cellular level—then progress to the clinical level, or the patient's "bedside." Scientists are increasingly aware that this bench-to-bedside approach to translational research is really a two-way street.[35]

The notion of translational research is applicable to research in interprofessional health care education and practice. Education-to-practice is also a two-way street. Observations and research in practice can inform education and training. Observations and research in education and training can inform practice.

REFERENCES

1. Argyris C, Schon D. *Theory in Practice: Increasing Professional Effectiveness.* Jossey-Bass, San Francisco; 1974.
2. Fawcett J. *Analysis and Evaluation of Nursing Theories.* Philadelphia: FA Davis; 1993.
3. National Heart, Lung, and Blood Institute (NHLBI). Request for Information (RFI): Public Comment on Development of a Funding Opportunity Announcement on Translating Discoveries in the Basic Behavioral and Social Sciences. Notice Number: NOT-HL-08-114. Released March 27, 2008. Available at: http://grants.nih.gov/grants/guide/notice-files/NOT-HL-08-114.html. Accessed September 17, 2008.
4. Pelligrino E. *Interdisciplinary Education in the Health Professions: Assumptions, Definitions, and Some Notes in Teams.* Educating for the health team. Conference report of the Institute of Medicine. National Academies Press, Washington, DC; 1972.
5. Baldwin D. The evolution of interdisciplinary education. In: Holmes D, ed. *Interdisciplinary Education as a Prelude to Interdisciplinary Practice (or Vice Versa).* Proceedings of the 4th Congress of Health Professions Educators. Washington, DC: Association of Academic Health Centers; 1997.
6. Ducanis A, Golin A. *The Interdisciplinary Health Care Team: A Handbook.* Rockville, MD: Aspen Publishers; 1979.

7. World Health Organization. *Learning Together to Work Together for Health.* Report of WHO study group on multiprofessional education for health personnel: The team approach. Technical report series 769. Geneva: WHO; 1988.

8. Centre for the Advancement of Interprofessional Education. *Interprofessional Education: A Definition.* London: Centre for Advancement of Interprofessional Education; 2002.

9. Drinka T, Clark P. *Health Care Teamwork: Interdisciplinary Practice and Teaching.* Westport, CT: Auburn House; 2000.

10. Barr H, Koppel I, Reeves S, Hammick M, Freeth D. *Effective Interprofessional Education: Argument, Assumption & Evidence.* Oxford: Blackwell; 2005.

11. Oandasan I, Reeves S. Key elements for interprofessional education. Part 1: The learner, the educator, and the learning context. J Interprof Care. 2005;19 Suppl 1:21–38.

12. Wakefield M. Capitalizing on our currency. *Nursing Outlook,* 1998;46(2):89–90.

13. Walker P, Baldwin D, Fitzpatrick J, et al. Building community: developing skills for interprofessional health. *Nurs Outlook.* 1998;46(2):88–89.

14. Uys LR, Gwele NS. *Curriculum Development in Nursing: Process and Innovation.* New York: Routledge; 2005.

15. Hall P, Weaver L. Interdisciplinary education and teamwork: a long and winding road. *Med Educ.* 2001 Sep;35(9):867–875.

16. Hirokawa R. A rose by any other name? Examining the differences between multidisciplinary and interdisciplinary health care teams. In: Swanson E, Valentine A, eds. *Redefining Education in Primary Care: Teaming Communities, Practitioners, and Educators.* Washington, DC: Association of Academic Health Centers; 1999.

17. Klein J. *Interdisciplinarity: History, Theory, and Practice.* Detroit, MI: Wayne State University Press; 1990.

18. Senge P. *The Fifth Discipline.* New York: Doubleday Press; 1990.

19. Tresolini C, Pew-Fetzer Task Force. *Health Professions Education and Relationship-Centered Care.* San Francisco, CA: Pew Health Professions Commission; 1994.

20. D'Amour D, Oandasan I. Interprofessionality as the field of interprofessional practice and interprofessional education: an emerging concept. *J Interprof Care.* 2005;19:8–20.

21. Baker D, Gustafson S, Beaubien J, Salas E, Barach P. *Medical Teamwork and Patient Safety: The Evidence-Based Relation.* Literature Review. AHRQ Publication No. 05-0053. Rockville, MD: Agency for Healthcare Research and Quality; 2005.

22. Braithwaite J, Travaglia JF. *Inter-professional Learning and Clinical Education: An Overview of the Literature.* Canberra: Braithwaite and Associates and the ACT Health Department; 2005.

23. Hammick M, Freeth D, Koppel I, Reeves S, Barr H. A Best Evidence Systematic Review of Interprofessional Education. Available at: http://www.bemecollaboration.org/beme/pages/reviews/hammick.html. Accessed February 14, 2008.

24. Reeves S, Zwarenstein M, Goldman J, et al. Interprofessional education: effects on professional practice and health care outcomes. *Cochrane Database of Systematic Reviews,* 2001, Issue 1.

25. Health Canada. *Interprofessional Education for Collaborative Patient-Centered Care: Final Report*. Available at: http://www.hc-sc.gc.ca/hcs-sss/hhr-rhs/strateg/interprof/summ-somm_e.html. Accessed February 14, 2008.

26. Kohn L, Corrigan J, Donaldson M, eds. *To Err Is Human: Building a Safer Health System*. Washington, DC: National Academy Press; 2000.

27. Pizzi L, Goldfarb NI, Nash DB. Crew resource management and its applications in medicine. In: Shojana KG, Duncan BW, McDonald KM, et al., eds. *Making Health Care Safer: A Critical Analysis of Patient Safety Practices*. Rockville, MD: U.S. Department of Health and Human Services, Agency for Healthcare Research and Quality; 2001:501–510.

28. Phillips DC, Soltis J. *Perspectives on Learning*, 4th ed. New York: Teachers College Press; 2003.

29. Schunk D. *Learning Theories: An Educational Perspective*, 4th ed. Upper Saddle River, NJ: Prentice Hall; 2003.

30. Clark P. What would a theory of interprofessional education look like? Some suggestions for developing a theoretical framework for teamwork training. *J Interprof Care*. 2006;20:577–589.

31. Ryder M. Instructional Design Models. University of Colorado Denver, School of Education. Available at: http://carbon.cudenver.edu/~mryder/itc_data/idmodels.html. Accessed February 14, 2008.

32. Scott WR, Davis GF. *Organizations and Organizing: Rational, Natural and Open Systems Perspectives*, 6th ed. Upper Saddle River, NJ: Prentice Hall; 2006.

33. Cannon-Bowers JA, Tannenbaum SI, Salas E, et al. Defining competencies and establishing team training requirements. In: Guzzo RA, Salas E, eds. *Team Effectiveness and Decision-making in Organizations*. San Francisco, CA: Jossey-Bass; 1995:333–380.

34. D'Amour D, Ferrada-Videla M, Rodriguez L, Beaulieu M. The conceptual basis for interprofessional collaboration: core concepts and theoretical frameworks. *J Interprof Care*. 2005;19:116–131.

35. Zerhouni EA. Statement on NIH: Enhancing Clinical Research before the Subcommittee on Health, Committee on Energy and Commerce, United State House of Representatives on March 25, 2004. Available from www.hhs.gov/as/testify/t040325a.html. Accessed September 17, 2008.

CHAPTER 5

Issues Related to Interprofessional Assessment

Brenda M. Coppard, PhD, OT, FAOTA
Gail M. Jensen, PhD, PT, FAPTA
Teresa M. Cochran, PT, DPT, GCS, MA
Caroline Goulet, PhD, PT

INTRODUCTION

In an era of increasing calls for accountability, assessment of interprofessional education (IPE) and its outcomes are needed. The scholarship of engagement that has interprofessional groups of students learning from one another is a rich area for research. Constructs inherent in IPE are similar to those measured in service learning experiences. This chapter outlines the issues surrounding assessment of IPE and offers suggestions for selecting assessment approaches and tools.

Over the next few decades the United States will face radical changes in the demographic profile of health care consumers, and health care work shortages are predicted. The clashing of these two phenomena will require health care professionals to enact flexibility, respect for each other, and interprofessional knowledge and skills to deliver client-centered care.[1] Such forces impose a fundamental question to educational reformers: How willing are they going to be to challenge the existing medical hegemony?[2] Because of the complexity of health care needs and their relationship to health care provision, one profession in isolation is not likely to meet a client's goals.[3] Thus a push for IPE developed. Proponents of IPE have attempted to provide evidence on the processes and outcomes of IPE.[4] So how is IPE assessment conceptualized and implemented? This chapter provides an overview of IPE assessment issues: what to assess, what approaches and tools are available, and directions for future IPE assessment.

IPE AND SCHOLARSHIP OF ENGAGEMENT

IPE experiences offer a rich opportunity for the scholarship of teaching, learning, and assessment and the scholarship of engagement. Boyer maintained that[5]

> the scholarship of engagement means connecting the rich resources of the university to our most pressing social, civic, and the ethical problems, to our children, to our schools, to our teachers, and to our cities. Campuses would be viewed by both students and professors not only as isolated islands, but staging grounds for actions ... ultimately the scholarship of engagement also means creating a special climate in which the academic and civic cultures communicated more continuously and more creatively with each other. . . .

Sandmann maintains that documentation is needed when one undertakes community engagement.[6] The process of the design and methodology of evaluation and documentation of community engagement is needed to demonstrate outcomes related to stakeholders (e.g., students and the community). Any adaptations made in the design or planned process of collaboration with the community or partners must be documented to track the outcomes produced by such changes. Such careful tracking of changes increases the opportunity for others to understand the methods used and the complexity of variables in community engagement. "Adaptations made in the process of collaboration with the community or partners are provided as evidence of reflective scholarship," Sandmann explains.[6] Adaptation and reflection are crucial because most community contexts have few of the controls of traditional research. Raising new questions based on one's past engagement and highlighting best practices that emerge from community collaboration are needed. Outcomes should be described in relationship to the stakeholders: the community, students, institution and units, profession, and faculty members. Such outcomes can be used not only for assessment purposes but to seed further scholarship of engagement.

IPE ASSESSMENT QUANDARY

Compared with other forms of professional education, IPE is more complex, and subsequently assessment methods and approaches do not have clearly defined parameters.[7] Such uncertainty may be uncomfortable for some educators and academics who seek direct cause-and-effect relationships. For example, there is the potential for multiple interaction effects between the learner with their peers, teachers, preceptors, administrative personnel, and patients, and this makes measurement of effects challenging.[7] The relationship between IPE and outcomes are delineated in Stone's representation in Figure 5-1.

Onwuegbuzie argues that teamwork and interdisciplinary education rely on overcoming disciplinary barriers and relaxing some of the more rigidly held beliefs about research paradigms, including the dichotomy of the quantitative–qualitative divide.[8] The validity and quality of IPE assessment are only as good as the measurement tools used. Stone advocates for the reconceptualization of research control when measuring outcomes in this area[7]:

The question of evaluation purpose must be applied—is it to support and measure the progress of student skills, knowledge and attitudes? Or is it to control for the effect of a "treatment" on a group by excluding "extraneous" and possibly confounding factors? The latter is rarely a feasible possibility in the applied settings with which most of us work, in fact Kember [see ref. 9] declares that "genuine control is impossible" in this sort of context. Then challenge then, is to accept the higher levels of uncertainty associated with less controllable systems.

Although evaluation of IPE can be challenging, there are research approaches and resources to use. Educational theory can also influence assessment. For example, knowledge of adult transformative education theory by Mezirow emphasizes becoming more reflective and critical, becoming more open to others' perspectives, and being more accepting and less defensive of new ideas.[10,11] These attributes are not solely needed for IPE but for professional lifelong learning as well. Curiously, such attributes are currently perceived as deficiencies in higher education.[7] For example, the Educational Testing Service captured student proficiency in critical thinking, and results revealed that 77% of college seniors were not proficient in critical thinking.[12]

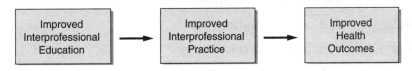

Figure 5-1
The relationship between interprofessional education, practice, and improved health indicators.[7]
Adapted from Stone N. Evaluating interprofessional education: the tautological need for interdisciplinary approaches. *J Interprof Care*. 2006;20:260–275.

Sophisticated approaches to IPE assessment integrate methods that inquire about the learning processes and the measurements of achievements and outcomes. Let's explore some of these approaches and constructs to be measured.

What Should Be Measured?

What should be measured in IPE experiences? Freeth and colleagues published a systematic review of IPE evaluations, project commissioned by the Learning and Teaching Support Network Centre for Health Sciences and Practice in the United Kingdom.[13] The authors expanded Kirkpatrick's four-level model of educational evaluation (Table 5-1) to a six-level model shown in Table 5-2. Commonly, IPE assessment measures include (a) students' reactions to IPE experiences, (b) students' changes in attitudes and perceptions, (c) students' and practitioners' acquisition of knowledge or skills, (d) behavioral changes made in professional practice based on IPE experiences, (e) changes in organization and care delivery, and (f) benefits to patients, clients, or communities.[13]

This systematic review included a report of the examples of the IPE programmatic goals.[13] Typically, these goals included improving interprofessional collaboration, improving quality of care, and improving collaboration and care. Teaching and learning methods reported in the review included guideline development or improvement, exchanging information, sharing experiences between participants, small group discussions, lectures, seminars, problem-solving activities in IPE groups, practice-based learning in IPE clinic placements, and role plays. Generally, learners were active in the learning process, and motivation to learn was usually garnered through a problem or work-related task. Reflection on practice and values was a common way to promote social interaction among different professions.

Table 5-1. Kirkpatrick's Model of Educational Outcomes

1. Reaction: To the education experience

2. Learning: Acquisition of skills and knowledge

3. Behavior change: Applying learning to practice

4. Results: In relation to intended programmatic outcomes

Source: Kirkpatrick, DL. Evaluation of training. In: Craig R, Bittel L, eds. *Training and Development Handbook*. New York: McGraw-Hill; 1967.

Table 5-2. Freeth and Colleagues' Model of Outcomes of Interprofessional Education[13]

1. Reaction: Learners' views on the learning experiences and its interprofessional nature

2a. Modification of attitudes/perceptions: Changes in reciprocal attitudes or perceptions between participant groups; changes in perception or attitude toward the value and/or use of team approaches to caring for a specific client group

2b. Acquisition of knowledge/skill: Including knowledge and skills linked to interprofessional collaboration

3. Behavioral change: Identifies individuals' transfer of interprofessional learning to their practice setting and changed professional practice

4a. Change in organizational practice: Wider changes in the organization and delivery of care

4b. Benefits to patients/clients: Improvements in health or well-being of patients/clients

Source: Freeth D, Hammick M, Koppel I, et al. A critical review of evaluations of interprofessional education. UK Centre for the Advancement of Interprofessional Education, 2002. http://www.caipe.org.uk/resources. Accessed May 6, 2008.

An interprofessional teamwork model was developed by Fertman and coworkers to promote interprofessional practice in rural areas.[14] Their four-pronged approach conceptualized a team as having context, structure, process, and outcomes (Table 5-3). This model can be modified to specific IPE endeavors and guide the planning of learning experiences and assessment endeavors.

What Approaches and Tools Are Available to Measure Outcomes?

What types of approaches and tools are currently available and applicable to IPE outcomes? A paucity of IPE assessments for health profession students exists. IPE experiences may be looked at as a component of a learning activity rather than exclusively assessed. For example, nursing and medicine faculty members developed standards to measure students' clinical, teamwork, and communication skills during an IPE experience.[15] An objective structured clinical skills examination and role play assessment were used as assessment approaches for the interprofessional group of students.

Table 5-3. Interprofessional Team Conceptual Model[14]

Context	Process
• Rural communities	• Team leadership
• Disease prevention and health promotion	• Information sharing
• Diverse professional cultures	• Collaboration/consensus
• Health care system and community relationships	• Problem solving
• Team rewards	• Conflict resolution
• Performance feedback	• Developmental stages
• Decision making	
Structure	**Outcomes**
• Team as individuals	• Evaluation and accountability
• Team as professionals	• Team maintenance and enhancement
• Team as a collaborative unit	

Source: Fertman CI, Dotson S, Mazzocco GO, et al. Challenges of preparing allied health professionals for interdisciplinary practice in rural areas. *J Allied Health.* 2005;34:163–168.

The IPE aspect of a learning experience can use various approaches. Such approaches for assessment include service-learning measures, self-assessment, questionnaires, and health indicator outcomes.

Service-Learning Measures

Interprofessional service-learning educational experiences may be assessed using measures of service learning. Some of the constructs of service learning are the same or similar to constructs of IPE, and this allows for use of assessment measure across both areas. IPE experiences that immerse students in the community have similarities to students engaged in community service-learning projects. Bringle, Phillips, and Hudson published a book entitled, *The Measure of Service Learning—Research Scales to Assess Student Experiences.*[16] This book contains a compilation of scales and measures of key constructs associated with service learning as listed in Table 5-4. Such constructs include motives, values, moral development, self, self-concept, student development, attitudes, and critical thinking.

Table 5-4. Measures of Service Learning Constructs[16]

Construct	Measure
Motives and values	Volunteer Functions Inventory Motivation to Volunteer Scale Public Service Motivation Scale Survey of Interpersonal Values Personal Social Values
Moral development	Defining Issues Test Sociomoral Reflection Objective Measure Prosocial Reasoning Objective Measure Revised Moral Authority Scale Ethics Position Questionnaire Visions of Morality Scale
Self and self-concept	Self-Esteem Scale Community Service Self-Efficacy Scale Self-Efficacy Scale Confidence Subscale of the Erwin Identity Scale Interpersonal Reactivity Index Texas Social Behavior Inventory Hope Scale Dean Alienation Scale Selfism Social Avoidance and Distress Scale
Student development	Student Developmental Task and Lifestyle Assessment Learning of Self Understanding Scale Problem-Solving Inventory Career Decision-Making Self-Efficacy Scale
Attitudes	AIDS Caregiver Scale Civic Action Community Service Involvement Preference Inventory Community Service Attitudes Scale Global Belief in a Just World Scale Life Orientation Test Revised Universal Orientation Scale Social Dominance Orientation Scale Civic Attitudes

(Continues)

Table 5-4. Measures of Service Learning Constructs[16] *(Continued)*

Construct	Measure
Critical thinking	Watson-Glaser Critical Thinking Appraisal
	Scale of Intellectual Development
	California Critical Thinking Skills Test
	Cornell Critical Thinking Test

Source: Bringle RG, Phillips MA, Hudson M. *The Measure of Service Learning—Research Scales to Assess Student Experiences.* Washington, DC: American Psychological Association; 2004.

Self-Assessment

Self-assessment measures relate to explicit learning goals. Self-assessment underpins the formation of mindful practice or the ability "to listen with attentiveness to patients' distress, recognize their own errors, refine their technical skills, make evidence-based decisions, and clarify their values so they can act with compassion, technical competence, presence and insight."[17] Methods to use self-assessment include field notes and focus groups; transcriptions of journals, essays, and web discussions; interprofessional computer conferencing; and videotape critiques.[4,18,19]

Questionnaires

The Interdisciplinary Education Perception Scale (IEPS) is an 18-item perception and attitudinal scale developed by Luecht and colleagues.[20] IEPS measures perceptions of students' interprofessional experiences relative to their own profession and other health professions. The four factors measured are: (a) professional competence and autonomy, (b) perceived need for professional cooperation, (c) perception of actual cooperation and resource sharing within and across professions, and (d) understanding the value and contributions of other professionals/professions. Psychometric development of the tool was conducted by Luecht et al.[20] and furthered by Hayward, Powell, and McRoberts.[20,21]

When choosing assessment tools, one has options. One can select an established tool or make an adaptation to an existing tool. Each option has advantages and disadvantages.

The main advantage of using an established tool is that it takes less time to incorporate into research than does adapting original tools. Many existing tools have some psychometric development completed, and thus one can make decisions based on its reliability and validity measures. The disadvantage of using an existing tool is that it may not exactly match what is to be measured.

Adaptations of original measurement tools are often used to assess IPE experiences. Validity and reliability issues emerge from such modifications. Adapting an existing tool may be more appropriate to answering a specific research question than the original scale. When adaptations are made, a pilot of the modified tool should be completed and appropriate revisions should be made. An example of modifying an existing tool was the creation of the Attitudes Toward Community Health Scale, reported by Rose and coworkers.[22] The authors adapted the Attitude Toward Research Scale.[23] The adapted scale was reviewed by three doctorally prepared faculty, and reliability testing equaled a 94.4% agreement within a 2-week test–retest design. The instrument was not tested for validity or reliability. When such tools are adapted, it is best to plan studies to measure validity and reliability so that the tools can be refined and used by others.

Health Outcomes and IPE

Measuring IPE's effect on health outcomes needs to be captured. Changes in health indicators because of IPE is not documented well in the literature. A critical need exists for outcome data so that IPE may garner funding and serve as a credible goal of educating health professions students. Zwarenstein et al. completed a search of 1,042 articles, but none of the studies met their inclusion criteria.[24] Despite the narrow inclusion criteria for their systematic review, there is growing evidence of IPE's impact on health outcomes in relationship to a variety of conditions. Although a direct cause and effect can rarely be claimed, there are indications that IPE is positively impacting health outcomes. For example, Edwards and Smith reported that IPE activities in eastern Tennessee resulted in an increase in employment in clinics associated with IPE and a decrease in the number of deaths from all causes and from cardiovascular deaths in IPE counties over a period of 5 years.[25]

Litaker et al. compared 157 patients with hypertension and diabetes mellitus.[26] Some received care from a physician only and other received care from a team of a nurse practitioner and physician. Results showed significant improvements in mean glycosylated hemoglobin levels and higher satisfaction with care from a team of nurse practitioner and physician than treatment solely from a physician.

In a randomized control sample of 144 people with Parkinson's disease, outcomes demonstrated that patients with Parkinson's disease declined significantly over 6 months. However, a short duration of multidisciplinary rehabilitation improved mobility.[27]

Future Directions of IPE Assessment

Measuring best practices in IPE is needed. Best practices can be conceptualized from two perspectives: single case and multiple cases. For example, best practices can be generated from reflecting on and analyzing what went well, what barriers were present, how the barriers were addressed, and what outcomes were achieved from a particular IPE experience or proj-ect. Likewise, best practices can be gleaned from analyzing multiple cases. For example, Jensen and Royeen identified rural best practices across 15 Quentin N. Burdick Rural Health Interdisciplinary Programs funded by the U.S. Public Health Service.[28] All projects dealt with specific areas of rural health and interprofessional training. They found that "best practice projects use multiple reflective tools including journal entries, team-based community projects, media portfolios, and qualitative tools for data collection such as interviews, focus groups, participant observation, and field notes."[28]

Researchers must continue to establish and develop assessment tools. Psychometric development of such tools will garner acceptance of outcomes from a quantitative perspective. When such tools are implemented across IPE endeavors, it offers the possibility of cross-case analysis.

A longitudinal design of IPE influences on professionals and practice is needed. Many IPE outcomes are gathered at the end of a program or experience, and researchers may miss capturing the important outcomes that occur over time. For example, the following questions are appropriate for a longitudinal study design:

- Does IPE affect one's practice and employment choices throughout a career trajectory?
- Does IPE affect how one engages in precepting professional students?
- How are health outcomes affected by interprofessional practice?

IPE assessors should consider both qualitative and quantitative measures to capture diverse aspects of the IPE experience. Listed below are various examples of research questions that lend themselves to both qualitative and quantitative research methods:

Qualitative

- How are decisions made in IPE teams?
- What pedagogies support IPE initiatives?
- What institutional infrastructures best support IPE efforts according to institutional category?
- How do stakeholders of IPE describe the impact on the community/individual/patient?

Quantitative

- How do attitudes/values/perceptions change with IPE experiences?
- What is the student profile of students who engage in IPE?
- How many IPE program completers were there for the project?

CONCLUSION

IPE is rooted in the scholarship of engagement. The complexity of human interactions is inherently involved in IPE. Despite a continued interest in IPE and a growing need to provide measures and outcome evidence for IPE effectiveness, there is a paucity of literature that concludes the effectiveness of IPE. Despite the current evidence, we must continue to formulate methods to measure IPE. Thus mixed methods (i.e., qualitative and quantitative approaches) must be considered to measure the process and outcomes of IPE.

REFERENCES

1. Humphris D, Hean S. Educating the future workforce: building the evidence about interprofessional learning. *J Health Serv Res Policy*. 2004;9:24–27.
2. Cameron A. New role developments in context. In: Humphris D, Masterson A, eds. *Developing New Clinical Roles: A Guide for Health Professionals*. London: Churchill Livingstone; 2000:7–24.
3. Walsh CL, Gordon MF, Marshall M, et al. Interprofessional capability: a developing framework for interprofessional education. *Nurse Educ Pract*. 2005;5:230–237.
4. Dalton L, Spencer J, Dunn M, et al. Re-thinking approaches to undergraduate health professional education: interdisciplinary rural placement program. *Collegian*. 2003;10:17–21.
5. Boyer EL. The scholarship of engagement. *J Public Serv Outreach*. 1996;1:11–20.
6. Sandmann LR. When doing good is not good enough! Good to great: the scholarship of engagement. Paper presented at the National Extension Director/Administrator Conference, February 2003, Fort Lauderdale, Fla.
7. Stone N. Evaluating interprofessional education: the tautological need for interdisciplinary approaches. *J Interprof Care*. 2006;20:260–275.

8. Onwuegbuzie A. Why can't we all get along? Towards a framework for unifying research paradigms. *Education.* 2002;122:518–530.

9. Kember D. To control or not control: the question of whether experimental designs are appropriate for evaluating teaching innovations in higher education. *Assess Eval Higher Educ.* 2003;28:89–101.

10. Meziorow and Associates. Understanding transformation theory. *Adult Educ Quart.* 1994;44:222–232.

11. Mezirow J, et al. *Learning as Transformation.* San Francisco, CA: Jossey Bass; 2000.

12. Association of Colleges and Universities. *Liberal Education Outcomes: A Preliminary Report on Student Achievement in College.* Washington, DC: Association of American Colleges and Universities; 2004.

13. Freeth D, Hammick M, Koppel I, et al. A critical review of evaluations of interprofessional education. UK Centre for the Advancement of Interprofessional Education, 2002. (http://www.caipe.org.uk/resources. Accessed May 6, 2008.

14. Fertman CI, Dotson S, Mazzocco GO, et al. Challenges of preparing allied health professionals for interdisciplinary practice in rural areas. *J Allied Health.* 2005; 34:163–168.

15. Morrison SL, Steward MC. Developing interprofessional assessment. *Learn Health Soc Care.* 2005;4:192–202.

16. Bringle RG, Phillips MA, Hudson M. *The Measure of Service Learning—Research Scales to Assess Student Experiences.* Washington, DC: American Psychological Association; 2004.

17. Epstein R. Mindful practice. *JAMA.* 1999;282:833–839.

18. Becker EA, Godwin EM. Methods to improve teaching interdisciplinary teamwork through computer conferencing. *J Allied Health.* 2005;34:169–176.

19. Fulmer T, Hyer K, Flaherty E, et al. Geriatric interdisciplinary team training program. *J Aging Health.* 2005;17:443–470.

20. Luecht RM, Madsen MK, Taugher MP, et al. Assessing professional perceptions: Design and validation of an interdisciplinary education perception scale. *J Allied Health.* 1990;19:181–191.

21. Hayward KS, Powell LT, McRoberts J. Changes in student perceptions of interdisciplinary practice in the rural setting. *J Allied Health.* 1996;25:315–327.

22. Rose MA, Lyons KJ, Miller KS, Cornman-Levy D. The effect of an interdisciplinary community health project on student attitudes toward community health, people who are indigent and homeless, and team leadership skill development. *J Allied Health.* 2003;32:122–125.

23. Selby M, Tuttle DM. Teaching nursing research by guided design: a pilot study. *J Nurs Educ.* 1985;24:250–252.

24. Zwarenstein M, Reeves S, Barr H, et al. Interprofessional education: effects on professional practice and health care outcomes [Review]. *Cochrane Database of Systematic Reviews,* 2000, Issue 3.

25. Edwards J, Smith P. Impact of interdisciplinary education in underserved areas: health professions collaboration in Tennessee. *J Prof Nurs.* 1998;14:144–149.

26. Litaker D, Mion L, Planavsky L, et al. Physician-nurse practitioner teams in chronic disease management: the impact on costs, clinical effectiveness, and patients' perception of care. *J Interprof Care*. 2003;17:223–237.
27. Wade D, Gage H, Owen C, et al. Multidisciplinary rehabilitation for people with Parkinson's disease: a randomized controlled study. *J Neurol Neurosurg Psych*. 2003;74:158–162.
28. Jensen GM, Royeen CB. Improved rural access to care: dimensions of best practice. *J Interprof Care*. 2002;16:117–128.

CHAPTER 6

Shaping the Future: Strategies for Promoting Interprofessional Health Professions Practice in Rural and Underserved Communities

Victoria F. Roche, PhD

INTRODUCTION

The pressing public health issue of practitioner shortages in rural communities is not unique to 21st century health care. Health professions scholars have been writing about the shortage for several decades, with some attributing the start of our current crisis to an early 20th century shift in the philosophy and practice of medical education to favor large, urban-centered enterprises with an emphasis on specialty care.[1] Significant study has recently been focused on identifying factors that influence the selection of practice careers (most commonly, but not exclusively, medical practice) in rural and/or underserved communities.[2–11] There is general agreement that growing up in a rural community, having a positive view of small-town life, coming to a health professions education program with an intent for general practice and a desire to foster close professional relationships with patients, and engaging in thoughtfully constructed rural community practice experiences as a student or resident all predispose to the selection of rural practice. Rural career selection appears to be negatively influenced by such things as a sense of personal and professional isolation; a perceived lack of continuing education opportunities; a sometimes overwhelming work load due to un-avoidable understaffing, disadvantageous salary, or service reimbursement systems; and concerns related to spousal employment and the quality of school systems.

Brooks et al.[5] distinguished the influence of personal characteristics, attributes, and dispositions related to rural medical practice that were formed before beginning a professional medical education program ("nature") from those that could be shaped by the medical school experience ("nurture") and found that both could be motivators for recruitment. Although their study was focused on physician recruitment, the lessons learned are readily applicable to other health professions disciplines. Their retrospective review of a decade of literature (1990–2000) revealed that the nature factors of rural upbringing and a propensity for rural practice before entering medical school correlated most strongly with recruitment into this type of practice. Retention in a rural community was more strongly correlated with the nurture-related elements of a rural health-focused curriculum and engaging in high-quality rural rotations, particularly during the residency years. A well-constructed rural residency experience allows practitioners to experience rural life firsthand for a protracted period of time, thus prompting familiarity and confidence in the value of small-town living[10] that was viewed as more important to retention than feeling prepared for medical practice itself.[12] A perhaps unintended benefit of having urban practitioners exposed to rural communities during their schooling through high-quality rotation experiences is the opportunity for enhanced interprofessional collaboration and networking with rural colleagues because of a better appreciation of the needs and challenges of rural practice.

Crandall et al.[3] categorized motivation for entering rural medical practice into four models. The affinity models encompass much of what Brooks and collaborators termed nature-related factors (rural background, a priori interest in rural practice, etc.). Crandall and coworkers claim that the nurturing strategies implemented by academic institutions can reinforce interest that is already a student's professional disposition, but probably does not do much to entice those without the intrinsic desire for rural community life and work.

Crandall's practice characteristic models move beyond inherent practitioner interest by emphasizing the nonsalary aspects of rural practice that must be in place to both initially and persistently engage the practitioner. Issues important to all health professionals, such as adequate technical support, helpful colleagues, and reasonable work schedules that permit time for family and the development of outside interests, fall into this domain. These issues, as well as those related to spousal employment and the education of children, must be proactively addressed if those with an affinity for rural practice can expect to be fulfilled and happy in it. The economic incentive models address salary and service reimbursement issues and call for an end to unjust health care financing practices that serve as disincentives to enter or stay in a rural health practice. Scammon and coworkers[4] also noted the significant challenges rural physicians face when attempting to secure fair reimbursement for services through Medicare and Medicaid, difficulties common to all professions seeking federal reimbursement for health care services rendered. The rural providers interviewed for their study talked of having such patients "shipped out" to them from less remote sites and alluded to the need for a systematic overhaul to provide structured referral processes and adequate reimbursement for quality care. Sempowski[6] also spoke to the need for reimbursement models featuring differentiated fees and/or bonuses for providing service to underserved communities.

The last of Crandall's rural practice-impacting domains was termed indenture models.[3] The indenture models include programs that require a set period of practitioner service in rural communities in exchange for financial support for schooling. Given the large debt load faced by graduates from almost any health professions education program, it is often assumed that the scholarship support and loan repayment benefits offered to practitioners in selected primary care-focused disciplines (including medicine, nursing, physician assistant, dental health, and mental health) by the National Health Service Corps (NHSC) would be strong rural practice recruitment and retention motivators, but the literature does not bear this out. With the possible exception of the Indian Health Service (IHS), where NHSC return-of-service physicians stayed in IHS practice 3 to 4 years beyond their required period of service,[9] many investigators found that NHSC practitioners most commonly either stay for the minimum time period to repay health education loans[3,6,13–16] or opt for an early buyout from their service commitment.[6] For example, in 1992 Pathman[13] and colleagues reported that, at 8 years, only 29% of NHSC physicians practicing in rural/underserved communities remained in their original practice community compared with 52% of non-NHSC rural practitioners, and 80% of the NHSC physicians who left their "home" community moved out of the rural setting entirely. The Pathman study is cited often in more current physician education literature,[4–6] indicating that its findings are still relevant to present day medical practitioners, although Cullen et al.[18] suggests that retention could be enhanced if longer service commitments were required. Scammon and coworkers[4] inferred that placing NHSC practitioners lacking the intrinsic commitment to underserved/ rural health in rural communities may actually provide a disservice to those communities, because the practitioners may be "ill suited to the environments into which they move." Others have noted that integration of the practitioner and his or her family into the rural community is crucial for career satisfaction and success in a rural setting.[3–5,17] If practitioners do not value or appreciate rural life, there may a risk for superficial relationships with rural patients and/or less-than-optimal holistic care.

As noted previously, although the preponderance of the literature in this area is focused on physician education and practice, most of the key issues identified are related more to personal disposition than educational pathway and should therefore be relevant to practitioners from other health professions disciplines.

STRATEGIES FOR PROMOTING PRACTICE IN RURAL AND UNDERSERVED COMMUNITIES

By all accounts, taking a balanced approach to the recruitment and retention of rural health care practitioners appears central to the success of meeting the future health care needs of citizens in rural/underserved America. This balance can be achieved by admitting students with "natural" characteristics that predispose to the selection of a rural/underserved practice and then providing appropriate "nurturing" experiences to reinforce and sustain that interest. The following sections describe specific programs and strategies implemented at Creighton University within the past 5 years that were designed or could be used to reinforce and sustain health professions student motivation to elect careers of service to rural and/or disadvantaged communities.

Interprofessional Pre-Matriculation Program

The Health Sciences at Creighton University has long dedicated efforts and resources to encourage students from traditionally underserved communities to prepare for health professions careers. Historically, the University has participated in educational outreach efforts supported by the Health Resource Service Administration (HRSA), the American Association of Medical Colleges, and Robert Wood Johnson's Health Professions Partnership Initiative[19] as well as local programs such as the Minority Youth Conference and Focus on the Health Professions. In 2005 the School of Pharmacy and Health Professions (SPAHP) collaborated with the

University's Health Science Multicultural and Community Affairs office (HS-MACA) to launch an academic enrichment and success program for educationally disadvantaged students who have been accepted into the School's Doctor of Pharmacy program. Entitled the School of Pharmacy and Health Professions Pre-Matriculation Program, students from rural/underserved backgrounds, many of whom come from secondary school systems ill-equipped to provide advanced coursework in math and science or which lack honors or placement programs that would allow students to refine interests, hone skills, and demonstrate capabilities, qualify for inclusion.[3]

When conducting file reviews of program applicants, the Pharmacy Admissions Committee and the Office of Admissions counselors make note of applicants from educationally disadvantaged backgrounds whose academic credentials are solid but not exceedingly competitive in a rigorous pharmacy education marketplace. When evaluating students, the committee members and counselors consider students to be educationally disadvantaged if they have had life experiences resulting in hardship that could realistically be expected to have adversely effected learning or academic performance as measured by preprofessional course grades, honors, scholarships, and so on. Characteristics such as being a first-generation college student or nontraditional in terms of age and background and/or completing preprofessional coursework at a community college are also considered. Evidence of high potential for success in a rigorous, values-focused health professions education program is essential and can come from testimonials from teachers and counselors provided in letters of recommendation, scores on the standardized Pharmacy College Admission Test (PCAT), and a dedication to professionalism and service evidenced through school-sponsored and extracurricular activities.

Out of a pool of over 1,300 applicants, the Pharmacy Admissions Committee selects up to 10 educationally disadvantaged individuals they believe have the potential to be outstanding pharmacists, even though their academic performance as measured by grade point average and/or PCAT scores may be less competitive than that of applicants from less disadvantaged backgrounds. Ten students represent twice the number the program can support each year and provide a pool of candidates sufficiently large to permit a competitive selection process as well as to ensure the availability of qualified alternates in the event one or more invited applicants decline. These students are notified that they are being considered for admission through the SPAHP Pre-Matriculation Program and are invited to an on-campus interview. During their interview day the students engage with their fellow applicants in orientation and information sessions, meet faculty and current students, and become familiar with the campus but also have special interviews with HS-MACA professionals and the prematriculation students from previous years. At the conclusion of the interview, the academic and professional potential of the Pre-Matriculation Program candidates are holistically reviewed by a selection committee comprised of the Chair of the Pharmacy Admissions Committee, the Associate Vice President for Health Sciences Multicultural and Community Affairs, selected HS-MACA staff, and the Senior Associate Dean for the School of Pharmacy and Health Professions. Through a consensus process, up to five candidates are offered admission contingent upon the completion of an 8-week summer academic enrichment program that involves coursework in biology, chemistry, mathematics, reading, and writing designed to shore up basic skills. Formal instruction in the principles and practices that promote academic success, as well as cultural competency, is also requisite. Students accepting this offer are told that although their academic costs, including books, are covered by the University, they are responsible for their travel and living expenses. The students' out-of-pocket expenses vary depending on their Omaha-based living arrangements (e.g., whether they live with family members, elect roommates, etc.), whether they own and operate a vehicle, and whether they must return to their hometown between the conclusion of the summer enrichment program and the start of the fall semester.

The philosophy of the SPAHP Pre-Matriculation Program mirrors that of the more familiar federally funded, postbaccalaureate Health Careers Opportunity Program. The summer enrichment phase of the Pre-Matriculation Program takes place immediately before the beginning of the fall term of the first professional year. Pharmacy students participate with selected postbaccalaureate students seeking admission to Creighton's medical and dental programs, which provides an early opportunity for interprofessional networking and relationship building. The program begins with a day-long orientation designed to put students at ease and establish a foundation for interprofessional camaraderie. The program goals and requirements are reviewed, and participants are given information on financial aid and the campus-based academic and counseling support services available to them. It is important to note that the University offers prematriculation programs in medicine and dentistry but that the purpose and scope of those programs are distinct from those of the SPAHP Pre-Matriculation Program.

Over the course of the following week participants take a series of tests to determine their baseline knowledge about content and concepts important for success in the pharmacy curriculum. Results from pretesting are used by the faculty of the College of Arts and Sciences, who teach the prematriculation courses, and the staff in the SPAHP's Office of Academic and Student Affairs and HS-MACA to counsel students about the students' particular strengths and areas of concern and to direct students to appropriate resources within the university and school to increase their chance for success. Students are given the opportunity to participate in individual or small-group tutoring sessions and/or may seek individual assistance from course instructors. The School's Office of eLearning and Academic Technology administers a basic computing and technology assessment to the pharmacy participants and uses the results to design technology skill development seminars. The remainder of the time is spent in class, shadowing pharmacist mentors from a wide variety of practice areas, securing tutoring assistance and/or studying independently or in groups, and becoming familiar with the school, the university faculty and administrative staff, and the city of Omaha.

At the conclusion of the 8-week program the students are expected to have gained a solid foundation in the preprofessional fundamentals essential for success in the Doctor of Pharmacy program, understand the university system and be fully aware of all resources available to support and assist them, have made friends and established interprofessional networks, and feel at home in the Creighton and Omaha communities. With their comfort and confidence levels heightened, they should be able to "hit the ground running" as their first professional year begins. As of 2007, all seven pharmacy students who were accepted into the SPAHP Pre-Matriculation Program have successfully completed the summer enrichment experience and are on track in their professional program of study. In 2008, the SPAHP Pre-Matriculation Program will be expanded to include the disciplines of occupational therapy and physical therapy, which will further augment the interprofessional character of the experience.

Recognizing that outstanding potential can be compromised by inadequate financial support, particularly at a private institution where tuition costs are higher than those charged by public institutions, the School has made scholarship monies available to prematriculation program "graduates." Student performance in the six required prematriculation program courses is the basis for determining the awards, and in the first year of its implementation, the two students who completed the program were both offered tuition scholarships that will be maintained as long as they remain in good academic standing. The Dean's Office is making efforts to keep the scholarship support significant (e.g., full or half tuition scholarships) in order that these originally educationally disadvantaged students are motivated to excel, graduate, and return to communities in need of their expertise and commitment.

Interprofessional Structured Cultural Immersions

As noted above, it is well recognized that health professions curricula have the power to shape and sustain student interest and commitment to practice in rural and underserved communities. Structured experiences of a significant duration (e.g., something more than an isolated or superficial exposure) with dedicated professional mentors, coupled with opportunities for interprofessional collaboration and reflection, serve to expose students to the joys and the challenges of rural life and allow them to make informed decisions about whether the opportunities and rewards inherent in rural practice are a good fit with their own values and personal/professional goals. Scammon and coworkers[4] stated that student engagement in meaningful service activities to rural/underserved populations while in school can be predictive of their ultimate practice choice. This realization should motivate institutions to thoughtfully and deliberately make room for service-learning courses and extracurricular service experiences within health professions curricula that have traditionally been content intense, rigid, and lock step.

Interprofessional Short-Term Immersions

At Creighton University, students are presented with a multitude of opportunities to engage with rural Native American communities through structured service-learning experiences. Our School's Office of Interprofessional Scholarship Service and Education (OISSE) is the focal point for extracurricular service involvement, including service to and with Native peoples, and offers two 3-day immersions in these rural reservation communities, each over 3 consecutive weeks. Students from our School's three health professions programs (occupational therapy, physical therapy, and pharmacy) as well as those from nursing, medicine, and dentistry are encouraged to participate, ensuring a true interprofessonal experience. Those who opt for an immersion are exposed to the rich cultural heritage of the Omaha and Winnebago people, are able to compare and contrast health services provided at the IHS (Winnebago) and tribally-run (Omaha) health care facilities, and build community through their interprofessional shadowing and practice experiences on-site. Participants begin to establish an interprofessional community of learners as they dialogue about their professions and experiences during the 3-hour commute to and from the reservations. Students reflect on experiences and, through required pre- and postexperience assessments on cultural and interprofessionalism awareness, are able to measure the effect of the immersion on their professional growth, including their understanding of professional roles and responsibilities, the importance of collaboration and team-based care, cultural competency, and career inclinations.

Students not able to commit to a 3-day immersion experience may elect to participate in guided community engagement and service activities with native patients, children, elders, and others through the School's Native American Interest Group, which is highly focused on rural, reservation-based populations. A service experience is a requirement of the physical therapy program, and many students elect to work within rural communities, very often beyond the minimum required number of hours.

Interprofessional Rural Health Training

Over the past decade, OISSE has been the recipient of numerous HRSA grants offered through the Quentin N. Burdick Program for Rural Interdisciplinary Training.[17,20] These grants, and the public health needs they were designed to address, have benefitted from the close, collaborative working relationship previously established between the SPAHP and the native communities, which were true partners in defining the spectrum of experiences in which the student trainees would participate. The students, numbering slightly over 1,300, came from our school's three health professions programs as well as from social work, occupational therapy assistant, and physical therapist assistant programs offered by other higher education institutions in the Omaha area. The consortium approach was important in that it allowed involvement from institutions that, on their own, would not have been able to engage their students in career-shaping service outreach of this type and expanded and enriched the interprofessional nature of the experience for all. The time of individual student involvement in reservation-based training ranged from 1 month to 1 year, depending on the curriculum and restrictions of each participating health professions program and the service options elected by each student.

The goals of the program, which, in part, were to address the social injustice of barriers to care, stimulate serious interest in careers with rural/underserved communities, and build a sustained health care capacity within the partnering communities, were successfully met. Themes that emerged from an assessment of student learning published in 2004 by Mu et al.[20] included recognition of the critical importance of interprofessional and collaborative interactions in the provision of care and an enhanced respect for the rural community. All 111 students in this study reported significantly more positive perceptions of interprofessional practice posttraining as compared to pretraining, and the extent of the pre- and postexperience perception difference was directly correlated to time spent in the communities. According to Mu et al., some members of the study cohort have gone on to establish practices in underserved communities.[20]

The shared commitment to working through the challenges (both anticipated and unanticipated) of establishing an interdisciplinary training program of this complexity and magnitude also helped build a sustained trust between all partners. This, in turn, facilitated further collaboration in the provision of additional health care services and in the education of students who were not associated with the training grants, such as those electing the short-term immersions described above.

Service-Learning Course Immersion in Pharmacy and Occupational Therapy

A 2-credit-hour service-learning-based elective course on Native American culture and health has been offered to Creighton pharmacy students for the past 4 years[21]and was broadened in 2007 to include occupational therapy. The goals of the course are multiple and include the stimulation of (a) awareness and thoughtful analysis of Native American health care beliefs, traditions, disparities, and needs through interaction with native health care professionals and healers; (b) reflective thinking about issues related to course content and experiences through journaling; (c) a desire to advocate for underserved populations; (d) decisions to elect an IHS Commissioned Officer Student Training and Extern Program experience, clinical rotation, and/or career; and (e) the concept of vocation in directing one's life's work. The target service communities are Chinle and Tsaile, Arizona, located within the Navajo Nation. The interprofessional Creighton-based faculty team has worked very closely with IHS practitioners in these communities in constructing the course to ensure that the needs of both the University and the various native communities (health care and civic) are met.

This elective course is a blend of classroom- and community-based learning experiences. Before the service-learning component of the course, students study the multiplicity of native cultures and explore the common and unique morbidities and health challenges that plague native communities. They engage with native and non-native health care practitioners serving native people in rural and urban communities and discuss barriers to care, social welfare challenges including poverty and its associated individual and community dysfunctions, and the use of traditional foods to maintain health. Discussion with various tribal elders and spiritual leaders has provided insight into the role of spirituality and ceremony in health, and the opportunity to dialogue with leaders of sovereign nations has clearly demonstrated the power of political advocacy. Students prepare for these discussions through assigned readings and by conducting research on a specific Native American health issue in preparation for an in-class, professionally presented seminar.

The high point of the course is the week-long cultural immersion experience in Chinle/Tsaile. Students live and work within the community and are guided in their daily activities by IHS health professional mentors. Students are housed individually or in pairs by an IHS health care practitioner, which provides them the opportunity to talk through the day's events and the impact they have had on their developing professional disposition. Students divide their time learning more about Navajo history and experiencing its culture, providing needed service to elders living in remote areas of the reservation (chopping wood, cleaning/repairing hogans, providing basic health assessments, etc.) under the guidance of a public health nurse or community health representative, and working closely with IHS pharmacists in Chinle, Tsaile, and Pinon. There are multiple opportunities for students to engage in interprofessional dialogue, networking and learning, socialize informally with Chinle citizens, and share meals, conversation, and cultural aspects of daily life with native families. While working in the pharmacies or rehabilitation clinics within the various health care facilities, students observe the extent of interprofessional dependence and collaboration that underpins IHS practice, the commitment to patient welfare and optimal care outcomes through routine and individualized patient counseling, and the holistic care realized from the proactive collaboration between IHS practitioners and the resident medicine man. They spend time at the end of each day recording reflections in course journals, thinking critically about the uplifting and troublesome experiences they had that day, and considering aspects of vocational prompting related to a career serving tribal people.

A high percentage of course enrollees have gone on to elect additional learning experiences with the IHS, including summer Jr. COSTEP experiences (32%), elective IHS advanced practice rotations (68%), and IHS residencies and/or careers (11%).[21] Two pharmacy program graduates are currently employed in an IHS or tribal hospital, two others are considering a change to IHS employment, and five pharmacy students yet to graduate have either firmly committed to or are on track for an IHS career. These results support the findings of others that high-quality, structured "nurturing" experiences embedded within a health professions curriculum can motivate students to action relative to electing practice with rural/underserved populations.

Web-based Health Professions Education in Pharmacy and Occupational Therapy

It has been well documented that students in health professions and other doctoral level academic programs can learn effectively through a distance when online courses are appropriately structured, managed, and facilitated.[22-27] Keys to lasting learning in high-quality distance education center around the development of interactive and engaged learning communities utilizing reliable and user-friendly web-based tools; nurturing trusting relationships among and between students and faculty so that students feel motivated, connected, and cared about; and thoughtfully orchestrating an online classroom environment that is both structured and flexible.[28-30]

In 2001 Creighton University became the first pharmacy program in the United States to offer an online, entry-level pathway to the Doctor of Pharmacy degree,[31] and, to date, we remain the only such program in existence. For the first time in history, students were able to access the didactic coursework required to earn a degree in pharmacy from their home communities. Laboratory and early experiential coursework is completed on campus during brief summer intensives and, to the extent possible, high-quality required and elective advanced practice experiences are completed in or around the students' home towns.

Before program launch, definitive steps were taken to ensure that distance students and faculty were well prepared for a positive and enduring learning experience. Resources were dedicated to substantially augment faculty numbers, and an extensive faculty development initiative was implemented to inform on the pedagogical elements and techniques essential to high-quality online learning. An Office of Information Technonlogy and Learning Resources (OITLR, now the Office of eLearning and Academic Technologies) was established and has grown to encompass 17 professionals skilled in such areas as e-learning and learning assessment, instructional design, website development, graphic arts, academic technology, programming, technical support, and distance education student support. An internal advisory board of faculty and key professional support staff informs the program leadership on all issues related to quality assurance, and an external advisory board is now being constructed to stimulate creative thinking about the future of web-based distance education within the School.

From the beginning, the School committed to implementing e-learning strategies considered "best practices" in distance education. In the early stages of program planning faculty worked with an assigned team of OITLR and Health Sciences Library professionals to establish course websites that were well organized, consistently structured, and easy for users to navigate. Educational mentors with content expertise were hired to assist faculty in keeping the distance cohort engaged in course content and on track for success. To supplement the learning resources available on the course website, audio and video from the classroom-based versions of didactic courses are now made available to distance learners through streaming technology. Faculty and mentors are available to distance learners through e-mail, instant messaging, and telephone, and robust conferencing software is available for web-based chats, examination reviews, and to facilitate other student–student, student–faculty or student–mentor interaction.

Web-based learners have some flexibility related to when they access course materials but must keep up with lessons because they have the same course assignment due dates and, in general, take examinations at the same time as their campus-based colleagues.[32] Examinations are proctored and taken at certified testing centers or other School-approved locations, such as a university, college, or public library. Most faculty members administer electronic exams that run through a secure browser that prevents access to functions, applications, and materials other than the examination. Students experiencing technical difficulties of any kind can access a highly responsive School-run Help Desk that operates 48.5 hours per week. A technology "hot line" dedicated to online exam support is also available, and examination "Plan B"s have been officially established for each course in the rare event of technology failure. Such contingency plans have involved faxing hard copies of the exam to proctors or identifying an alternate date for the examination.

All web-based matriculants must meet the same academic prerequisites and performance standards as those admitted to the campus-based program but must also be well versed in technology, self-disciplined, mature, and focused. Our experience over greater than 6 years has shown that the distance cohort quickly establishes a united and fully collaborative learning community, in some ways more tightly knit than the cohort studying on campus. They are intensely supportive of one another and reach out regularly through electronic study groups, online discussion boards or chats, collaborative sharing of student-developed learning resources, and, if classmates live in the same community, face-to-face interactions to help all in their class do their best work. They communicate proactively with the instructors and the educational mentors hired by the School to help guide student learning, take great pride in their profession, have joined and taken leadership roles in student professional organizations, and are loyal to and appreciative of the University for providing this unique opportunity to fulfill their career aspirations. Three classes of entry-level distance Doctor of Pharmacy graduates have performed at levels statistically equivalent to or higher than the campus-based cohort on externally validated case-based assessments of each ability-based outcome established for pharmacy graduates and on the standardized pharmacy licensing examination (NAPLEX). Several of these graduates have been accepted into high-quality pharmacy residency programs, whereas others have readily found employment in all facets of the pharmacy profession.

With our e-learning support systems established and fully functional and with a proven track record for success, our School is now poised to focus a segment of our distance health professions education program on rural and underserved communities. Several participants in the distance Doctor of Pharmacy program have come from rural areas but were not specifically recruited for that reason. The School is now beginning to track matriculants who come from, and return to, rural communities, and there are some positive indicators that the program may indeed be able to meet this societal need. For example, the greatest number of matriculants over the distance Doctor of Pharmacy program's 7-year history have come from Nebraska, Missouri, and Minnesota. In addition, 13 students who matriculated in 2001 came from towns of 2,500 or fewer, and 8 of those (61.5%) accepted employment in rural communities when they graduated in 2005.

The specific vision for using our expertise for social good has evolved over the past 2 years and is now under serious discussion and planning. The program's director is committed to this plan of action, which also has the support of the dean and key administrators in the School. The aforementioned external advisory board will include a member who can advise School faculty and administrators on the specific health care needs of rural/underserved populations and challenge us to consider how best to interest qualified students living in these communities in seeking their professional practice degrees through our distance programs. Scholarship support will be secured to support distance students from underserved communities, and they will be made aware of federal loan repayment programs for which they may qualify.

In 2008, the School will expand its web-based degree program options to offer the entry-level Doctor of Occupational Therapy (OTD) degree to a select group of students studying at the University of Alaska at Anchorage (UAA). The didactic component of Creighton's campus-based OTD curriculum will be provided to UAA learners utilizing technologies secured and/or developed to facilitate the web-based delivery of the didactic Doctor of Pharmacy curriculum. All laboratory-based OTD coursework will be offered on-site at UAA by Creighton faculty. The state of Alaska has a sufficient number and variety of rural clinical education sites to support the experiential component of the OTD curriculum, and students enrolled in this web-based program will complete the clinical component of their degree in their Alaskan home communities.

Health professions recruitment and retention studies have shown that students often practice in communities similar to where they have trained.[1,10,20] Allowing distance students who are firmly rooted in their rural communities to obtain their health professions education without disrupting families and/or leaving the area where they are established should go a long way toward augmenting the cadre of qualified providers in underserved areas. As previously noted, rural health professions practice is often interprofessional by nature, and students receiving clinical education in this environment gain important exposure to interprofessional health systems, role models, and mentors. In addition, if you maintain residence in your rural community for most of your professional education, retention becomes less of an issue.

CONCLUSION

Addressing the health care needs of citizens in rural and/or underserved communities is a social mandate that demands the full and immediate attention of the academy. Health professions education programs of all types can do much to contribute to the solution by (a) establishing admission policies targeting learners from these communities and (b) facilitating their entry into degree programs through initiates such as the interprofessional prematriculation program and web-based entry level degree offerings. Likewise, academic institutions offering health professions degrees should (re)design curricula to require exposure to high-quality interprofessional service-learning immersions and/or interprofessional practice and training opportunities in rural settings. All these tactics have been shown to be motivators for practice in underserved communities and, if properly constructed, can promote interprofessional cooperation and collaboration. The lessons learned from the strategies and initiatives presented in this chapter, which were designed to promote interprofessional understanding and teamwork and cultivate sustained interest in practicing in underserved communities, are broad enough to be applicable to health professions programs of all types. It remains the responsibility of each health professions-based school and college to critically examine their mission, program structure and constituency, and design opportunities and implement strategies that foster a committed and sustained interest in interprofessional rural/underserved practice.

REFERENCES

1. Slack MK, Cummings DM, Borrego ME, Fuller K, Cook S. Strategies used by interdisciplinary rural health training programs to assure community responsiveness and recruit practitioners. *J Interprof Care.* 2002;16:129–138.
2. Hostetter CL, Felsen JD. Multiple variable motivators involved in the recruitment of physicians for the Indian Health Service. *Rural Health.* 1975;90:319–324.
3. Crandall LA, Dwyer JW, Duncan RP. Recruitment and retention of rural physicians: issues for the 1990s. *Rural Health Pol.* 1990;6:19–38.
4. Scammon DL, Williams SC, Li LB. Understanding physicians' decisions to practice in rural areas as a basis for developing recruitment and retention strategies. *J Ambul Care Marketing.* 1994;5:85–100.
5. Brooks RG, Walsh M, Mardon RE, Lewis M, Clawson A. The roles of nature and nurture in the recruitment and retention of primary care physicians in rural areas: a review of the literature. *Acad Med.* 2002;77:790–798.
6. Sempowski IP. Effectiveness of financial incentives in exchange for rural and underserviced area return-of-service commitments: systematic review of the literature. *Can J Rural Med.* 2004;9:82–89.
7. Adams ME, Dollard J, Hollins J, Petkov J. Development of a questionnaire measuring student attitudes to working and living in rural areas [Electronic version]. *Rural Remote Health.* 2005;5:1–10. http://www.rrh.org.au/articles/subviewnew.asp?ArticleID=327. Accessed May 6, 2008.
8. Shannon CK, Baker H, Jackson J, Roy A, Heady H, Gunel E. Evaluation of a required statewide interdisciplinary rural health education program: student attitudes, career intents and perceived quality [Electronic version]. *Rural Remote Health.* 2005;5:1–10. http://www.rrh.org.au/articles/subviewnew.asp?ArticleID=408. Accessed May 6, 2008.
9. Brown SR, Birnbaum B. Student and resident education and rural practice in the Southwest Indian Health Service: a physician survey. *Fam Med.* 2005;37:701–705.

10. Meyer D, Harnel-Lambert J, Tice C, Safran S, Bolon D, Rose-Grippa K. Recruiting and retaining mental health professionals to rural communities: an interdisciplinary course in Appalachia. *J Rural Health*. 2005;21:86–91.

11. Charles G, Bainbridge L, Copeman-Stewart K, Art ST, Kassam R. The Interprofessional rural program of British Columbia (IRP*bc*). *J Interprof Care*. 2006;20:40–50.

12. Pathman DE, Steiner BD, Jones BD, Konrad TR. Preparing and retaining rural physicians through medical school. *Acad Med*. 1999;74:810–820.

13. Pathman DE, Konrad TR, Ricketts TC III. The comparative retention of National Health Service Corps and other rural physicians. *JAMA*. 1992;268:1552–1558.

14. Pathman DE, Konrad TR, Ricketts TC III. Medical education and the retention of rural physicians. *Health Serv Res*. 1994;29:38–58.

15. Rosenblatt RA, Saunders G, Shreffler J, Pirani MJ, Larson EH, Hart LG. Beyond retention: National Health Service Corps participation and subsequent practice location of a cohort of rural family physicians. *J Am Board Fam Pract*. 1996;9:23–30.

16. Stone VE, Brown J, Sidel VW. Decreasing the field strength of the National Health Service Corps: will access to care suffer? *J Health Care Poor Underserved*. 1991;2:347–358.

17. Jensen GM, Royeen CB. Improved rural access to care: dimensions of best practice. *J Interprof Care*. 2002;16:117–128.

18. Cullen TJ, Hart LG, Whitcomb ME, Rosenblatt RA. The National Health Service Corps: rural physician service and retention. *J Am Board Fam Pract*. 1997;10:272–279.

19. Houtz LE, Kosoko-Lasaki O. Creighton collaborative Health Professions Partership. *Acad Med*. 2006;81:S28–S31.

20. Mu K, Chao CC, Jensen GM, Royeen CB. Effects of interprofessional rural training on students' perceptions of interprofessional health care services. *J Allied Health*. 2004;33:125–131.

21. Roche VF, Jones RM, Hinman CE, Seoldo N. A service-learning elective in Native American culture, health and professional practice. *Am J Pharm Ed*. 2007;71:129–137. Article 129.

22. Williams SL. The effectiveness of distance education in allied health science programs: a meta-analysis of outcomes. *Am J Dist Ed*. 2006;20:127–141.

23. Hollis V, Madill H. Online learning: the potential for occupational therapy education. *Occup Ther Int*. 2006;13:61–78.

24. Gallagher JE, Dobrosielski-Vergona KA, Wingard RG, Williams TM. Web-based vs. traditional classroom instruction in gerontology: a pilot study [Electronic version]. *J Dent Hyg*. 2005;79:1–10.

25. Alsharif NA, Roche VF, Ogunbadeniyi AM, Chapman R, Bramble JD. Evaluation of performance and learning parity between two required on-campus and web-based medicinal chemistry courses [Electronic version]. *Am J Pharm Ed*. 2005;69:33–43. Article 33. www.ajpe.org.

26. Coma Del Corral MJ, Guevara JC, Luquin PA, Pena HJ, Mateos-Otero JJ. Usefulness of an internet-based thematic learning network: comparison of effectiveness with traditional teaching. *Med Inform Internet Med*. 2006;31:59–66.

27. Billings DM, Connors HR, Skiba DJ. Benchmarking best practices in web-based nursing courses. *Adv Nurs Sci.* 2001;23:41–52.

28. Young S. Student views of effective online teaching in higher education. *Am J Dist Ed.* 2006;20:65–77.

29. Thomas RC Jr. Supporting online students with personal interaction. *Educause Quart.* 2005;1:44–51.

30. Chao T, Saj T, Tessier F. Establishing a quality review for online courses. *Educause Quart.* 2006;3:32–39.

31. Malone PM, Glynn GF, Stohs SJ. The development and structure of a web-based entry level Doctor of Pharmacy pathway at Creighton University Medical Center [Electronic version]. *Am J Pharm Educ.* 2004;68:Article 46. www.ajpe.org/aj6802/aj680246/aj680246.pdf

32. Johnson K. Reality from a virtual education. *J Pharm Soc Wisc.* 2006;3:55–56.

CHAPTER 7

Interprofessional Collaboration: Addressing the Needs of the Underserved Geriatric Population

Ann Ryan Haddad, PharmD
Joy D. Doll, OTD, OT

INTRODUCTION

Much has been discussed and written about the boom in the older adult subset of our population. All trends indicate that the older adult population will not only increase in numbers but also in diversity and education. With increases in education levels, clients demand more of the health care system, but health disparities are expected to widen with minority groups facing increasing challenges in access of appropriate care. Today, almost one-third of older adults live on a low income, with the percentages increasing for minority older adults.[1] For example, in 2004 the average income for a white older adult was $215,000, whereas an African-American older adult accrued an average of $26,300.[2] These financial factors influence not only the ability to receive care but also the ability to access support services or address any long-term care needs that may arise. Research shows that individuals without health insurance or who are underinsured do not attend regular physician visits and tend to seek health care only when they are acutely ill, causing increased cost and drain on health care resources.[1,2]

As people age the risk of developing a chronic disease increases, and many older adults face the challenge of dealing with more than one chronic condition. Approximately 60% of older adults 65 and older report having five or more chronic diseases, about 30% are obese, and only 22% engage in regular exercise.[1] In 2002 and 2003 the most common chronic medical conditions for older American adults 65 years and older, in rank of prevalence, were hypertension (51%), arthritis (48%), all categories of heart disease (31%), any cancer (21%), diabetes (16%), and sinusitis (14%).[3] With the increase of chronic conditions, not only do health costs rise but management of these multiple conditions becomes more complicated. Older adults may find themselves on multiple medications, each required to manage a specific chronic condition, draining resources and complicating the ability for individuals to manage their own care. The cost of multiple prescriptions also complicates the health care picture. In 2003, 14% of Medicare costs went to cover prescription drugs, which did not account for out-of-pocket expenses or coverage by private insurers.[3] Average yearly out-of-pocket expenses for Medicare recipients with a prescription drug expense with no other insurance was $1,353, whereas those with Medicare coverage plus any private insurance was $892 per year.[4] An Administration on Aging report noted average health costs in 2003 for older Americans were $2,142 for insurance, $920 for drugs, $678 for medical services, and $158 for medical supplies.[5] The combination of income disparities, multiple health conditions, lack of physical activity, and high costs of medications leaves many older adults unable to access appropriate care.

GERIATRIC POPULATION AS UNDERSERVED

With the compelling statistics of the health status of the geriatric population, the health care system must mobilize to address the unique health concerns of older adults. The health care industry stands at a crossroads in the choice to prepare students for the future and to be prepared to treat older adults or continue to let the gaps in service grow, increasing disparities. According to the Institute of Medicine's Workshop on Disability in America, most older adults will develop some sort of disability, and the report predicts that as more older adults live longer, society as a whole will feel the effects of disability.[6] With the vast needs of the geriatric population, the health care system today may not be adequate to address chronic disease and quality of life issues for older adults. Working under this basic assumption, considering the geriatric population as an underserved population is not difficult. So the question bears to be asked, if the geriatric population is currently underserved and the situation will only become more dire as the population grows, what systems need to be in place to ensure quality of care for all of the geriatric population? As health care professionals, we know the challenges older adults face but have not developed the appropriate systems to adequately address them.

Today, many older adults "age in place" or reside in their own homes, facing the challenge of managing a chronic disease without much support. These older adults are often called community-dwelling elders. Even if a family caregiver is available, that individual might not have a health care background to make informed, appropriate decisions and to assist the older adult. Barriers to quality of life may emerge due to simple developmental changes that occur with aging, such as changes in vision that could lead to the inability to drive. Simple issues like transportation have a major impact on the health status of an older adult by preventing access to medical appointments, to the local pharmacy, and to other health-related needs.

Management of the health concerns for aging persons is challenging, and with the growth of the older subset of the population, the health care system faces both strain and challenge in addressing these issues. In long-term care facilities, older adults receive constant care from an interprofessional team of health care providers, which assists with disease management. But for older adults living in the community, health care professionals face a real challenge in assisting them to manage chronic disease and disability. Many factors, including disability status, family support system, access issues, and the growing older adult population, affect health status of older adults. This calls on the health care field to look to health promotion and disease prevention strategies to encourage "older (and younger) adults to take a more active role in maintaining health and forestalling disease and disability."[7]

COMMUNITY DWELLING ELDERS

Today, a variety of health care services exists for older adults, ranging from independent living facilities to full-care, skilled nursing facilities to hospice. Despite stereotypes of older adulthood and expansion of long-term care, 93% of older adults reside in the community.[8] The number of older adults residing in the community calls on health care providers to explore ways to address health care issues within these environments. Supportive services exist for older adults, such as senior centers, but the unique needs of baby boomers, the generation moving into elder years, call for more creative and active options attractive to a wide socioeconomic status. With an understanding of chronic disease, health care practitioners readily know the implications on future ability to participate in activities of daily living and how to educate elders to manage and delay the onset of these issues. Health care providers are being called to increase community-based care to address these needs. Healthy People 2010 established goals related to developing community-based health care services.[9] Healthy People 2010 identifies that health care professionals need to "[i]ncrease the quality, availability, and effectiveness of educational and community-based programs designed to prevent disease and improve health and quality of life."[9] This response seems so simple, but the health care system faces many challenges in reaching older adults in the communities in which they reside.

Community-based care is both complicated and not well defined in health care. This makes its implementation especially challenging. This is especially true for geriatric care, but slowly strides are being made. Recently, the American Geriatrics Society Task Force on the Future of Geriatric Medicine identified five goals to enhance geriatric health care:[10]

1. To ensure that every older adult receives high-quality, patient-centered health care
2. To expand the geriatrics knowledge base
3. To increase the number of health care professionals who use the principles of geriatric medicine in caring for older persons
4. To recruit physicians and other health care professionals into careers in geriatric medicine
5. To unite professional and lay groups in the effort to influence public policy to continually improve the health and health care of seniors

The Task Force noted that geriatric medicine cannot achieve these goals alone. To meet these goals, a collaborative effort of partners, agencies, government, and organizations is necessary.[10]

According to the Center for Healthy Aging, a division of the National Council on Aging, the only way to adequately address health in older adults is through partnerships between health care entities and community-based organizations.[7] One recommendation is using the model of an academic–community partnership in which an academic institution uses its resources to address the needs of older adults while promoting health professions education through real-world clinical experiences. Academic–community partnerships exist to benefit both entities, with academic institutions providing invaluable resources to communities and communities providing opportunities for student learning and research. Partnerships between academic institutions and communities provide "a strong framework for meeting educational and community goals."[11] Later in this chapter, the authors propose some suggestions to assist academicians in the health sciences work to address the needs of community-dwelling elders and begin to train the health care practitioners of tomorrow to begin transitioning the health care system to a community-based model.[12]

ADDRESSING HEALTH NEEDS OF OLDER ADULTS

With the growing older adult population and the shortages of health care providers, interprofessional practice is a method for addressing the unique needs of older adults and ensuring quality care.[13] With the complexity of the needs of older adults, one health care provider alone cannot adequately address the health care needs of an individual and collaborative care ensures that multiple needs can be addressed efficiently and effectively. Although far from adequately meeting needs, the health care system has begun transitioning from solely delivering health care in the traditional primary care and acute care settings to "increasingly address health promotion, maintenance of functional ability, and quality of life issues that rely on a much broader basis than traditional health care has embodied in the past."[13] Collaborative care is a necessary component of addressing the multifaceted and complicated nature of chronic disease in older adults who often face multiple chronic conditions.[12] According to Hornby and Atkins, collaboration "requires working at the interface of a number of different boundaries" and is a foundation to interprofessional practice.[14]

Among academic–community partnerships, collaboration among health care educators becomes necessary to address the complicated nature of addressing health issues in a community setting. Facing insurmountable challenges complicated by issues such as socioeconomic status and social problems, some academicians in the health professions have found that collaborative work is the only pathway to finding adequate and appropriate solutions to address the problems at a community level.[11] Furthermore, the recognition of the value of student learning in a realistic and collaborative environment has led to community engagement opportunities that provide a new avenue in health professions education as evidenced by groups such as the Community-Campus Partnerships for Health, who focuses on community-based learning for health professions students.

CURRENT GERIATRIC MODELS

Although considering the geriatric population as underserved might be uncommon, the idea that there needs to be a system in place to address the unique needs of older adults is not. Academic institutions have adopted effective research models for addressing the underserved needs of older adults. An extensive literature review with key words of "geriatric, interprofessional, projects, faculty, development, models, interdisciplinary/interprofessional education/practice" revealed exemplar programs focused on geriatrics. Exemplar programs exist in academic health centers that have explored the role that health care practitioners should play to meet the needs of geriatric clients. Geriatric education centers (GECs) exist to promote quality health care practitioners in the area of geriatrics following a collaborative model based within an academic–community partnership. Currently, there are 50 GECs nationwide that take a multidisciplinary approach to geriatric education for health care professionals, including continuing education, curricular development, and faculty training.[15] These centers provide unique training focusing specifically on the geriatric population, building on the skills of practitioners and ensuring quality geriatric care. GECs are a part of the federal Health Resources and Services Administration's Title VII programs.

An example of an academic institution's approach to addressing the needs of the geriatric population is the Medical University of Ohio (now known as the University of Toledo) that developed the PROMISE Institute (Providing Resources, Opportunities, and Mentorship in Interdisciplinary Service and Education). The PROMISE Institute provides educational opportunities for faculty and students to work in interdisciplinary teams in the provision of culturally competent health promotion to underserved urban and rural older adults. The teams developed and conducted health assessments and provided health promotion recommendations and education to medically underserved older adults in a variety of settings. These settings included an urban senior center serving a large Hispanic clientele, an urban low-income senior housing facility, and a rural assisted living facility. The directors of the PROMISE Project noted that staff at these sites recognize the cost benefit of the services provided because most of the sites cannot provide such services to their clients due to limited budgets and staff. Site staff expressed appreciation for the opportunity to help students gain a better understanding of the older clients they serve.[16]

Another unique example of geriatric interdisciplinary practice is the Idaho State University Senior Health Mobile program, which provides interdisciplinary health services by students and faculty to older adults in rural southeast Idaho. Examples of services provided include medication management, fall prevention, home safety inspection, hypertension screening, comprehensive health assessments, strengthening, diabetic management, wellness education, and referral and follow-up. Students and faculty provided services in community senior centers, the motor home, or client's home. The Health Mobile program directors also surveyed the 123 participating students using the Interdisciplinary Education Perception Scale (IEPS).[17] The IEPS is an 18-item perception and attitude inventory intended to assess perceptions of students participating in interdisciplinary activities. There are four components within the IEPS:

1. Professional competence and autonomy
2. Perceived need for professional collaboration
3. Discernment of actual cooperation and resource sharing within and among disciplines
4. Knowing the value and contributions of other professionals or professions[22]

They discovered changes in students' perceptions, pre- and postinterdisciplinary activities, for professional competence and autonomy as well as perception of actual cooperation and resource sharing within and across professions and understanding the value and contributions of other professionals and professions. The program directors noted the need to assess student perceptions of interdisciplinary geriatric practice because students' perceptions "influence the ability to meet the needs of a changing society."[18] The directors also challenged academia to use creative models like mobile health care to provide services to older clients where they live, especially considering recent health care reform and community-based care initiatives.

A final project example, identified in the literature, was a faculty- and student-driven interdisciplinary geriatric health program developed by the College of Health Professions, Medical University of South Carolina in collaboration with the Charleston Area Senior Citizens Center. The faculty and students from the department of health information administration developed and administered a health status and health educational needs survey to 159 seniors who were representative of the center's 8,000 older clients (seniors living in a HUD apartment building next to the center, attending the daily lunch program, and members of the center's community chapters). Most respondents lived alone, had annual incomes less than $10,000, and did not have a high school diploma. Common health issues included arthritis (65%), hypertension (41%), and pain related to arthritis (35%). This health program focused on development of a needs assessment survey, evaluation of service utilization at local senior centers, to stay healthy, proper nutrition, and dealing with arthritis. Faculty and students from occupational therapy, physical therapy, and health professions education developed and presented educational programs based on the interests and needs of the respondents, planning and implementation of health-screening and educational programs, and development of appropriate interventions for underserved older adults in the community.[19]

Common threads identified through each of these three highlighted projects include (a) establishing collaborative relationships with community partners who provide services to underserved older adults, (b) identification of health and educational needs of the older adults, and (c) provision of interdisciplinary services onsite whether it is the senior center, client's home, or assisted living community. From the faculty and student standpoint, each of these projects provided opportunities to develop interdisciplinary teams in practice, education, and research. Activities through academic–community partnerships benefit all involved. Ideally, faculty are able to model appropriate and effective interdisciplinary team skills and behaviors in addition to their own unique clinical practice skills, students have access to clinical opportunities in unique patient settings (often their own living environment), and clients have health care professionals who are interested and willing to provide care and listen to them without rushing them along. Community partners are also able to provide more comprehensive services to the clients for whom they provide care.

FACULTY DEVELOPMENT IN GERIATRICS

There are many challenges to providing interprofessional education within academic institutions, linked to everything from time or scheduling logistics to the lack of understanding about the definition and purpose of interprofessional care. Even successful program models in interprofessional care continue to struggle with the common difficulties associated with interprofessional work. Faculty development in the areas of geriatrics and interprofessional education and practice helps promote quality in service delivery and ensures that the complicated nature of the interprofessional work effectively addresses the needs of geriatric clients.

Several faculty development initiatives to promote interprofessional collaboration have been identified by Steinert[20] and Ulian and Stritter[21] that can be specifically applied to geriatric outreach. Overarching themes in these development initiatives include promoting change at the individual and organizational levels, focusing content on interprofessional education and patient-centered practice, and implementation of a model of interprofessional education and collaborative practice. Changes at the organizational level include changing how faculty are evaluated and rewarded, provision of resources to meet faculty needs, and promotion of faculty mentoring or networking. On the individual level, faculty development programs should address views and beliefs that could negatively affect interprofessional education and collaboration and develop knowledge and skills for interprofessional teaching and practice.

Most academicians with interests in geriatric health care have, at some point in their careers, clinical and academic, practiced in environments that foster interprofessional teams. This is common in long-term care facilities, assisted living facilities, and geriatric assessment centers where input from all members of the team is vital in providing appropriate care for geriatric patients. From this standpoint, faculty interested in collaborating with interprofessional teams providing care for older adults have developed the skills, attitudes, and behaviors needed to effectively work and participate in an interprofessional team.

The complicated dynamics of interprofessional health care education and practice requires a significant investment by faculty and exploration in how to sustain such opportunities both for student learning and community impact. Faculty development is one piece of the puzzle of interprofessional education and collaboration to promote sustainability and buy-in for faculty, students, and the community members served. Harris et al.[22] describe various elements of sustainability for multidisciplinary health professions education in communities based on results of the Community Partnerships in Health Professions Education, a 5-year program funded by the W.K. Kellogg Foundation. The program involved several institutions in seven states. Information on facilitating factors and barriers for multidisciplinary education was derived from pre- and postsurveys of faculty and students, site reports, and site visits. Facilitating factors for service program sustainability were "leadership, complementary missions, curriculum that mirrors clinical community practice, partnership boards, and faculty development." Barriers to sustainability were "professional identities and territorial boundaries, structural differences, costs, and unclear goals." Those institutions with successful projects had leaders who were collaborative, advocated across disciplines, and held influential positions either at the state or university level. Institutions with missions focused on providing service to the underserved also met with greater success in their community partnerships. Student teams that learned together through their interactions with real patients and cases were also found to be successful, especially when faculty could be role models at their own interdisciplinary practice sites.[22]

Significant funding ($6 million) to each institution by the W.K. Kellogg Foundation for the Community Partnerships in Health Professions Education necessitated "change from outside in" as site reports indicated 63 policy changes occurred within involved institutions to maintain important components of the Community Partnerships in Health Professions Education initiatives. The substantial external financial support facilitated changes that increased the likelihood for successes. Partnership boards comprised of members from the community as well as the academic institution was also identified as a positive sustainability element. Projects with more positive outcomes had partnership boards with a greater percentage of community members. Successful faculty development programs focused on a case study model involving campus and community-based faculty and community members. The departmental structure of academic institutions can create barriers for multidisciplinary education. The various health disciplines may have distinct philosophies, identities, and values.[22]

Structural differences that affected the Kellogg examples were scheduling or calendars for the various disciplines and curriculum structure. Increased costs associated with educating students in the community were costs for "housing, transportation, faculty and staff salaries, and lost revenue from decreased services at health clinics." These extra costs can also pose a barrier for the institution and community partner. Unclear goals and mismatched expectations of either the institution or community partner may negatively impact sustainability of projects.[22]

The described facilitating and sustainability factors and potential barriers are important for any interprofessional team to consider when developing geriatric health care initiatives. It is extremely beneficial to have established relationships or contacts with members of the community-partner agencies, understand what their priority health care needs are and the timeline under which they may be operating and devise plans to meet these needs that are acceptable to the community partner.

BEST PRACTICES FOR ACADEMIC SETTINGS

With the geriatric subset of the population being underserved, academic institutions can play a powerful role in addressing need and preparing health professions students. Based on the comprehensive literature review and successes and challenges noted across interprofessional programs geared toward geriatrics, academic settings can enact some best practices to address the needs of community-dwelling elders. All these best practices fall under the assumption that academic settings will adequately assess the unique community needs and build programs based on community-driven needs and not academic demands. Recommendations for best practice follow:

1. The underserved geriatric population must be treated by an interprofessional health care team. According to the Geriatrics Task Force, several core attributes and competencies focus on the interprofessional team in geriatric patient care by providing coordinated care through team communication, sharing responsibility for processes and outcomes, respecting all team members, and ensuring that patient needs are thoroughly addressed.[14]

2. Faculty members are called to work in interprofessional collaboration to develop strategies and educational opportunities for health professions students while meeting geriatric community members' needs. Faculty across the health professions are called to model interprofessional behaviors to encourage students to engage in interprofessional practice as an innate part of their practice context. One example is to form a geriatrics work group within the academic institution that includes an interprofessional group of faculty tasked at addressing needs of geriatric community members and incorporate student learning objectives. The geriatric work group creates an action plan for interprofessional community-based experiences involving geriatric clients. The action plan may revolve around the identified needs of the community partners, incorporating input from community partners into initiating programs to meet health care needs, and assessment of community partners, clients, and students after program implementation.

3. Faculty development is the key to sustained interprofessional geriatric education in academic settings. To initiate and sustain interprofessional geriatric education, faculty development programs may focus on the vast opportunities available for scholarship on their interprofessional teaching and practice, developing interprofessional team processes, and identifying faculty mentors across disciplines to guide junior faculty.

4. Health professions geriatric education must take place in the community setting. Interprofessional experiences are most genuine in the community setting and demonstrate to students the need to transition health care services beyond traditional health care delivery models. Incorporating these types of experiences into didactic classes in the earlier professional years may also help prepare students for their final clinical year. It provides them with glimpses of what they will encounter in their professional careers.

CONCLUSION

Academic institutions can utilize their resources in faculty and students to build interprofessional teams across health disciplines to meet the needs of community partners. Through collaboration with their community partners, geriatric teams or work groups can create innovative programs to address unmet needs of geriatric clients. While meeting the needs of geriatric clients, health professions students are also immersed in authentic community-based health care. These experiences, for many, are their first face-to-face encounters with real patients. Interprofessional community-based opportunities enhance their professional education and allow them to develop as professionals who, in turn, embrace the interprofessional team philosophy. This chapter identified key aspects necessary to promote the development of a strong community-based initiative and some of the challenges faced in implementing nontraditional health care. Yet, the outcomes and ability to meet community needs with an interprofessional community-based care model far outweigh the challenges.

REFERENCES

1. Federal Interagency Forum on Aging Related Statistics. Older Americans Update: Key Indicators of Well-Being, 2006. Available at: http://www.agingstats.gov/update2006/default.htm. Accessed February 6, 2007.
2. Administration on Aging. A Statistical Profile of Black Older Americans, 65+. Available at: http://www.aoa.gov/PRESS/fact/pdf/Attachment_1302.pdf. Accessed February 6, 2007.
3. Foster W, Levine S. National Council on Aging: Widening the Net of the Medicare Benefit. Available at: https://www.ncoa.org/Downloads/NCOACaseStudy%2Epdf. Accessed February 8, 2007.

4. Stagnitti MN. Statistical brief no. 125. Outpatient Prescribed Medicine Expenses by Source of Payment and Insurance Status for the Medicare and Non-Medicare Populations, 2003. Medical Expenditure Panel Survey. Agency for Healthcare Research and Quality. May 2006. Available at: http://www.meps.ahrq.gov/mepsweb/data_files/publications/st125/stat125.pdf. Accessed April 4, 2007.

5. Greenberg S. A Profile of Older Americans: 2005. Administration on Aging. U.S. Department of Health and Human Services. Available at: http://www.aoa.gov/PROF/Statistics/profile/2005/2005profile.pdf. Accessed April 4, 2007.

6. Field M, Jette AM, Martin L. *Workshop on Disability in America—A New Look.* Washington, DC: Institute of Medicine; 2006.

7. Collaborative Care for Aging Well. *Promoting Partnerships.* Washington, DC: National Council on Aging; 2006.

8. Hertz RP, Baker CL. Elders in the Community: Predicting Those in Need of Care. Available at: http://www.pfizer.com/pfizer/download/health/pubs_facts_elderscommunity.pdf. Accessed February 6, 2007.

9. U.S. Department of Health and Human Services. *Healthy People 2010.* 2nd ed. With Understanding and Improving Health and Objectives for Improving Health. 2 vols. Washington, DC: U.S. Government Printing Office, November 2000.

10. American Geriatrics Society Core Writing Group of the Task Force on the Future of Geriatric Medicine. Caring for older Americans: the future of geriatric medicine. *J Am Geriatr Soc.* 2005;53:S245–S256.

11. Plowfied LA, Wheeler EC, Raymond JE. Essential ingredients of effective academic-community partnerships. *Nurs Educ Persp.* 2005;26:217–220.

12. Seifer SD. Building and sustaining community-institutional partnerships for prevention research: findings from a national collaborative. *J Urban Health.* 2006; 83:989–1003.

13. Clark PG. Service-learning education in community-academic partnerships: implications for interdisciplinary geriatric training in the health professions. *Educ Gerontol.* 1999;25:641–660.

14. Hornby S, Atkins J. *Collaborative Care: Interprofessional, Interagency and Interpersonal* 2nd ed. Williston, Vermont: Blackwell Publishing; 2000.

15. National Association of Geriatric Education Centers. Legislative Priorities. Available at: http://www.nagec.org/legislative/default.asp. Accessed February 8, 2007.

16. Jepsen Thomas J, Kopp Miller B. The PROMISE Institute: an opportunity for interdisciplinary and community collaboration. *OT Pract.* 2005;10:16–20.

17. Luecht RM, Madsen MK, Taugher MP, Petterson BJ. Assessing professional perceptions: design and validation of an Interdisciplinary Education Perception Scale. *J Allied Health.* 1990;19:181–191.

18. Hayward KS, Kochniuk L, Powell L, Peterson T. Changes in students' perceptions of interdisciplinary practice reaching the older adult through mobile service delivery. *J Allied Health.* 2005;34:192–198.

19. Wager KA, Trickey BA, Mitcham MD, Brotherton S. An interdisciplinary educational approach to assessing the health care and health educational needs of the elderly in a South Carolina community. *J Allied Health.* 1998;27:202–207.

20. Steinert Y. Learning together to teach together: interprofessional education and faculty development. *J Interprof Care.* 2005;5(Suppl 1):60–75.

21. Ulian J, Stritter F. Types of faculty development programs. *Fam Med.* 1997; 29:237–241.

22. Harris DL, Henry RC, Bland CJ, Starnaman SM, Voytek KL. Lessons learned from implementing multidisciplinary health professions educational models in community settings. *J Interprof Care.* 2003;17:7–20.

SECTION 2

Community Context

CHAPTER 8

The Librarian Is Out: Role of the Librarian in Rural Health Outreach

Siobhan Champ-Blackwell, MSLIS
Teresa L. Hartman, MLS

INTRODUCTION

According to the Medical Library Association, "medical librarians provide health information about new medical treatments, clinical trials and standard trials procedures, tests, and equipment to physicians, allied health professionals, patients, consumers, and corporations. They help physicians provide quality care to patients, help patients find information, answer consumers' questions, and provide information to the health care industries."[1] Medical librarians are strong partners in the treatment of illness and the maintenance of good health for health care professionals and for health consumers as well. The New York Public Library recently became the first public library to be designated as a "Resource Library" of the National Network of Libraries of Medicine, agreeing to promote and offer materials and outreach to improve health information access to the citizens of the state of New York.

Despite this, medical librarians are not typically looked upon as resources when institutions plan their outreach efforts. Services for underserved populations, especially in inner city and rural settings, focus on access to health care: blood pressure and diabetes checks, cancer screens, and immunizations. These efforts typically leave out or do not sufficiently emphasize the important piece on access to health information. Perhaps this is because "the predominant perception of libraries is as a place to borrow printed books."[2]

BACKGROUND: THE RURAL SETTING

Rural health professionals face different situations than their metropolitan colleagues, including a smaller number of fellow practitioners spread throughout a wider geographical area. According to the National Rural Health Association,[3] one-fourth of the U.S. population resides in rural areas, but they have access to about 10% of physicians. Barriers to access for health care services by rural residents include shortage of health care providers, lack of transportation, lower levels of income, inadequate insurance coverage for care, and limited availability of health care services.[4] The shortage of health care providers and other barriers to access to services for rural residents present a challenge to communities to find ways to provide equitable access to health care.

INFORMATION NEEDS OF RURAL HEALTH CARE PROFESSIONALS

"To study the phenomena of disease without books is to sail an unchartered sea; while to study books without patients is not to go to sea at all."[5] To understand the information needs of rural health care professionals, first let us explore the fundamental needs they face. Liverman et al.[6] identified three levels of information need for all health care providers[6] based upon the work of Osheroff et al.[7]:

1. Information that is needed for decision making and that is already known by the health professional (currently satisfied needs);
2. Information that is not known by the health professional but that he or she recognizes as being applicable to the decision-making process (consciously recognized needs);
3. Information that is important to the circumstances at hand but that the health professional does not realize is applicable (unrecognized needs).

Item 3 might include information that the provider knows about but mistakenly does not see as useful, but also includes that information that is unknown to the provider that would be useful if she or he had access to it.

In addition to these basic information need levels, Quiram et al. listed seven key information needs for both rural and urban public health personnel identified through a 1997–1998 series of discussions with the Washington State public health workforce[8]:

1. Tools and resources that facilitate contact with experts
2. Legislative updates
3. Data set content information
4. Resources for outcome measures and benchmarks
5. Scheduling software
6. Templates for common applications
7. Databases that offer knowledge-based information

The information needs of rural providers are not so different from the needs of any health provider; what is different are some of the barriers to access to the needed information.

Josephine Dorsch, in a literature review done in 2000, identified several common behaviors of all health professionals when accessing health information, including the underuse of information and reliance on colleagues over "bibliographic sources." She also noted additional barriers unique to rural professionals: "isolation, lack of library services, and inadequate access to information."[9] Both urban and rural professionals rank colleagues high on their preferences as information resources, and both also rank medical literature high, especially their own personal library. However, rural professionals rely more on textbooks from their personal library, whereas urban professionals turn to journals.[9] This results in urban professionals having a greater access to more current evidence-based research than their rural counterparts. "Evidence based medicine is the conscientious, explicit, and judicious use of current best evidence in making decisions about the care of individual patients. . . . By best available external clinical evidence we mean clinically relevant research. . . . External clinical evidence both invalidates previously accepted diagnostic tests and treatments and replaces them with new ones that are more powerful, more accurate, more efficacious, and safer."[10] Without access to the current research, rural professionals are less able to follow evidence-based medicine practices that allow them to remain current in proven diagnostic and treatment protocols.

In a study comparing the information-seeking behaviors of nursing students with those of clinical nurses, it was found that "considerably more nursing students used electronic databases and the Internet for health information than clinical nurses."[11] The clinical nurses also turned to human resources at a higher frequency, with use of a human resource being attributed to time constraints. "The leading sources of information for rural physicians . . . in order of frequency: colleagues, medical meetings, journals, books, and libraries. . . . A colleague thus served as an easily accessible source, usu-ally saving the time and effort required to consult books and journals (even those in the inquiring physician's private collection). Physicians said they knew whom they could trust to give reliable information and to maintain confidentiality."[12]

BARRIERS TO ACCESS

Dorsch[9] notes a lack of library services as a barrier to rural professionals, but the problem is not so much a lack of services as it is a lack of *knowledge* of ser-vices. Dee and Stanley in their interviews with clinical and student nurses found that both groups did not feel confident with their ability to make use of any library, even a public library, and were unsure what resources would be available to them there.[11] In a study done by Andrews et al., which demon-strated rural primary care practitioners relied on print resources above online information, the authors speculate the reason for this "could be the result of a general lack of awareness of user-friendly sources."[13]

In a rural setting, access to the tools identified is limited by the barriers of time and distance, including the digital divide. In 1997, statistics presented on rural Internet access at a Joint Commission on Accreditation of Healthcare Organizations' presentation found that "while web capacity was 100 percent for health agencies serving populations greater than 500,000, it was only 65 percent for health agencies serving populations less than 25,000."[7] Not only is access an issue, but so is speed. "Connection speed is a more important factor in Internet use than experience."[14] If there is access at the workplace, connection speed does *not* appear to be an issue: "at work, the broadband gap between rural and non-rural Americans is small and not statistically significant; 72% of rural workers who have online access at work have high-speed connections, compared with 75% of urban and suburban online workers."[15]

ROLE OF THE MEDICAL LIBRARIAN

So far in this chapter, information needs of and barriers to access to health in-formation faced by rural providers have been identified. Creating an inter-professional health care team that includes a medical librarian is an important step toward helping to overcome the disparities in access to health information that rural providers face. "Knowledge has to reach the point where it is needed and be available when it is needed."[16] Effective use of the medical librarian allows this process of efficient delivery of information to occur. Librarians are trained in locating and evaluating information and are able to conduct a better and faster search than someone who does not search for health information as a profession. There are specific roles the librarian can play in overcoming barriers.

Earlier in the chapter, three levels of information needs were identified: currently satisfied needs, consciously recognized needs, and unrecognized needs.[6] Librarians are experts in accessing information and use that expertise to increase awareness of available resources, while assisting with locating needed information and training providers to use information resources in their daily practice. Most health care providers have enlisted the aid of a medical librarian at least once in their studies to assist in a search of the literature. Although this is a vital task librarians are experts in, it is only one of many in which they have training and expertise.

Medical librarians can identify and supply continuing education opportunities for rural providers, including distance education, and can teach continuing education courses. Training health professionals to find and access full-text knowledge databases for patient care information needs can assist the professional in having quick access to needed information at their fingertips.

A librarian can be invaluable in assisting with information needs surrounding the accreditation process.[17] "Knowledge-based information" resources are critical in patient care and clinical decision making. The management of knowledge-based information resources falls under the responsibility of the medical librarian.

The isolation a rural professional faces carries over into a lack of support for information technology. Often, the medical librarian is able to translate technology requirements for information seeking into a seamless bridge. Librarians set up the infrastructure within their own institutions; they understand the technology requirements for databases and other tools used to access information and can help to ensure a rural site has the necessary technology to support their desired tools.

Often, students who are sent out on rural rotations have direct access to their university's medical library and medical librarians. They can take advantage of access to databases and resources their home institution supplies them with and are better informed on these resources with the assistance of a medical librarian.

ACCESS TO A MEDICAL LIBRARIAN

It is often difficult for a rural provider to know how to locate a librarian, even when they come to understand the need for a librarian as part of the inter-professional team. Health professionals work with or near one of the 1,279 Critical Access Hospitals in the United States, very few of which have onsite librarians.[3] Providers have many tools they can use to learn how they can access library services in their geographical area. The National Network of Libraries of Medicine provides services to providers in the United States through regional medical libraries and by funding outreach efforts of network libraries and through programs such as Loansome Doc, a document delivery program. In addition, individual libraries offer outreach as a part of the mission of their institution.

Librarians have created fact sheets outlining ways professionals can locate possible library services, such as "Need a Library?" by the Hospital Libraries Section of the Medical Library Association.[18] Most major health and medical libraries have a customer service page specifically outlining their service population. The National Library of Medicine's Loansome Doc program provides free online access for locating a library that will provide document delivery to unaffiliated customers, though the document delivery service often has fees associated with it due to publisher limitations on journal access. A health care professional can register for a Loansome Doc account through the National Library of Medicine's website, and once that account is set up, articles found while searching PubMed or the National Library of Medicine's "Gateway" can be ordered online through Loansome Doc.

Once a library is identified as a service provider, rural health professionals are encouraged to communicate with the library frequently and should know the primary contact librarian or department that is assigned outreach duties. They can involve the library in planning and committee meetings so future information needs can be anticipated and resources budgeted and ordered in time. They can work with the library to identify secondary and tertiary service sources to aid in rapid information delivery in emergencies.

COLLABORATION IS THE ANSWER

The problems of access to health information have been identified, and the many roles the medical librarian can fill to overcome those challenges have been discussed. The rest of this chapter outlines examples of ways specific libraries and librarians have become part of the interprofessional health care team.

The University of Utah's Spencer S. Eccles Health Science Library outreach efforts began over 30 years ago. The program provides library services to those considered "unaffiliated" and also specifically targets three groups: staff, students, and providers associated with the Utah AHEC program; staff of the Utah Department of Health; and staff with the University of Utah Health Sciences Center.[19] The National Library of Medicine and the National Network of Libraries of Medicine have been involved in several collaborative efforts with medical libraries in the West Coast and "four corners" states to increase access to health information for providers serving Native American clients, through the Tribal Connections and the Tribal Connections Four Corners projects. These are just a few examples of many outreach efforts medical librarians have been involved in to provide services to rural and unaffiliated providers. Most programs also add in consumer health information outreach efforts. Partnering up with public libraries and community organizations in their geographical areas has led to numerous training sessions of public library staff and programs on health information resources offered to the public across the country.

An example of a collaboration that addresses public health workforce information needs is the Partners in Information Access for the Public Health Workforce. The site's mission statement is, "Helping the public health workforce find and use information effectively to improve and protect the public's health."[20] Medical librarians are represented by 4 or more of the 12 agencies that work together to create and maintain this quality resource.

EXPANDED EXAMPLE

To understand how a medical librarian can be a colleague in rural outreach and interprofessional practice, an example is elaborated, based on the experiences of the authors. There are many similar examples of partnership and outreach that have and continue to take place across the United States.

The mission of the National Network of Libraries of Medicine is to "advance the progress of medicine and improve the public health by providing all U.S. health professionals equal access to biomedical information and by improving the public's access to information to enable them to make informed decisions about their health."[21] The National Network of Libraries of Medicine consists of eight regional medical libraries and thousands of network members. The regional medical libraries administer and coordinate services in their geographical areas. Their outreach efforts are especially aimed at providers who work at locations unaffiliated with a biomedical library.

In 2001 the University of Utah Eccles Health Sciences Library was awarded the 5-year contract to become the National Network of Libraries of Medicine, MidContinental Regional Medical Library. As a part of that contract, Eccles included a position that was new to the National Network of Libraries of Medicine infrastructure: community outreach liaison. That position was subcontracted to Creighton University's Health Sciences Library/Learning Resource Center and has remained there through the renewal of the contract into the year 2011. In the first 5 years of the contract (2001–2006) the position was partially funded by the Creighton University Health Sciences Library/Learning Resource Center, and the community outreach liaison was also part of the outreach team for the Creighton library.

Creighton University is a Jesuit institution that includes as a part of its mission the promotion of justice. Providing increased access to health information for underserved populations has been a part of the Health Sciences Library/Learning Resource Center mission as a way to fulfill that mission. The community outreach liaison partnered with several departments at Creighton to support the outreach efforts of those departments, including the Health Sciences Multicultural and Community Affairs Department and the Office of Interprofessional Scholarship, Service and Education. In addition, the Creighton University Medical Center's "Partnership in Health" office includes the library in their outreach efforts. An exploration of the partnership between Creighton University's Office of Interprofessional Scholarship, Service and Education and the Health Sciences Library/Learning Resource Center demonstrates numerous ways a medical library can support and partner with health providers to create a health professional outreach team.

The Office of Interprofessional Scholarship, Service and Education has a long-standing relationship with the Omaha Tribe of Nebraska, located in Macy, Nebraska. The Tribe operates the Carl T. Curtis Health Education Center, which includes a clinic, nursing home, and the Four Hills of Life Wellness Center. The Office of Interprofessional Scholarship, Service and Education coordinator served as a link between the Health Sciences Library/Learning Resource Center and the Omaha Tribe by arranging a visit for the community outreach liaison and the outreach librarian to meet the administrators of the Carl T. Curtis Health Center. The Carl T. Curtis Health Center is not affiliated with Creighton University. This means that the Health Sciences Library/Learning Resource Center is limited by publisher restrictions on what kind of online access the staff at the health center can have.

However, the community liaison returned to the center and offered a training session to providers on how to access and search the National Library of Medicine's free online resources, such as PubMed. The providers also joined an informal listserv of health information around minority and public health issues, which eventually became the "Bringing Health Information to the Community" web log.[22]

In the summer of 2004 the community outreach liaison was invited to be part of the team that attended the eHealth Summer Institute held by the Center for Collaborative Research at Thomas Jefferson University in Philadelphia. The institute's objectives were to "provide occupational and physical therapists and speech-language pathologists with the knowledge and skills to develop web-based health programs for individuals in communities that are underserved."[23] The community outreach liaison attended the Institute with the Creighton University physical therapist who held a clinic at the Carl T. Curtis Center and with the occupational therapist for the Omaha Tribe of Nebraska. This team put together a website to be used by the Omaha Tribe as a resource in understanding health issues they face.

The next step in this process occurred when the Office of Interprofessional Scholarship, Service and Education applied for a grant from the National Library of Medicine to develop a "healthy Internet café" at the Wellness Center for the Omaha Tribe. This café will include a computer lab that will be open to all members of the Omaha Tribe and will make use of the eHealth website to create and expand on resources specific to health concerns of the Omaha Tribe.

As stated earlier, the digital divide includes both access to the Internet and speed of access. Although speed is not an issue for rural workplaces that have Internet access, it is a problem for rural residents. By the end of 2005 only 24% of rural residents had high-speed Internet access in their homes.[15] Having the Internet café available at the Wellness Center, which serves as a community meeting place, will increase the availability of Internet access for members of the Omaha Tribe.

When the Office of Interprofessional Scholarship, Service and Education applied for the National Library of Medicine grant, they included the library director, the outreach librarian, and the community liaison in the planning and goal-setting meetings to ensure that health information access issues were effectively included. The outreach librarian was also written into the grant, and she will be offering classes and trainings at the café, should the grant be awarded.

GLOBAL REACH

Rural health professionals have many opportunities to use the technical, information access, and knowledge management skills of a medical librarian. For example, it is common for rural health professionals to be assigned additional duties because of the low number of providers available for assignments. In such a situation, a rural professional is able seek out the assistance of the medical librarian to help ensure the success of the project or event. If the duty is to write a grant, the librarian could assist with statistics, bibliographic resources, locating examples of awarded grants to use as models, or editing the application for reading level assessment. If the duty is to explore and/or implement an ethics committee, the medical librarian could assist with locating information resources on clinical and organizational ethics issues, creating a list of potential ethics professional consultants, locating anecdotal and peer-reviewed evidence on success of other ethics committees in similar settings, and becoming a member of the ethics committee once it is established. If the duty is to develop policies to implement health information technology plans within the clinical setting, the librarian can search for forums and summits that would assist with background information and identify model plans for review. These hypothetical examples illustrate how the knowledge management, information access, and technology skills of the medical librarian can add to an interprofessional health care team's success.

A real-world example of how a rural health professional used a medical librarian when faced with an additional duty is described in an article by Ford.[24] Ms. Ford was serving as a volunteer for Unite for Sight at the Buduburam Refugee Camp in Ghana. Ms. Ford discovered that she needed to act not only as a nurse promoting eye care to the refugees in the camp but also as a train-the-trainer, creating curriculum on eye care for others to follow. She contacted her university medical librarian with her information need. The medical librarian was able to search and evaluate relevant resources and e-mail them to her for her education and use.

Another example demonstrating how medical librarians assist with information needs in a user-friendly manner is illustrated in the National Library of Medicine's free, full-text resource, MedlinePlus. Medical librarians at the National Library of Medicine locate and maintain health topic pages, such as the page on Rural Health Concerns,[25] linking to credible full-text resources and including direct links to subject and date-specific PubMed subject searches, all in the interest of making information access as seamless as possible for users.

Medical librarians have been successfully involved with health profession student education, particularly while students are on rotation. The goal is to support students as they work toward becoming lifelong seekers of information and education. As the students find themselves in unfamiliar networks trying to use their familiar information resources, medical librarians assist with locating quality information sources both inside and outside the academic arena, allowing students to expand their information-seeking skills as they anticipate the time after graduation when they must set up their own information resource pathways. Librarians counsel students to consider the high cost of information access while budget planning for their future professional practice life, just as they would consider other costs as basic as office space rental and furniture. As they seek out library resources and librarians for assistance in using information resources, the students model good information-seeking behaviors to their rural preceptors, most of whom have access to the academic library as a benefit of their mentorship.

ACADEMIC SETTINGS

Two examples illustrate how medical librarians support students on rotation. The first is based at the University of Nebraska Medical Center, where a librarian from the McGoogan Library of Medicine is assigned as liaison to the family medicine clerkship rotation that takes place every 2 months. The librarian is among the lecturers during orientation day, demonstrating how to search available information resources, and then assists students who request to check out a laptop to use while in the field. After the students arrive at their assigned locations throughout Nebraska, the librarian remains involved as their primary information contact, assisting with accessing full-text resources and locating alternate methods to access the Internet if the network at the rural hospital or clinic is restricted. Additional outreach is being conducted by librarians in the User Services Department through a program called "Nebraska Go Local."[26] Librarians have created a database of web links to Nebraska health facilities and health support groups so that Nebraska consumers and health professionals can easily locate them using MedlinePlus. The University of Nebraska Medical Center as an institution supports both of these programs, which take hundreds of hours per year to successfully conduct.

The second example is at the Creighton University Medical Center, where the education coordinator librarian from the Creighton Health Sciences Library/Learning Resource Center is assigned as liaison to the nursing program. Serving undergraduate, graduate, and nursing faculty, the librarian travels off campus a couple of times a year to conduct onsite training sessions, supporting the nursing program rotations that take place at a rural community hospital. The nursing liaison librarian remains accessible to students and faculty through e-mail and phone support and partners with the community hospital's librarian for education events and resource access. Additional support for this outreach program is evident through an upgraded hospital library's computer lab, ongoing training for the hospital librarian, and funds for increased information resources on site (personal communication, 2007).

CONCLUSION

The examples presented in this chapter should serve as models for rural interprofessional health care teams seeking more time and cost-efficient ways to locate vital information while facing access and time barriers in their practice. Whether acting proactively or on an as-needed basis, medical librarians are human links to health information sources. Providing necessary access to quality health information resources to interprofessional health care teams fits the unique skill set of medical librarians. Including librarians in their role of information locators enables rural health care providers more time to attend to the health care needs of their population.

REFERENCES

1. Medical Library Association. Medical Librarianship: A Career Beyond the Cutting Edge. Available at: http://www.mlanet.org/pdf/career/eng_cutting_edge_05.pdf. Accessed October 6, 2006.
2. Tenopir C. Perception of library value. *Library J.* 2006;December 15. Available at: http://www.nrharural.org/go/left/about-rural-health/what-s-different-about-rural-health-care. Accessed May 12, 2008.
3. National Rural Health Association. What's Different About Rural Health Care? Available at: http://www.nrharural.org/about/sub/different.html. Accessed November 6, 2006.
4. Mu K, Chao CC, Jensen GM, Royeen CB. Effects of interprofessional rural training on students' perceptions of interprofessional health care services. *J Allied Health.* 2004;33:125–131.

5. McGoogan LS. A volunteer librarian's progress. *Nebr Med J.* 1979;64:276–278.
6. Understanding the information needs of health professionals. In: Liverman CT, Ingalls CE, Fulco CE, Kipen HM, eds. *Toxicology and Environmental Health Information Resources: The Role of the National Library of Medicine.* Washington, DC: National Academy Press; 1997:70.
7. Osheroff JA, Forsythe DE, Buchanan BG, Bankowitz RA, Blumenfeld BH, Miller RA. 1991. Physician's information needs: Analysis of questions posed during clinical teaching. *Annals of Internal Medicine* 114:576–581.
8. Quiram B, Meit M, Carpender K, Pennel C, Castillo G, Duchicela D. Rural public health infrastructure: a literature review. In: Gamm L, Hutchison L, eds. *Rural Healthy People 2010: A Companion Document to Healthy People 2010.* Vol. 3. College Station, TX: The Texas A&M University System Health Science Center, School of Rural Public Health, Southwest Rural Health Research Center; 2003.
9. Dorsch JL. Information needs of rural health professionals: a review of the literature. *Bull Med Libr Assoc.* 2000;88:346–354.
10. Sackett DL, Rosenberg WM, Gray JA, Haynes RB, Richardson WS. Evidence based medicine: what it is and what it isn't. *BMJ.* 1996;312:71–72.
11. Dee C, Stanley EE. Information-seeking behavior of nursing students and clinical nurses: implications for health sciences librarians. *J Med Libr Assoc.* 2005; 93:213–222.
12. Dee C, Blazek R. Information needs of the rural physician: a descriptive study. *Bull Med Libr Assoc.* 1993;81:259–264.
13. Andrews JE, Pearce KA, Ireson C, Love MM. Information-seeking behaviors of practitioners in a primary care practice-based research network (PBRN). *J Med Libr Assoc.* 2005;93:206–212.
14. Fox S. *Digital Divisions.* Washington, DC: Pew Internet & American Life Project; 2005. Accessed September 4, 2006.
15. Horrigan J, Murray K. *Rural Broadband Internet Use.* Pew Internet & American Life Project; Feb. 2006. Available at: http://www.pewinternet.org/pdfs/PIPRural-Broadband.pdf. Accessed May 6, 2008.
16. Brice A, Muir Gray JA. What is the role of the librarian in 21st century healthcare? *Health Info Libr J.* 2004;21:81–83.
17. Bandy M. Librarian's Guide to a JCAHO Accreditation Survey. Available at: http://www.mlanet.org/resources/jcaho.html. Accessed December 10, 2006.
18. Need a Library? Unaffiliated People. Available at: http://www.hls.mlanet.org/needlibrary.html. Accessed November 6, 2006.
19. McCloskey KM. Library outreach: addressing Utah's "digital divide." *Bull Med Libr Assoc.* 2000;88:367–373.
20. Partners in Information Access for the Public Health Workforce. Available at: http://phpartners.org/. Accessed September 4, 2006.
21. About the National Network of Libraries of Medicine. Available at: http://nnlm.gov/about/. Accessed September 4, 2006.

22. Champ-Blackwell S. Bringing Health Information to the Community. Available at: http://library.med.utah.edu/blogs/BHIC/. Accessed September 4, 2006.
23. Lyons KJ, Swenson-Miller K, Corman-Levy D. JCHP to conduct eHealth summer institute. *Health Policy Newsletter*. 2004;17.
24. Ford VB. *Akwaaba!* I am welcome! *Reflections on Nursing Leadership*. 2006;32:first quarter.
25. MedlinePlus Rural Health Concerns. Available at: http://www.nlm.nih.gov/medlineplus/ruralhealthconcerns.html. Accessed December 1, 2006.
26. MedlinePlus GoLocal Nebraska. Available at: http://cuhsl.creighton.edu/login?url=https://www.refworks.com/Refworks/?WNC=true. Accessed January 10, 2007.

Addressing Culture While Building the System: Leadership Challenges in Interprofessional, Interagency Rural Health Networks

Jane Hamel-Lambert, MBA, PhD
Caroline Murphy, PhD

INTRODUCTION

Developing rural health networks to facilitate integration across community-based organizations and university partners is a viable strategy for improving physical, allied, and mental health care services for children and families. Typically, health care services are isolated by profession and care is weakly coordinated across providers of various disciplines, which is potentially confusing and burdensome to families. The divide between services runs deepest in our distressed and disadvantaged rural communities, where health professional shortages, mental health professional shortages, unemployment, and stigma regarding mental health all contribute to growing health disparities. Developing integrated, interprofessional health care teams can be accomplished in rural communities when agencies join together to form rural health networks, leveraging the resources and expertise of individual partners to improve access and quality of care. Specifically, rural health networks can foster interdisciplinary collaboration, reduce fragmentation, and increase access to quality, comprehensive, and coordinated care in rural communities. Whereas a shared vision for change is a necessary starting point, leadership that respects regional culture, corporate culture and climate, and the value of the participatory process is critical when transforming our health care system.

BACKGROUND

For decades, experts have debated the essence of effective leadership. Efforts have extensively examined the role of personality traits,[1] the role of the situation,[2] and cognitive abilities[3] in delineating what makes a leader effective. Not surprisingly, there is sufficient support for each dimension to value its influence. The next challenge is to integrate the multiple dimensions, including characteristics of the leaders and followers, agency-specific and historical culture, and the interplay among those variables into a comprehensive model of leadership that informs the development and selection of our nation's leaders.[4]

Developing effective leadership is critically important to transforming our health care system according to the agenda set forth in the President's New Freedom Commission[5] and further expounded by the Institute of Medicine.[6-8] Specifically, Crossing the Quality Chasm[6] calls on our nation to transform our current health delivery system along the lines of six guiding aims: "health care should be safe, effective, patient-centered, timely, efficient, and equitable" (p. 5). The report then defines quality health care as consumer driven and calls for professionals to collaborate across disciplines, to coordinate health information, and to communicate with families. Achieving this vision requires system integration; system integration requires leadership.

In the child mental health arena, the number of systems involved in caring for a child with complex needs expands beyond health and mental health providers. Minimally, this requires the involvement of professionals from education, and, potentially, it includes professionals from social services and juvenile justice. Also, religious leaders, coaches, community stakeholders, and family members all participate in addressing the challenges confronting child and family well-being. Finally, the socioeconomic and sociopolitical factors in rural areas can further complicate the delivery of quality health care and social services.

Together, the President's New Freedom Commission[5] report and the *Report of the Surgeon General's Conference on Children's Mental Health: A National Action Agenda*[9] delineate action steps to transform how health care is delivered in our nation. The vision is appealing. Both call for a health care system in which mental health is valued and families and consumers contribute to health care decisions. Both visions demand the elimination of health disparities, stress the importance of accelerating the path from bench to bedside, and encourage the use of telehealth to facilitate improvements in quality and access.

The Surgeon General's report[9] recognized numerous sectors involved in helping parents care for children with behavioral and developmental problems. Providing a parent perspective, Dr. Simpson noted, "Multiple barriers to access and communication difficulties among the multiple systems exist; parental involvement, family satisfaction, preferences, and quality of life are often disregarded"(p. 19). In addition to addressing barriers and communication failures essential to improving care, the conference put forth the following recommendations[6] (pp. 18–27):

> *In Primary Care: increase mental health training of primary care physicians, screen for developmental, socio-emotional and mental health problems, and improve linkages;*
>
> *In Schools: improve mental health training for educators to improve the identification of children with behavioral and mental health problems, increase utilization of screening programs, and screen for emotional and behavioral disorders similarly to vision and hearing screenings; and*
>
> *In Child Welfare: do comprehensive assessments rather than screening for problems and improve access to evidence-based treatments and assessments.*

The message is consistent: (a) Integrate mental health knowledge and services into all systems that serve children, and (b) train teachers, childcare providers, parents, doctors, and others to recognize mental health issues and create easy access to services so that early recognition is linked to quality care. The accomplishment of these goals calls for coordination among health professionals and integration of services across sectors. Developing a rural health network to facilitate integration across professionals and systems is a potential strategy to facilitate access to quality services.

System integration requires collaboration. Sadly, because our health education programs are typically "siloed" (exist in their own disciplinary silo) and reinforce professional boundaries, providers are often ill-prepared to offer comprehensive care, coordinated and delivered by interprofessional teams.[7] In large urban tertiary care centers, interprofessional teams are simply staffed by pulling health care providers from internal departments. In contrast, in rural communities where there are significant health professional shortages, if interprofessional teams are constructed, they are very likely multiagency teams, which further compound the challenge of providing co-ordinated care. Care coordination and the exchange of information across agencies requires considerable administrative time for copying information, sending it, and documenting the sharing of records (nonreimbursable activi-ties), and often it is not efficient, such that exchanged information is not typ-ically available at the time the patient is being seen, reducing the value of that information itself. Consequently, caretakers are typically responsible for re-porting what the last provider said to the next provider, which may or may not be accurate or believed by the next provider.

Not surprisingly, when interdisciplinary collaboration hinges on inter-agency cooperation, leadership challenges emerge. Agencies are constrained by different mandates and missions, requiring a constant visioning of collabo-rative solutions that create benefit for multiple partners. In addition to agency-specific culture, the regional cultural invariably influences the process.

This chapter describes our experience developing a rural health network in southeast Ohio, the Appalachian region of our state. Historically, rural health networks evolved to countermanaged care pressures. Typically, the in-tegrated health systems that emerged were well positioned to financially ne-gotiate managed-care contracts, but few were "highly integrated, either clinically or functionally . . . and few involved community participation" (pp. 40–42).[10] Our network strives for a coordinated, collaborative model of care whose sustainability is anchored in jointly planned clinical and functional in-tegration among partners focusing on improving access to quality physical health, mental health, and allied health services for families.

Composed of consumers, 13 community agencies, and five departments from three colleges within our university, our rural health network brings to-gether a diverse group representing consumers and multiple professions: early childhood programs, counseling, social work, nursing, medicine, psychology, speech-language pathology, and education. Funding for the development of our rural health network initially came from Health Re-source Service Administration's Quentin N. Burdick Program for Rural Interdisciplinary Training (D36HP03160) and subsequent support was awarded by Health Resource Service Administration's Office of Rural Health Policy's Rural Health Network Development Planning Grant Program (P10RH06775) and Office of Rural Health Policy's Rural Health Network Development Grant Program (D06RH07920).

Consistent with the leadership literature, the evolution of our rural health network has been influenced by characteristics of our leaders and our part-ners, the culture and climate of partner agencies, and our regional culture.

First, we highlight the Appalachian culture of the region, commenting on its influence on our network's development. Next, we explore the concepts of corporate culture and climate, which operate both within and between agencies. Finally, we describe the participatory leadership process we engaged in to establish our network's structure and strategic plan.

REGIONAL CULTURAL

Although Appalachian Ohio counties account for over one-third of the state's total number of counties, this area, with its unique strengths and needs compared with other regions of the state, remains an underserved and understudied portion of the state. The unique social, economic, and political characteristics of Appalachian culture likely have a significant influence on health care utilization and, specifically, utilization of mental health services.

Strength of the Appalachian Family

The values of people indigenous to Appalachia often are characterized by individualism, faith, modesty, strong familial ties, and a sense of place that ties them to their geographical and familial homes.[11] The region was geographically and socially isolated from industrialized portions of the country throughout much of the 19th and 20th centuries.[12,13] Thus people indigenous to the region were self-sufficient and often handcrafted all their food, clothing, shelter, and technological needs. Much of this self-reliance remains today, as several descriptive studies have found that many people from Appalachia continue to be notably independent and modest, to value solitude and privacy, and to be proud hard-working individuals.[11,12,14] Indeed, the Appalachian community provides a sense of safety and security, wherein differences are accepted within its cultural boundaries.

The evolution of our rural health network's development has respected the Appalachian values that are embodied not just in our institutional partners, but in the people representing those agencies, most of whom hail from the region. This strong sense of culture, acceptance, and belonging has contributed favorably to our developing interprofessional, interagency rural health network. Incorporating the strong regional sense of family, hard work, and acceptance into our transformational efforts has been critical in fostering interagency collaborations and relationships.

Just as family often is viewed as the hub of Appalachian culture, it is a central value that our partners infuse into our network. Initially, prospective partners struggled to understand (a) how their affiliation with the network would or would not threaten their primary allegiance to their home agencies, and (b) how it would benefit the consumers they served. Routinely, this dilemma resolved when the partners could see the link between their role in the network and the possible benefits to be gained by belonging to the group. Once in, mirroring our regional style of putting others' needs first, our partners often put their own agencies' needs behind those of other partners.

Ultimately, the pride and responsibility our partners feel toward the network is an expression of our cultural values. Although not necessarily explicit, this core value creates a common language fostering interagency collaboration and a sense of connectedness between the partners. Building the sense of connectedness between our partners creates a commitment to work collaboratively because we are a "family."

Further, building on the self-reliance inherent in much of the Appalachian culture, our network has a fundamental goal of empowering the family to be an equal participant in the process of transforming how a community delivers mental health care to young children. To achieve this goal, we found it quite beneficial to enlist parent involvement at different stages of network development activities, adopting the philosophy of community-based participatory research.[15]

Community-based participatory research is a philosophy that equitably involves all partners in the analysis, planning, and interpretation of community problems. Furthermore, it involves a commitment to designing actionable interventions or responses to what is learned through broad stakeholder analysis. By utilizing the views and values of all stakeholders, the effectiveness of proposed solutions to community-identified problems are potentially magnified because they have been designed for the people, by the people. This participatory approach to community evaluation and change deviates from traditional research and evaluation strategies that establish evidence-based practices in highly controlled environments and then aim to translate those models into communities with rich cultures and historical traditions. Community-based participatory practices resonate with Appalachian culture, which intuitively respects that authority of the family in health decisions and behaviors. Interestingly, our community-based organization partners have surpassed our university-affiliated partners in creating an infrastructure that values consumers at a level equal to the professionals in planning and evaluation of the services they offer. Because our community agencies have active parent advocacy groups, our collaborative partnerships have readily established linkages to consumers who are comfortable participating in planning and evaluation processes.

Building Trust

The Appalachian region is one rich in natural resources such as coal and lumber. Mining politics and practices during the industrial revolution of the late 1800s and early 1900s, however, forced many Appalachian families into severe and chronic poverty. Although large absentee corporations bought much of the land in Appalachia, they refused to locate their headquarters in the region. Thus, rather than having widespread employment opportunities in these corporations, indigenous Appalachians often were left with rare yet dangerous and extremely low-paying jobs to work the land that no longer belonged to them. The subsequent regional economic distress prevented improvements to infrastructure such as the building of roads, schools, and social service agencies, which caused many communities to be extremely isolated well into the latter half of the 20th century.[12,13] Therefore people indigenous to Appalachia often have felt particularly taken advantage of and thus have developed a sense of distrust toward those not from the region (i.e., "outsiders").

It is important to note that much of the pessimism and distrust for "big business" or "outsiders" that is often used to characterize people from Appalachia is an artifact of the region's loss of ownership of its indigenous property and rich resources. Clearly, building trust among stakeholders, especially families, must be a top priority in developing a rural health network for mental health, especially in an area such as ours.

This has important implications for interprofessional and especially interagency collaborations. In our experience, this plays out most prominently in "town-grown" politics, or those between local agencies and those partners associated with our local large, land-grant state university. Significant tensions can exist when a mismatch is perceived between the needs and values of the community and those of the university. There also is significant concern in our region that health and mental health professionals being trained at the university—who often hail from areas outside of the Appalachian region—have no means by which they can truly understand local families' experiences. For example, a recent study found that Appalachian parents were more concerned about relationship and trust issues with their child's mental health professional than were non-Appalachian parents of the same socioeconomic status living in the same underserved rural areas.[16]

These tensions almost certainly exist in any university–community partnership, but we found it to be especially beneficial in our region to engage in open dialogue about our perceptions and expectations of our roles as professionals, whether working for the university or for community agencies, and how to come together to best meet the needs of the community. We found that only through ongoing and open dialogue can we as a group of interagency professionals continue to challenge ourselves to move beyond stereotypes and misnomers so that history is not recapitulated. Our leadership closely monitors processes underlying network activities to identify patterns of subgrouping, exclusionary language and behavioral dynamics, as well as monitoring who is befriending key leaders, because power dynamics can often be played to the advantage of individual partner interests. Dysfunctional patterns are labeled and explored openly, underscoring our continued commitment to developing a rural health network that functions as a change agent within our community.

CORPORATE CULTURE AND CLIMATE

There are multiple levels of culture to consider when developing interagency partnerships, especially in a rural Appalachian area, where barriers to children's mental health care likely are more formidable than in other rural areas.[16] Beyond the regional culture, however, one must consider the corporate culture issues that are agency- and or system-specific (e.g., early education, mental health). Organizational climate and culture have been marked as indicators of an agency's "openness to innovation" and can be used as indicators of an agency's readiness to change.

Together, organizational culture and climate comprise the social context in which changes and innovations are adopted. Hemmelgarn and colleagues[17] discussed this issue in their examination of corporate culture within community mental health agencies that service children and families: "In a broad sense, organizational culture provides a social context that invites or rejects innovation, complements or inhibits the activities required for success, and sustains or alters adherence to the protocols that compose the organization's core technology" (p. 77).

Within any one agency, corporate culture comprises the agency's shared beliefs and norms. Employees learn what is valued within the agency through its culture. Relatedly, the climate of that agency is experienced in the degree to which employees feel appreciated, rewarded, and comfortable to adopt innovations and to engage in change processes without fear of negative consequences. Organizational social context for our rural health network then becomes an extraordinarily complex concept because the "organization" comprises multiple professionals from varied disciplines, many of which may have very different cultures and corporate climates (e.g., for-profit vs. nonprofit, university-based vs. community-based).

Organizational culture cannot be divorced from regional culture. One cultural phenomenon that has influenced both the regional and organizational contexts is the ethic of neutrality, a communication style wherein individuals are motivated to keep the peace between themselves and others.[18] To preserve relationships, conflicts are not challenged or questioned. For consumers, many of the families in our area have expressed their frustration in feeling unheard or confused when seeking mental health care for their children. Because of this ethic, however, they frequently do not question their health providers. Within the network, we also experienced this phenomenon when professionals from various agencies do not readily voice their concerns or agency needs so as to not disrupt network development activities. In "holding their cards too close," however, both the family members and the professionals engaging in this ethic are left feeling devalued and unheard.

We argue that it is a critical leadership activity in health network development to create a climate that is respectful of each agency's culture in building the network's interagency social context that best sets the stage for open, engaging, and safe collaborations. In part this is accomplished as trust builds over time, but a commitment to keeping processes transparent has proven critical. Such processes include fully disclosing concrete details, like which agencies are getting money in grant budgets, to more reporting more subtle dynamics, like who is talking to whom between formal meetings. Because decisions are jointly authored by network members, the distribution of resources is jointly determined (as is the plan) and imbalances are intentional and not reflective of favoritism or bias. Maintaining this transparency between community-based organization and university partners, who at time are competitors, network leaders can minimize the degree to which professionals feel compelled to keep the peace among each other. Setting a norm of full disclosure permits individual partners to assert their agency's needs in our developing network.

PARTICIPATORY LEADERSHIP: STRUCTURE AND STRATEGY

Creating a structure and a strategy was critical in establishing an identity and direction for our rural health network. It seemed relatively naive to believe that simply sitting partners together in a room would result in a new way of doing business together. Indeed, there was ample evidence in our community of acronym-based initiatives that set out to accomplish much but often digressed into meetings where members attended to see and be seen. Although a strategy without a formal structure may have held the collaborative partnership together for the immediate project, we invested in building a formal structure to establish a collective identity that would knit together our interagency partnership beyond our first accomplishments. To achieve this, our rural health network legally filed articles of incorporation with the state of Ohio, designed a governance structure and elected a board of directors, and wrote bylaws regulating the conduct of the board. Once in place, the board of directors appointed a president of the corporation. All these activities emerged from a democratic, participatory process involving all our members.

Ultimately, our rural health network challenges the traditional boundaries between agencies and providers in our community by asking partners to "reassemble" resources to create innovative solutions to improve access and quality in health care delivery. Creative integration of human resources, both individual providers and intangible assets such as professional expertise, occurs only when the membership agrees on the problem to be solved and shares a vision for the future. In our experience, the leadership style that supported the successful development of the structure and strategy of the network was participatory and transformational.[19]

One of the earliest participatory decisions our network made was to refine our mission and to pursue the goal of improving the delivery of health and mental health care to young children in our community. From a broad range of concerns, we chose to focus on this issue because of its importance to our partners. Even though the process of refining our focus was participatory, involving partners from all groups (e.g., the community and university, parents and professionals, administrators and direct care providers) and our membership could articulate the direct benefits that our revised mission had for multiple partners, the decision had the indirect consequence[20] of relegating partners with research and training missions to a position of lesser importance than those with service missions. Indeed, this decision made explicit differences between our partner agencies that may not have been clearly understood.

Once we set our course of action, accepting that the degree of commitment (e.g., time, personnel, resources) by a partner was determined by how well aligned our project was, that partner's mission and mandates was a formative step. Accepting that not everyone would buy into every project to the same degree sounds intuitive, but somehow it was surprising that there was no expectation of equal contribution. Rather, there was a high degree of respect afforded institutional differences as well as enthusiasm about the synergy that could arise from combining members' individuals strengths. This was reflective of the Appalachian cultural values of focusing on the strengths of the "family" and accepting differences among "family members."

In an effort to lead a transformational journey, resources have been committed to cross-training participants, so community agencies without granting experience have participated in grant-writing workshops, clinicians and consumers have attended training in community-based participatory research, and both consumer and community-based organizations are credited and participating in professional conference posters and presentations. Individual growth and development is nurtured through targeted activities addressing each person's professional areas of interest (e.g., training in fetal alcohol syndrome, autism) or leadership skills (e.g., executive mental health leadership, team development, management). This focus offers something to the individual participant and to the agencies those people represent. Taken together, we are transforming our communities' capacity to better meet the needs of children and families.

Ideally, the formative rural health network will facilitate our members' efforts to work collaboratively across traditional boundaries previously set by state policies, preservice educational models, and traditional patterns of service delivery. As if granting permission to the membership, the formal structure allows our partners to reassemble our collective resources, thus creating innovative solutions to improving quality and access to health care. An organization with this degree of flexibility was aptly described by Kaplan and Norton[21] as a "Velcro organization" (p. 102), one in which strategy and structure morph in response to internal and external changes. Similarly, an interagency network strives for innovation by reconfiguring its resources, a process whose complexity is rooted in agency-specific culture and interagency relationships.

Strategy creates the path between "now" and the vision. Agreeing on what to do is often easier than agreeing on how to accomplish the change. The importance of jointly planning the rearrangement of existing resources and being committed to new practice patterns ideally should be crafted so that conflict between the agencies is minimized. Left unchecked, conflict will derail a collaborative process. Threats to the collaborative process can take the form of personal or agency-specific gains and ulterior motives, though they more commonly include undisclosed resentment or dissatisfaction regarding how decisions are made.

A jointly authored strategy accomplished through engaging partners in a participatory process may take longer to create than one proffered by an autocratic leader; however, the resulting pathway is more likely to reflect the membership values and to respect the constraints imposed by individual agency mandates. In addition, the participatory leadership style protects the network from succumbing to the empty vessel fallacy: "Change agents and others who introduce an innovation often commit the empty vessels fallacy by assuming that potential adopters are blank slates who lack a relevant experience with which to associate the new slates who lack a relevant experience with which to associate the new idea" (p. 240).[20] To the extent that partners honestly represent their motivations for collaborating, openly share their experiences and knowledge, and value the contributions of others, the innovative solutions put forth by the network will fit with the community's needs and will be sustainable. Each partner should strive to clearly articulate their role as well as their responsibility to the network. Such clarity reinforces the trust among the partners, and refines the shared vision for change and the path to reach that goal.

More significantly, when change is jointly authored, what emerges is a common language that further substantiates the identity of the network membership. As interdisciplinary partners work cooperatively on clinical projects (i.e., in an integrated assessment clinic or in a primary care practice with colocated mental health services), members learn to speak each other's language. Participating in the process of change builds the common ground, anchoring a communication structure that bridges subtle discipline-specific differences. Effective interdisciplinary integration is accomplished when providers can pose targeted questions to professionals that are anchored by a core understanding of the discipline-specific assumptions and practice preferences.

Managing change within a system requires change agents to become a part of that system. In so doing, the historical tensions that led to the current state of tension within the system can too easily be recapitulated. In our experience, we have found that it is critical to respect history without recapitulating or legitimizing such tensions. When managing these change processes, leaders must continually question their assumptions and self-monitor reflexive behaviors, noting when leadership style and interactions with individual partners vary. Further, leaders must be closely attuned to what motivates some interactions to be easy and others to be distant. Although variability in interactions is natural, reflection on the factors that contribute to these changes can illuminate the alliances that are building as well as the historical tensions that are being inadvertently reinforced. As with many of the leadership challenges discussed in this chapter, we found that through open and ongoing discussion about the process of our network's development, potential barriers to collaboration are attenuated allowing the system to evolve.

The experiences we shared in this chapter highlight the importance of valuing the people over the project. Indeed, the potential for transforming a health delivery system lies in transforming the potential of its people. The capability to set professional development goals for each partner that pushes that person's potential out along a horizon is the essence of transformation leadership. Done effectively, this sparks interactions throughout all levels of the system, such that the system will unfold and expose possibilities that otherwise lay hidden in job description and hierarchical power structures. The leadership of our rural health network looks for evidence of partner strengths and interests through the participatory processes and aims to set in motion opportunities that facilitate growth at the individual level, but also foster the development of the network as a whole. "The leaders will know that the best form of leadership will build followers into disciples who take responsibility not only to accept a vision, but to expand that vision even further than their leaders anticipated" (p. 89).[22]

LINK TO INTERPROFESSIONAL EDUCATION AND LEADERSHIP DEVELOPMENT

Thus far, we discussed the leadership challenges associated with meeting the national call to transform health delivery systems in our rural Appalachian region of Ohio. We enjoyed a wealth of professional and consumer expertise as we developed our rural health network. Our commitment to transformational leadership processes does not stop at the professional service level; we are also committed to fostering educational programs that prepare preservice professional for interprofessional, interagency collaboration.

Our preprofessional training programs expose trainees to interprofessional training opportunities, not only to optimize the likelihood that interprofessional, interagency partnerships transform the way health care is delivered in rural communities but also to ensure that our health professionals are capable of delivery care through interprofessional, collaborative partnerships. Both interdisciplinary courses and interdisciplinary training rotations best prepare our future health, education, and mental health professionals to provide care to children. Professional socialization should no longer occur in isolation. "All health professionals should be educated to deliver patient-centered care as members of an interdisciplinary team, emphasizing evidence-based practice, quality improvement approaches and informatics"(p. 45).[7]

In the classroom, theory should be taught and applied to cases, and live real-world experiences should then be used to help students integrate their learning. Discussion of how real experiences contrast with what the theory holds creates a rich learning opportunity. Professional internships and training rotations that immerse professionals into settings optimally should include process training groups that allow for discussion of how team dynamics influence case management and outcomes. Additionally, interprofessional journal clubs are another mechanism for increasing awareness of definitive writings within various disciplines and for fostering dialogue between disciplines that increases an understanding of discipline differences and builds a comfort interacting with other professions. Layering in specific training experiences that addresses interprofessional differences and dynamics can readily be accomplished if the professional leadership behind the training programs hold these values.

Alternatively, accreditation programs and professional licensure requirements can adopt language requiring interprofessional training programs. Formal policies and infrastructure can effectively support the shift toward models of preprofessional training by requiring what only some value. Interprofessional training best prepares physical, allied, and mental health providers for delivery of quality care through coordinated systems.

CONCLUSION

The call for transformation change in our health systems also requires leadership development and mentoring as essential steps toward improving quality and access to health and mental health services in rural communities.[8,23] Much like there is a gap between the bench and the bedside because our providers struggle to translate evidence-based practice efficaciously, our vision for an equitable, quality health system for our nation will remain a vision on the page without leaders who can bring it to life. The transformation of our nation's health care system cannot take place without visionary leaders whose actions will bridge us from our fragmented models of health care delivery across the chasm to efficient, integrated, interprofessional systems of care.

REFERENCES

1. Zaccaro SJ. Trait-based perspectives of leadership. *Am Psychol.* 2007;62:6–16.
2. Vroom VH, Jago AG. The role of the situation in leadership. *Am Psychol.* 2007;62:17–24.
3. Sternberg RJ. A systems model of leadership. *Am Psychol.* 2007;62:34–42.
4. Avolio BJ. Promoting more integrative strategies for leadership theory-building. *Am Psychol.* 2007;62:25–33.
5. New Freedom Commission on Mental Health. *Achieving the Promise: Transforming Mental Health Care in America. Final report.* (DHHS Pub. no. SMA-033832). Rockville, MD: U.S. Department of Health and Human Services; 2003.
6. Institute of Medicine. *Crossing the Quality Chasm: A New Health System for the 21st Century.* Washington, DC: National Academy Press; 2001.
7. Institute of Medicine. *Priority Areas for National Action: Transforming Health Care Quality.* 2003. Available at: http://www.nap.edu/books/0309085438/html/41.html. Accessed August 17, 2005.
8. Institute of Medicine. *Quality Through Collaboration: The Future of Rural Health.* Washington, DC: National Academy Press; 2005.
9. U.S. Public Health Service. *Report of the Surgeon General's Conference on Children's Mental Health: A National Action Agenda.* Washington, DC: Department of Health and Human Services; 2000.
10. Rural Health Research Center. *Rural Health Networks: Forms and Functions.* Minnesota: University of Minnesota Press; 1997.
11. Duncan CN, Lamborghini N. Poverty and the social context in remote rural communities. *Rural Sociol.* 1994;59:437–461.
12. Beaver PD. Appalachian cultural systems, past and present. In: Keefe SE, ed. *Appalachian Mental Health.* Lexington, KY: University Press of Kentucky; 1988:15–23.
13. Couto R. (1994). *An American Challenge: A Report on Economic Trends and Social Issues in Appalachia.* Dubuque, IA: Kendall/Hunt.
14. Lohmann RA. Four perspectives on Appalachian culture and poverty. *J Appalachian Studies Assoc.* 1990;2:76–88.
15. Viswanathan M, Ammerman A, Eng E, et al. *Community-Based Participatory Research: Assessing the Evidence.* Rockville, MD: Agency for Healthcare Research and Quality; 2004.
16. Murphy CE, Owens JS. Parent's perceptions of barriers to children's mental health care in Appalachian Ohio. Poster presented at The Research and Evaluation Enhancement Project Health Disparities Forum, Columbus, Ohio, April 2006.
17. Hemmelgarn AL, Glisson C, James LR. Organizational culture and climate: implications for services and interventions research. *Clin Psychol Sci Prac.* 2006;13:73–89.
18. Andrews MM, Boyle JS. Competence in transcultural nursing care. *Am J Nurs.* 1997;97:16AAA–16DDD.

19. Bass B. *Transformational Leadership*. Mahwah, NJ: Lawrence Erlbaum Associates; 1998.
20. Rogers EM. *Diffusion of Innovations,* 4th ed. New York: Free Press; 1995.
21. Kaplan R, Norton D. How to implement a new strategy without disrupting your organization. *Harv Bus Rev*. 2006;84:100–109.
22. Bass B, Avolio B. *Improving Organizational Effectiveness Through Transformational Leadership*. London: Sage Publications; 1994.
23. Size T. Leadership development for rural health. *NC Med J*. 2006;67:71–76.

Community Organization Principles and Sustainable Interprofessional Health Care Practices

Mary Ann Lavin, ScD, RN, ANP, FAAN
Deborah E. Bust, BJ
Brenda Le, MSN, APRN-BC, RN, FNP
David C. Campbell, MD, MEd
Marvin Bostic, MS
Margaret M. Herning, PhD, PT
Elaine Wilder, PhD, PT
Claudia List Hilton, PhD, OT, SROT
Patricia D. Miller, MS, CCC-SLP

INTRODUCTION

Interprofessional practice and education traces its roots at the very least to the 1960s.[1] Much of this work took place within community settings. This article examines community organization principles in the development of interprofessional community-based practices, which also serve interprofessional clinical practice needs.

Community intervention,[2] empowerment praxis,[3,4] community coalitions,[5,6] and community development methods[7,8] are terms used to describe the interaction of health professionals with the community. Historically and philosophically, this terminology may be traced back to the community organization work of Saul Alinsky.[9] His grass roots approach, first articulated in the 1930s, developed and used community organization methods to encourage ordinary citizens to articulate their problems, establish their own priorities, develop plans that addressed these problems, and change the system.

By the 1960s community development efforts were being used not only in U.S. cities but in the developing world. Community leaders and members, supported by community organizers, brought potable water to villages and impoverished sections of large urban areas (personal observation, La Paz and Viacha, Bolivia, 1965–1968). Cooperatives were formed to ensure just market prices.[10,11] Today, community organization methods continue to be used nationally and internationally to address community and societal issue such as health care disparities,[12] needs of aging populations,[13] and high infant and child mortality rates.[14]

The purpose of this chapter is to report on the use of community development *principles* applied over the last 40 years in the establishment of three interprofessional health care practices. Use of the term "principles" is intentional in lieu of the term "model." For those who engage in community organization work, this distinction is important. "Principles" refer to fundamental truths or assumptions. "Models" refer to the application of structured or patterned behaviors that yield similar outcomes in a variety of settings. Principles guide the day-to-day human interactions of community organizers. Models tend to be abstract, hypothesizing relationships among people and outcomes that may or may not be related to the concrete needs of a community. Alinsky did not favor such approaches. He stated, "The greatest barrier between myself and would-be organizers arises when I try to get across the concept that tactics are not the product of careful, cold reason, that they do not follow a table of organization or plan of attack"[9] (p. 165). No structured theoretical framework or conceptual model is provided in this article. Rather, three stories are presented that manifest the human and communal principles enunciated by Alisky and others. Central to each story is the involvement of the community in shaping its own program and program priorities. One principle that flows vertically through each story: power. In Alinsky's words[9] (p. 51),

> *Power is the very essence, the dynamo of life. It is the power of the heart pumping blood and sustaining life in the body. It is the power of active citizen participation pulsing upward, providing a unified strength for a common purpose. Power is an essential life force always in operation, either changing the world or opposing change. Power, or organized energy, may be a killing explosive or a life-saving drug.*

Bolivia is the site of the first story.

THE BOLIVIAN STORY

Situated in the Andes at an altitude of about 12,000 feet, La Paz, the administrative capital of Bolivia, is the highest capital in the world. The official languages of Bolivia are Spanish, Aymara, and Quechua. Today, the city proper is home to approximately 835,000.[15] In 1965 it housed about 350,000 persons.

This is a story about a La Paz community, called Tembladurani. In 1965 the people of Tembladurani called for the creation of a tuberculosis prevention and treatment program. The community organization lessons learned then were responsible for the methods used 30 to 40 years later in rural and urban communities in the United States. The learner was a registered nurse from the United States, working within a Catholic parish called Cristo Rey in La Paz. At that time, the parish encompassed Templadurani.

The story begins in 1965 when the nurse arrived in La Paz to begin work in primary care and community health nursing in a parish that included Tembladurani. About the same time a young Bolivian social worker joined the parish and consultorio staff. After about 6 months, the social worker and the nurse both decided that what the consultorio really needed was a maternal and child clinic. This decision was based on the number of infant deaths witnessed and the lack of a comprehensive program to address the needs of infants and mothers. Being familiar with community development methods, the nurse–social worker team decided to present their idea at one of the area's outdoor town hall–type of meeting. Whereas Spanish was the primary language for the social worker, Spanish was the nurse's second language and the second language of most of the people who gathered for the meeting. Their primary language was Aymara.

The social worker addressed the group. She explained the concern about the number of infant deaths and the number of pregnancy complications in women who were not attended by clinic staff. The social worker explained that she and the nurse thought that a maternal and child clinic might help address this need, but they wanted the opinion of the community before moving forward with planning.

The address was met with silence. No one spoke. The social worker and nurse thought that the silence would be broken if they just waited. When the silence made the nurse too uncomfortable not to speak, the nurse said, "We really do want to hear your ideas, but we don't know how to interpret silence. We very much want to hear what you, the people, want. Help us understand." An Aymara woman stood. She spoke simply, slowly, and clearly. She said, "We don't need a maternal and child clinic; we need a clinic for *mal de pulmon*." (This means "bad lung," the most common cause being tuberculosis.) Surprised, the nurse asked, "Why do you think, given limited resources, that a tuberculosis clinic would be more important than a maternal child clinic?" Still standing, the Aymara woman stated with authority, "The man goes out from the home to work and gets *mal de pulmon*. When he gets *mal de pulmon*, he can't work. When he can't work, there is no money. When there is no money, there is no bread. When there is no bread, the family can't eat. When the family can't eat, the whole family dies. Therefore, a *mal de pulmon* clinic is more important than a maternal and child health clinic."

After that clear-cut prioritization of community needs, the social worker and the nurse informed those present that they would be working in the parish for about 3 more years. They asked the community if they would assume responsibility for seeing that the clinic continued after they left. They agreed. Today, the tuberculosis clinic in Tembladurani continues to see tuberculosis patients and has expanded to include primary care and maternal and child care. The clinic sees about 12,000 patients each year and serves as an educational site for medical and social work students. The consultorio, where the social worker and nurse worked, no longer exists.

The principles enunciated in this story are the importance of sharing experiences and may be summarized as follows:

- Respect for the community is essential.
- Listening to the community is a basic sign of respect.
- Community assessment is incomplete unless the members of a community, who best know their own health needs, are an integral part of the assessment and decision-making process.
- To access the information known to community members, the members themselves (not leaders, but ordinary citizens) need a forum to express their own assessment.
- Decisions made by the community are the basis for action.
- Community members remain committed to programs they help design.
- Interprofessional skills and services are needed when assisting a community to organize in the accomplishment of complex tasks.
- Community organization work is integrative.

In fact, community organization work is powerful because it is integrative. Support for this conclusion is beautifully expressed in the following quotation by Máire Dugan[16]:

Integrative power is the capacity to obtain what we need and want, in concert with others. This is the richest form of power because it is rooted in the most basic element of human nature. It also has the richest potential. Because human organizations are dynamic and organic, the whole can be greater than the sum of the parts. Integrative power thus transforms in a way that always adds to what existed before the change.

Washington County, Missouri is the site of the second story.

STORY OF HEALTH OUTREACH AND PREVENTIVE EDUCATION AND THE GREAT MINES HEALTH CENTER

This is a story of power and organization, which for Saul Alinsky are one and the same.[9] The narrative begins with a rural health outreach demonstration program called HOPE, an acronym for Health Outreach and Preventive Education. Because the name "HOPE" was and remains so meaningful to the community, the acronym is used through this story. Because HOPE is a story of the interaction between organization and power, it is appropriate to present this section in terms of its developmental stages: the setting, population-based assessment, community involvement, delineation of HOPE services, leadership, use of community health workers, HOPE outcomes, and the sustainability challenge and change.

Setting

The setting is Washington County, Missouri, a 749-square-mile area located in the foothills of the Ozarks. The area possesses great natural beauty, a national forest, and recreational areas. The land also poses a threat. Situated in the nation's Lead Belt, the Washington County Lead District was a leader in lead production.[17] Although the lead mines have closed, lead deposits, exposed in the soil, remain a source of risk for the residents, particularly infants and young children.[18] The lead poisoning rates in children less than age 6 in Washington County, although half the rate of the city of St. Louis, are still four to eight times greater than rural Missouri counties (e.g., Benton, Bollinger, and Wayne Counties) located outside the Lead Belt.[19]

Population-Based Assessment

The rural nature of the county was associated with poverty, health care provider recruitment, transportation, and water supply challenges. The people of Washington County possess a rich Scotch-Irish and French heritage. Many are also poor. At the time the story begins, 28% of the population lived at or below the 100% poverty level and 56% lived at or below the 200% poverty level. Unemployment more than doubled that of the state.

The geography and demographics of Washington County made it difficult to attract health care providers. Statistics for the county in 1991 were one physician for every 5,162 persons and one registered nurse for every 645 persons. Comparable figures for the state were one physician for every 512 persons and one registered nurse for every 127 persons.

Transportation was a challenge in that the county spanned 762 square miles. The interstate highway closest to the county seat was 55 to 60 miles away. Therefore there was some degree of geographic isolation, and, unlike many rural areas, the youth of Washington County preferred to remain in the country rather than move away. Given the size of the county, transportation to Potosi, the County seat, was also a problem for many, especially the poor and the elderly.

More than 80% of the population of Washington County depended on wells for their water supply. To determine if the well water contained adequate amounts of natural fluoride to protect teeth required laboratory testing. The water supply to cities in the County seat was not fluoridated. An estimated 73% of the eligible children did not participate in a state-funded fluoride sealant program.

More specific health issues were divided into maternal/child health, mental, and adult health concerns. The infant mortality rate in the county was higher than overall state levels. The adolescent pregnancy rate doubled that of the state. One-fourth of all pregnant women did not receive prenatal care. More than 25% of pregnant women smoked throughout pregnancy. Seventy-two percent of mothers were Medicaid participants, and 75% were WIC participants. Thirteen percent of infants were born with "abnormal conditions," defined as anemia, birth injury, fetal alcohol syndrome, respiratory distress syndrome, and meconium aspiration requiring assisted ventilation. Infant and child development evaluation services were needed.

In 1996 there were no providers delivering mental health services in Washington County. The Missouri Department of Mental Health estimated a 33% psychiatric need for the area. County schools reported special needs rates varying between 4% and 19% of the student population.

Excess mortality rates reflected adult health needs. Rates exceeded those of the state for deaths from all causes, motor vehicle crashes, work-related injuries, lung cancer, breast cancer, cardiovascular disease, and homicide. This information led to the derivation of preventive health strategies that included methods of implementing conflict resolution methods, gun safety in the home, motor vehicle accident prevention, heart healthy eating and exercise, safety strategies across the life span, smoking cessation education, and breast and cervical cancer screens.

Community Involvement

Although the above population-based needs assessment was important, it was not the only source of information used to identify the objectives and priorities of HOPE. A citizens advisory committee was formed to assist in the development of the project and its focus. Committee members consisted of recognized but informal community leaders, solicited from each of the small towns across the county. A series of citizen advisory committee meetings were held with an interprofessional team from Saint Louis University and Washington County to gather input and identify community needs and priorities.

An interprofessional team from Saint Louis University and Washington County informed the citizens advisory board of the results of the population-based assessment. Board members agreed with the interprofessional team that both on-site and outreach services were called for. Outreach services referred to the use of vans to deliver professional staff and equipment to schools and community centers within the county's small towns. Board members disagreed, however, with the interprofessional team's priorities, which were to provide healthy child screens, breast and cervical cancer screens, and health promotion/education. The board members' highest priorities were dental and mental health. Unfluoridated water and the presence of only one dentist in the county who accepted Medicaid patients made it obvious why dental health was the highest priority. Their reason for choosing mental health over physical health services required further exploration. When asked if they agreed with the Missouri Department of Mental Health estimate of a 33% psychiatric need for the region, they unanimously said "no." The percentage, the state agency indicated, was much too low. When asked for a more accurate percentage, one member responded 80% with all board members' heads nodding in agreement.

Depression was said to be the major problem. When asked for a cause of such widespread depression, they did not hesitate to answer "poverty." Their input into the planning process clarified HOPE's purpose, redirected its priorities, directly affected its budget, and gave the community a chance to voice what they needed and obtain it through work in concert with others. The services to be provided by HOPE listed in accord with the priorities identified by the citizens advisory board were as follows:

- Preventive dental health (oral health screens, x-rays, efforts to fluoridate wells, increase emphasis on the dental sealant program, and testing of well water for fluoride content)
- Mental health services (provided by postdoctoral fellows under the supervision of a psychologist from St. Louis Behavioral Medicine Institute, mental health social workers, and a psychiatric/mental health clinical nurse specialist from Saint Louis University)
- Healthy children and youth screens
- Breast and cervical cancer screens, with appropriate follow-up and referral when indicated
- Health promotion/education
- Infant and child developmental evaluations, with appropriate follow-up and referral when indicated

HOPE's 3-year budget totaled 1.2 million dollars, with 40% funded by the Bureau of Primary Health Care, Office of Rural Health Policy of the Health Resources and Services Administration and the remaining 60% funded by the in-kind services of the nine-member interprofessional consortium. Members of the consortium included Washington County Memorial Hospital, Saint Louis University (Schools of Nursing, Medicine, Social Work and Departments of Physical Therapy, Occupational Therapy, Communication Sciences and Disorders), St. Louis Behavioral Medicine Institute, Washington County Health Department, Missouri Bureau of Dental Health, two county-located dental offices, and a billing/management firm. The host organization was Washington County Memorial Hospital.

Leadership

A decision was made by the HOPE consortium to hire a Washington County resident to be the project director to capitalize on community leadership and involvement. The director selected was a strong formal and informal leader and a natural community organizer. Her strong commitment to health care and her educational background in journalism was fortuitous. She coordinated activities of the HOPE consortium, located building/office space, interviewed and hired community health workers, purchased all office and medical equipment, established Internet connectivity for HOPE through a partnership with the public school system, served as HOPE's chief financial officer, managed all day-to-day office activities, maintained ongoing communication among all members of the consortium and with the political leaders within the county, assisted with the development/submission of all government progress reports, and, most important, began building partnerships with other emerging groups in the community, whose members were uniting to improve the county's access to health care and health-related services. Her leadership and grant-writing role in the eventual transition of HOPE to a federally qualified health center was pivotal to its success.

Use of Community Health Workers

Three community health workers assisted with health education, contributed to the delivery of health care services to the community, and helped bridge communication gaps. Towns were often separated by miles. Not everyone had continual phone service due to interrupted or discontinued service. Some clients did not subscribe to phone service and relied on the telephones of neighbors. Direct person-to-person communication was needed to facilitate access to, delivery, and follow-up of health care services. Community health workers filled this gap. They also filled a communication gap in language that occurs at times between providers familiar with medical terminology and patients who speak in lay terms. Finally, they helped fill communication gaps that occurred between providers from urban St. Louis and patients from rural Washington County. In terms of a more specific job description, community health workers were hired to:

- Interact directly with adults, children, and families to identify and refer individuals for the available health services
- Provide support for persons with mental health disturbances
- Ensure follow-up services on patients with positive child/adolescent health screens, developmental screens, breast and cervical cancer screens, or treatment recommendations
- Assist with the set up of remote clinical examination sites in preschools, schools, churches, and community centers
- Meet with local groups and explain HOPE services and promote healthy living.

Before beginning their work, each community health worker completed a series of community health worker education classes at Saint Louis

University School of Nursing. As part of this educational program, they received extensive inservice training from

- A Saint Louis University faculty child development team on methods of screening children for developmental delays, indicative of the need for further evaluation by the child development team
- A Saint Louis University psychiatric clinical nurse specialist on communication and therapeutic communication methods, developmental theory across the life span, and conflict management/resolution
- Other HOPE providers on the community health worker role in implementing the purposes and methods of the grant and measuring its outcomes, the essentials of home visiting, health care record documentation and its legal implications, and providing for patient privacy and ensuring confidentiality.

Hope Outcomes

During its 3 years of funding, HOPE outcomes may be summarized as follows: 1,097 mental health visits, 138 mental health teleconsults, 990 healthy children and youth screens, 343 breast and cervical cancer screens, 115 child development evaluations, and 89 dental screens. Total health care encounters numbered 3,662. Sixty Saint Louis University students representing six professions (language and speech pathology, medicine, nursing and advanced nursing practice, occupational therapy, physical therapy, social work) contributed 953 clinical practicum days. They assisted in the delivery of direct care services and, with the community, planned and implemented 11 continuing professional education programs and 24 health promotion programs for county residents. Overall, HOPE was considered a success, but some direct patient care services yielded more health care encounters than others.

Although the community identified dental health as its highest priority, this service had the fewest number of patient visits. Reasons were that it soon became apparent that oral health assessments, even including x-rays, were of little value if the clients, with little money available for transportation, had to travel 80 to 90 miles for dental care. Therefore the focus turned to promoting dental health within the schools and collaborating with the Missouri Bureau of Dental Health to influence the County seat to fluoridate its water supply. The fluoridation initiative failed due to opposition from a few vocal community members.

The community's second highest priority, the provision of mental health services, met with the greatest success. It was the service with the most provider days (a psychiatric/mental health clinical nurse specialist, two postdoctoral psychologists with telehealth backup, and a social worker, for a total full-time equivalent of 0.40). It met the community's expressed need for service and for privacy, a factor especially important in small communities lacking the anonymity of city life. When clients entered the HOPE Office, no outside observer knew if they were entering for mental health or other services.

The reason for the success of the healthy children and youth screens was ease of access. Nurse practitioner services were provided to children, with parental approval, within the schools themselves, with the schedule being managed by the community health workers.

Breast and cervical cancer screens were less successful numerically, about one-third of the healthy children and youth screens. Despite relative ease of access, with the examination equipment being set up in community centers or church halls within small towns, access to large numbers was not nearly as easy as access to healthy children and youth screens within school settings. Also, the degree of follow-up entailed a greater investment of time in follow-up than the follow-up required by the healthy children and youth screens. Anonymous satisfaction with service ratings were high to very high.

The child development team provided evaluation, referrals, and follow-up for children who demonstrated possible delay or atypical patterns in motor skills, speech and language skills, hearing, sensory responses, play skills, or self-care skills. The team had the fewest number of encounters, attributable to several factors. First, the number of children with developmental delay represented a much smaller targeted population than the population targeted for healthy children and youth screens and for breast and cervical cancer screens. In addition, the clients were for the most part not self-referred but referred by community physicians, nurse practitioners, or community health workers. Unless the parent was also concerned, motivation to follow-up with a very thorough, videotaped assessment by a language and speech pathologist, occupational therapist, and physical therapist may have been difficult to sustain. Perhaps, too, parents may have feared having their child diagnosed with a development delay or feared that St. Louis providers would not understand Washington County parenting. Some parents and relatives who reported strong satisfaction with services provided indicated they feared that the presence of a development delay would be considered a sign of abuse and they would be reported to the Missouri Department of Family and Child Services for abuse. This fear may have been more widespread. Additionally, the actual number of referrals from primary care providers was disappointing, despite their continued verbal support and despite the fact that the child development team sent comprehensive and timely reports to the providers when referrals were made.

The low provider referral rate may imply that primary care providers do not have a comfortable script for informing parents that their child needs development evaluation, when the parents themselves had not identified a problem. There was a time when primary care providers were not comfortable asking questions about thoughts of harming self or others with patients who were depressed. There was a time when domestic violence was not a subject broached by primary care providers. Today, education efforts have paid off, and most primary care providers do not hesitate to inquire into these issues. Perhaps more provider education is needed, if parents of children with possible delays are to be appropriately referred.

Referrals from community health workers were less than anticipated, primarily because the amount of work entailed in assisting with healthy children and youth screens and with breast and cervical cancer screens had been underestimated, and there may have been some degree of reticence on the part of the community health workers to tell neighbor-parents that their child needed to be evaluated. It is also unclear why referrals were not obtained from schools in the area, because the child development team was well received when making visits to various local schools and child service providers, informing teachers of the available in-depth evaluation. Competition may have been one reason as the area schools did provide a form of child evaluation services by their own personnel at less cost than paying for the more detailed evaluation provided by HOPE's child development team. Given the number of actual and potential obstacles to seeking care, the 115 child development team actual encounters represent an accomplishment. When the grant ended, child development team services also ended. For a time, language and speech evaluation services were provided in Washington County by another health care facility from St. Louis. Those services also closed, within a relatively short period of time. The challenge of delivering high-quality child developmental evaluation services to at-risk rural populations remains.

Sustainability Challenge and Change

Although economically sustainable under Medicaid legislation from 1996 to 2000, HOPE was no longer economically sustainable once legislation required that all primary care services must be delivered in primary care offices. The legislation undercut funding for healthy children and youth screens in school settings and breast and cervical cancer screens in small community centers throughout the county. Without revenue from these services, mental health services were not viable. Although the faculty from Saint Louis University used the community development principles to establish HOPE, they did not anticipate that the community would surmount these seemingly insurmountable economic barriers. Faculty assumed the initiatives begun by HOPE would cease, but they underestimated the power of a community intent on the continuation of services they helped design.

The transition from HOPE to a federally qualified health center was facilitated greatly by a nonprofit agency formed in 1997: the Washington County Community Partnership. The purposes of the Partnership were to:

- Perform community assessments
- Identify local needs
- Create strategic plans
- Advocate for and promote physical and emotional wellness programs
- Pursue and administer state, federal, and private funding aimed at addressing targeted needs

As part of Missouri's Caring Communities program, its mission is to promote awareness of community strengths and needs, while working together to make a positive difference. From its inception, the Partnership team was sensitive to the critical access and health care issues of the county. The HOPE project director was a member of the Partnership team and eventually became its president.

When grant funding for HOPE ended and new Medicaid legislation prohibited the kind of outreach services HOPE was providing, other alternative methods were needed to carry on the mission of HOPE in serving the medically underserved population of rural Washington County. In response, the Partnership championed a local movement to improve access to health services for the low-income population on a permanent basis. Specific steps were taken. With the assistance of the Missouri Primary Care Association, a data collection effort resulted in a formal community needs assessment in the spring of 2001. A series of three community-wide public meetings were held to discuss the serious implications of county health indicators. The community decided to apply for a federally funded health center. The role of the community in "deciding" the direction to follow cannot be stressed enough. As was apparent in the Bolivian story and in the story of the formation of HOPE, decision-making lay with the people in the community.

Because the governance of a federally qualified health center and the by-laws of the Washington County Community Partnership were not consistent, a new legal entity was formed in 2002: the Great Mines Health Center. Volunteers, drawn from the earlier community-wide meetings, and members of the Partnership formed a planning committee for the new health center. The planning committee:

- Studied documentation from the HOPE experience
- Identified ongoing health access problems
- Collaborated with community leaders to address identified needs
- Ensured its integrated interprofessional (physician, nurse practitioner, mental health counselor, and health educator) approach to health care

The Partnership continued its collaboration with the Great Mines Health Center, even after the Center became functional. It provided guidance on improving productivity while eliminating potential duplication of services. It insisted on a new model of interprofessional, integrated services designed to improve access and continuity of care. The board of directors of the Great Mines Health Center elected as president the executive director of the Partnership who was the former HOPE project director. It seems evident that sustainability reflects not only a community's decision to act but also the capacity of the people within the community to lead.

Sustainable health care service must leverage dollars and human resources. For the Great Mines Health Center, leveraging began with the technical assistance provided by the Missouri Primary Care Coalition, which provided background data needed when requesting funds from sources other than federally qualified health center monies. These other funds included the following:

- Four years of funding from the Primary Care Resource Initiative for Missouri through the Missouri Department of Health and Senior Services
- Four years by the federal Delta Regional Authority to form collaborative technical networks among rural community health centers
- Three years of funding by the Missouri Foundation of Health safety net funds in support of mental health, primary care, and health education services
- A one-time appropriation for pharmaceutical program services, dental equipment/services, and furniture through the office of the Missouri Senator Kit Bond

- A three-year AmeriCorps Vista volunteer, who promoted the formation of an oral health coalition, fluoridation of city water supplies, and county-wide oral health screenings

These funds allowed the Great Mines Health Center to open 3 years before the receipt of federally qualified health center funding.

A functional governance structure is an essential component of successful community development programs. By federal mandate, 51% of the membership of board of directors of a federally qualified health center must be users of the health center. The user-majority board of directors meets monthly to develop and direct policy, monitor the financial position of the organization, and determine progress toward organizational goals. A key role of the consumer members is to bring the viewpoint, concerns, and needs of the target population to the board's attention, thereby assisting in programs and plans to best address ongoing community needs. The long-standing manifestation of community involvement in the design and development of the Great Mines Health Center greatly strengthened the application for federally qualified health center funding.

Sustainability requires community involvement in decision making and leadership to put into place the decisions made. It also requires persistence and determination. Four federally qualified health center applications were submitted before approval: December 2002, April 2003, December 2003, and December 2004. In January 2006 the Great Mines Health Center was officially designated a federally qualified health center. In 2007 the Great Mines Health Center established two outreach centers. Great Mines of Jefferson County is located in DeSota, Missouri. Its emphasis is the health care of children. Great Mines of St. Francois County is located in Farmington, Missouri. Its emphasis is health care of the elderly. Eleven years had passed since the funding of HOPE.

Inherent in the success of the Great Mines Health Center are three principles enunciated by Saul Alinksy.[20] The first principle is that the Great Mines Health Center is a people's program. Alinksy defines a people's program as any program the people themselves decide.[20] The second principle is that a people's program can only be brought to fruition through organization, where people find that the problems they thought were unique are common to many.[20] The recognition of common problems leads to a sharing of information, problem solving, compromise, and the use of power to fulfill the program they envision. The third principle is that of leadership, where the leaders refer to persons defined by the community as leaders and whom the community admires. Community or native leadership is so important that Alinsky states that "without the support and co-operative efforts of native leaders any such venture is doomed to failure from the beginning"[20] (p. 64). These principles were in place from HOPE's inception to the designation of the Great Mines Health Center as a federally qualified health center, and they remain in place today. The next story takes place in St. Louis, Missouri.

JAMES HOUSE HEALTH CENTER

The Bolivian story stressed the decision-making power of the community. The Washington County story stressed power and organization. This story about the James House Health Center stresses the power of human solidarity in creating health behavior change, and its story is ongoing. It is not a story of a highly efficient and competitive health care center. In fact, it is neither highly efficient, assuming that numbers of patients seen per hour is a measure of efficiency, nor competitive. In fact, it is a story analogous to Saul Alinsky's story of Butch, who was a leader of a community gang, admired by many.[20] Why was he admired? He helped people in the community. He even gave them cash, when needed. The newsboy, the narrator, was asked by a sociologist why Butch was appreciated more than a local welfare agency, especially because Butch had doled out only $25.00 to the agency's $150.00? The newsboy responded as follows[20] (p. 71):

> *You don't seem to understand. It isn't what you give that's so damn important, it's how you give it. They got that dough from Big Butch not just without a single snoop but with a pat on the back and real sympathy. When you go to Butch you're a human being. When you go to the Welfare, you're a . . . a . . . Well, they got a word for it—you're called a "case."*

The newsboy knew what he was talking about. Butch was "in solidarity" with the members of the community, and human solidarity is powerful. In fact, for many the democratization of Poland and even the collapse of the Berlin wall is attributed to the human solidarity movement championed by Lech Walesa and John Paul II, beginning in the late 1970s.[21] Human solidarity is not just a feel-good moment or series or moments, an experience, or an attitude appropriate only for volunteers. Once the notion of human solidarity is internalized, it remains a lifelong commitment to the human person, regardless of guise. It is the virtue epitomized in John Donne's poem *No Man Is an Island* and in Martin Luther King's song *We Shall All Be One*. Within the health care arena, it empowers both providers and clients alike, and, surprisingly, the most striking outcome is positive health care behavior change. The story of the James House Health Center is really only just beginning, but it is a story of human solidarity and behavior change with a center built on community organization principles. The description that follows includes the setting, population-based assessment, community involvement, delineation of James House Health Center services, leadership, James House Health Center outcomes, and the sustainability challenge.

Setting

James House Health Center is located within a residence for independent living elderly and people who are disabled. This residence, managed by a firm under contract to the St. Louis Housing Authority, is located within an area of north St. Louis that, although now depressed, has a history of having been home to many of the African-American business and professional class. Many who live in the building grew up in the neighborhood. The residence itself is a 10-story structure, with 150 one-bedroom and studio apartments. The building contains two large activity rooms, one frequently and the other seldom used. The seldom used activity room is located on the ground floor and is perfect for physical therapy activities, health fairs, and student–instructor conferences. Also on the ground floor is a five-room space that has been renovated to include a reception area, two examination rooms, a small laboratory room, and an office. Use of this space required the joint approval of the residents, represented by the tenants advisory board at the city-wide and residential levels and the approval of the management firm that operates the facility.

Organizational decisions to request the use of this space as a health center were made by a community–university partnership. Members of the partnerships included the St. Louis Housing Authority, which contracted with the Institute for Family Medicine, which in turn contracted first with the Saint Louis University School of Nursing and later with the University's Doisy College of Health Sciences. The basis for this decision included a population-based assessment and involvement of the community in the decision-making process.

Population-Based Assessment

Public housing communities are by definition low-income communities. Income data for elderly and disabled residents from 2005 to 2006 data reveal an average annual income of $9,310, well below the 2005 federally designated "low-income" level of $17,960 per year for a family size of one. Low-income communities are at risk of poor health outcomes.[22-26] Ninety-eight percent of the James House residents are Black. The association between low income and poor quality care is more pronounced among African-American populations.[24,27]

Health care racial disparities are present in the city of St. Louis. The age-adjusted hospitalization rates for diseases such as diabetes mellitus, heart disease, and stroke are higher for African-Americans than Whites in the city of St. Louis.[28] Assuming that a higher rate of hospitalizations represents poorer control of these illnesses, then these figures represent health care disparity. Increased use of secondary (early detection) and tertiary (disease complication) prevention methods is needed to address this disparity.

Community Involvement

Four steps were used in establishing the community–university partnership that became the James House Health Center. First, the director of the Institute for Family Medicine, the director of Resident Initiatives for the St. Louis Housing Authority, and the Saint Louis University School of Nursing representative met to discuss the overall project. Second, these three individuals toured six public housing residences designated for the elderly persons and those with disabilities. From these six, three residences were identified as having the most potential for the development of an on-site clinic. Third, health care needs as perceived by the residents of these three apartment buildings were solicited at town hall–type meetings. The following needs and priorities were expressed:

- Dental health services
- Mental health services
- Chronic illness services (diabetes, high blood pressure, poststatus stroke, obesity, asthma, management of therapeutic regimen, disability or age-associated mobility/balance problems, fall risk)

Interestingly, the priorities in the predominantly Black St. Louis City community were the same as the priorities in rural White Washington Country. The common denominator is neither race nor geography but unavailability of needed services for those in the lowest income brackets. The last step was to request permission to proceed with the James House Health Center from the city-wide tenant advisory board of the St. Louis Housing Authority, after having obtained approval from the James House tenants advisory board.

Delineation of James House Services

The resident request for dental health services is important. Poor dental health is associated with hand grip strength in the elderly,[29] oral and oropharyngeal squamous cell cancer,[30] cardiovascular disease,[31] and increased mortality.[32] Yet, the limited availability of dental health care among the poor discourages those who seek it. At the same time, the resources that are available are often unknown. The James House Health Center provides residents with a list of available dental health resources and facilitates the making and keeping of dental health appointments.

Psychiatric mental health services are more readily available to the Medicaid population in the city of St. Louis than in rural Missouri. Therefore the nurse practitioners at the James House Health Center do not provide direct mental health care services but provide supportive, referral, and coordination of care services.

Population-based advanced practice nursing adult care services are provided by two certified nurse practitioners. One practices under a collaborative agreement with the physician director of the St. Louis-based Institute for Family Medicine and assists with chronic diseases management, primarily diabetes mellitus, hypertension, obesity, asthma/chronic obstructive pulmonary disease, and acute self-limited illnesses. In addition to the supervision of nursing students in the care of community living elderly and disabled persons, the other nurse practitioner has established a practice to treat human responses to illness, such as ineffective management of therapeutic regimen, deficient health knowledge, noncompliance, fear, loneliness, risk for self or other directed violence, risk for infection, impaired verbal communication, and decisional health-related conflict. She also promotes health-seeking behavior. She functions as community organizer, strengthening the making of healthy choices and the creation of a healthier environment.

Each practitioner consults with or refers to interprofessional colleagues. For example, the patient's primary care providers are contacted when a change in the patient's condition warrants it. When regular patient services are required, home health agencies are contacted to provide professional or assistive care to residents, including shopping and housekeeping services and preparing daily medications. Collaboration with the Doisy College of Health Sciences Department of Physical Therapy has been productive.

Physical therapy is one of the most needed services within James House. In the spring of 2006, a physical therapy faculty member and physical therapy student provided the following weekly services:

- Collaboration with the nursing students in caring for particular resident needs
- Consultation on care of selected residents with long-standing disabilities. These consultations included a variety of professional activities.
- Evaluation of the resident's living capacity and performance
- Assessment of accessibility and special equipment needs within resident apartments
- Establishment of weekly treatment sessions to work on standing, ambulation, and balance along with range of motion, strength, and endurance
- Consultation with the nursing students at each session to obtain an update on the resident's condition
- End-of-semester conference with physical therapy and nursing students to review each resident's outcomes, home exercise instructions, and discharge-from-service plan
- Health record documentation of the initial plan of care, ongoing treatment sessions, and discharge-from-service plan

In the summer of 2006 the physical therapy faculty member accompanied by four physical therapy students distributed a flyer to invite residents to a weekly exercise class. Nursing faculty provided the initial screening of the residents and ongoing monitoring of the residents' blood pressure and heart rate. Each resident was given an elastic band for resistive exercises. Class sessions focused on flexibility and strengthening exercises followed by standing and ambulation balance activities. In the fall of 2006 the physical therapy faculty member, in collaboration with nursing students, repeated a weekly exercise class. The therapist also provided consultation on specialized needs of individual residents.

Although the physical therapy efforts were limited to a small number of residents, the experience provided an opportunity for students to identify special concerns of older adults who are poor and suffering with multiple health problems. It also provided numerous occasions for physical therapy to work collaboratively with nursing utilizing the expertise of each profession.

Such exchanges advanced the work of interprofessional education by allowing students to apply clinically what they learn didactically about the need for and advantages of interprofessional collaboration and better prepare them for the interprofessional world of practice they will enter upon graduation.

During the spring of 2007 James House became the pilot site for a new interprofessional course, offered to Saint Louis University entry-level students in their last semester (nursing, medical, occupational therapy, and physical therapy). Called Integrative Interprofessional Practicum Experience, this course was the first clinical practica offered by a new interprofessional curriculum. The students first conferred with the James House residents and then planned and presented to them two interactive presentations. One presentation involved a health fair approach, with booths established for residents to walk from one to another. Booths included activities on stress management, a cane/walker adjustment booth, blood pressure measurement, and blood sugar screening. Follow-up was provided, when indicated. The other presentation covered such topics as how to read food labels, exercise, and preparation of a healthy full-course meal. Approximately 45 people, or one-third of the resident population, attended each session.

Outcomes

During its first year, the Center initiated health records on 48% of the people who lived within the residence. Sixteen Saint Louis University public health nursing students and six senior community health project nursing students completed 197 nursing encounters and updated a fire disaster plan with the cooperation of the St. Louis Housing Authority and the St. Louis Fire Department. There were 227 patient encounters, of which 63% were served by Saint Louis University nursing faculty and the remainder by a nurse practitioner and physician of the Institute for Family Medicine. Saint Louis University's Department of Physical Therapy began organized exercise classes and were used as consultants in the care of individual patients. In 2006 the Institute for Family Medicine conferred upon Saint Louis University School of Nursing of the Doisy College of Health Sciences the first annual Community Champion Award in the health care organization category for its work in helping to initiate and expand clinical services in partnership with the St. Louis Housing Authority.

Results from the second year follow the same pattern in terms of the numbers of visits. What is becoming obvious, however, is that residents are becoming more actively engaged in health-seeking behavior. Examples include successful weight loss plans among those with diabetes, regular exercise programs among those who have had strokes, active participation in blood pressure management among those with hypertension, and increased interest in structured exercise programs (e.g., those offered by the YMCA).

Inherent in all above activities is professional and interprofessional competence and even more importantly a personal relationship with the residents that is built on respect for the humanity of the other person, acceptance of the other, trust, appreciation of the life experience of each, comfortableness with the setting, and lack of bureaucratic red tape. It is the "how to give it" and the "human being" factors about which the newsboy talked in the quotation that opened the section. Simply put, it is human solidarity.

Sustainability Challenge

At the writing of this article, it is not clear how the 2-year-old James House Health Center will continue to sustain itself, but then it also wasn't clear how the tuberculosis clinic in Bolivia was going to continue or how Washington County, Missouri was going to transform the HOPE model into a federally qualified health center, called Great Mines. What is clear is that the relationship between the residents and the providers at James House epitomizes the human element that is central to authentic, functional, and eventually sustainable community-derived health care programs.

LIMITATIONS OF REPORT

The limitations of this report are several. Because the purpose of these narratives was to report on the relationship between the principles of community organization that undergirded the success of health care centers, barriers and challenges encountered were not analyzed as thoroughly. In addition to the ones presented, notably factors most likely to have contributed to the relatively few infant and child development evaluation visits at the HOPE and the Great Mines Health Center, other difficulties were also faced. These included episodes of discouragement and disillusionment, interprofessional communication challenges, financial concerns, community health and safety issues that required intervention by center professionals, methods of ensuring student safety, and stress occasioned by a new interprofessional curriculum. Analysis of these factors, however, extends beyond the scope of this article and awaits future publication.

CONCLUSIONS

Several conclusions may be drawn from theses stories in addition to the principles enunciated within each. University health care professionals are in a unique position to partner with community to help meet community-identified needs. When partnering is sincere and when community priorities are addressed, the success of such programs are likely to exceed expectations. Crucial to such success even today is the application of community organization principles, first enunciated by Saul Alinsky. Whereas the bulk of clinical practica sites may need to be situated within established health care agencies, the role of the university in establishing its own sites in partnership with the community should not be overlooked or its educational impact underestimated. Learning within such sites extends beyond the teaching of clinical or even interprofessional competencies. It includes learning the meaning and value of human solidarity, the centrality of human change to life, and the happiness encountered in such pursuits.

Each victory will bring a new vision of human happiness, for man's highest end is to create—total fulfillment, total security, would dull the creative drive. Ours is really the quest for uncertainly, for that continuing change which is life. The pursuit of happiness is never ending—the happiness lies in the pursuit.[20] [p. xvii]

REFERENCES

1. Lavin MA, Ruebling I, Banks R, et al. Interdisciplinary health professional education: a historical review. *Adv Health Sci Educ Theory Pract.* 2002;6:25–47.
2. Griffiths R, Horsfall J, Moore M, Lane D, Kroon V, Langdon R. Assessment of health, well-being and social connections: a survey of women living in Western Sydney. *Int J Nurs Pract.* 2007;13:3–13.
3. Waitzkin H, Iriart C, Estrada A, Lamadrid S. Social medicine then and now: lesson from Latin America. *Am J Public Health.* 2001;91:1592–1601.
4. McMillan B, Florin P, Stevenson J, Kerman B, Mitchell RF Empowerment praxis in community coalitions. *Am J Community Psychol.* 1995;23:699–727.
5. Chen CM, Hong MC, Hsu YH. Administrator self-ratings of organization capacity and performance of healthy community development projects in Taiwan. *Public Health Nurs.* 2007;24:343–354.
6. Wynn TA, Johnson RE, Fouad M, et al. Addressing disparities through coalition building: Alabama REACH 2010 lessons learned. *J Health Care Poor Underserved.* 2006;17(2 Suppl):55–77.

7. Xaverius PK, Homan S, Nickelson PF, Tenkku LE. Disparities rank high in prioritized research, systems and service delivery needs in Missouri. *Matern Child Health J.* 2007;11:511–516.
8. Huang CL, Wang HH. Community health development: what is it? *Int Nurs Rev.* 2005;52:13–17.
9. Alinsky SD. *Rules for Radicals.* New York: Vintage Books; 1971.
10. Kelly C. Health care in the Mississippi Delta. *Am J Nurs.* 1969;69:758–763.
11. Rivera V. Rural cooperatives in Northern Guatemala. Center for Latin American Studies, University of California, Berkeley. Available at: http://socrates.berkeley.edu:7001/Events/fall2002/12-02-02-Rivera/index.html. Accessed September 9, 2007.
12. Pearson TA. Capacity for research in minority health: the need for infrastructure plus will. *Am J Med Sci.* 2001;322:243–247.
13. Minkler M, Frantz S, Wechsler R. Social support and social action organizing in a "grey ghetto": the tenderloin experience. *Int Q Community Health Educ.* 2005–2006; 25:49–61.
14. Perry H, Berggren W, Berggren G, et al. Long-term reductions in mortality among children under age 5 in rural Haiti: effects of a comprehensive health system in an impoverished setting. *Am J Public Health.* 2007;97:240–246.
15. Thomas Brinkhoff: City Population. Available at: http://www.citypopulation.de/Bolivia.html. Accessed September 9, 2007.
16. Dugan MA. Integrative power. In: Burgess G, Burgess H, eds. *Beyond Intractability.* Boulder: Conflict Research Consortium, University of Colorado, Posted October 2003. Available at: http://www.beyondintractability.org/essay/integrative_power/. Accessed September 9, 2007.
17. Western Historical Manuscript Collection—Columbia. Lead mining companies, Washington County, Missouri, records, 1809–1954 (C3893). Columbia, Missouri: University of Missouri Ellis Library. Available at: http://whmc.umsystem.edu/invent/3893.html. Accessed September 9, 2007.
18. Protecting Missouri's Natural Resources. Jefferson City, Missouri: Missouri Department of Natural Resources. Available at: http://www.dnr.mo.gov/env/pmnr/pmnr06-10.htm. Accessed September 9, 2007.
19. Fiscal Year 2003 blood lead testing data. Jefferson City, Missouri Department of Health and Senior Services. Available at: http://www.dhss.mo.gov/ChildhoodLead/FY03.pdf. Accessed September 9, 2007.
20. Alinsky SD. *Reveille for Radicals.* New York: Vintage Books; 1969:54–71.
21. CNN Perspectives Series. Lech Walesa: Polish Trade Union Leader, Dissident. Available at: http://www.cnn.com/SPECIALS/cold.war/episodes/19/interviews/walesa/. Accessed September 9, 2007.
22. Mechanic D. Population health: challenges for science and society. *Milbank Q.* 2007; 85:533–539.
23. Turrell G, Lynch JW, Leite C, Raghunathan T, Kaplan GA. Socioeconomic disadvantage in childhood and across the life course and all-cause mortality and physi-

cal function in adulthood: evidence from the Alameda County Study. *J Epidemiol Community Health*. 2007;61:723–730.

24. Gold R, Michael YL, Whitlock EP, et al. Race/ethnicity, socioeconomic status, and lifetime morbidity burden in women's health initiative: a cross-sectional analysis. *J Women's Health (Larchmt)*. 2006;15:1161–1173.

25. Rao SV, Kaul P, Newby LK, et al. Poverty, process of care, and outcome in acute coronary syndromes. *J Am Coll Cardiol*. 2003;41:1195–1956.

26. Rao SV, Schulman KA, Curtis LH, Gersh BJ, Jollis JG. Socioeconomic status and outcome following acute myocardial infarction in elderly patients. *Arch Intern Med*. 2004;164:1128–1233.

27. Trinacty CM, Adams AS, Soumerai SB, et al. Racial differences in long-term self-monitoring practice among newly drug-treated diabetes patients in an HMO. *J Gen Intern Med*. 2007. November, Volume 22, Issue 11, 1506–1513.

28. Hospitalization profile for St. Louis City residents by race. Jefferson City, Missouri: Missouri Department of Health and Senior Services the City of St. Louis 2000. Available at: http://www.dhss.mo.gov/ASPsHospitalization/MainRace.php?cnty=191&dtdb=hospprfgdbm&cndb=cntydb&urdb=hspurldb&lbdb=hlabldb&lbdbs=hlabldb&pth=/web/data2/. Accessed September 9, 2007.

29. Hamalainen P, Rantanen T, Keskinen M, Meurman JH. Oral health status and change in handgrip strength over a 5-year period in 80-year-old people. *Gerodontology*. 2004;21:155–160.

30. Rosenquist K. Risk factors in oral and oropharyngeal squamous cell carcinoma: a population-based case-control study in southern Sweden. *Swed Dent J*. 2005; 179(Suppl):1–66.

31. Montebugnoli L, Servidio D, Miaton RA, Prati C, Tricoci P, Melloni C. Poor oral health is associated with coronary heart disease and elevated systemic inflammatory and haemostatic factors. *J Clin Periodontol*. 2004;31:25–29.

32. Ajwani S, Mattila KJ, Närhi TO, Tilvis RS, Ainamo A. Oral health status, C-reactive protein and mortality—a 10 year follow-up study. *Gerodontology*. 2003;20:32–40.

Connecting Interprofessional Education to the Community Through Service Learning and Community-Based Research

Pamela J. Reynolds, PT, EdD

INTRODUCTION

"Interprofessional education requires collaborative practice settings where learners can be exposed to educational experience."[1] Establishing educational experiences through partnerships with the community agencies and organizations, such as free health care clinics, senior citizen centers, and after-school programs, is another venue in which to accomplish interprofessional education that broadens and enhances opportunities for students to provide quality collaborative care for the patient/client/service recipient. Methods of integrating interprofessional education into the community include service learning and community-based research. In the context of these pedagogies, the term *community* refers to local neighborhoods, the state, the nation, and the global community. The human and community needs are then defined by the community.[2] The national Community–Campus Partnerships for Health defines partnership as "a close mutual cooperation between parties having common interests, responsibilities, privileges and power."[3] Generally, community partners are organizations and agencies that deliver support services to underserved or marginalized populations. Development of community partnerships requires sensitive exchange of ideas across the cultural boundaries of the community partner organization and academic institutions such as universities and colleges. Outcomes and products of partnership between the academic institution and the community can inform community-based health care practices, and influence advocacy actions and health policy decisions (e.g., identifying population needs, defining services needed/provided, outcome assessment of current program[s]).

One of the purposes of this chapter is to define service learning and community-based research by identifying the characteristics they have in common with interprofessional education. An example of an interprofessional service learning course provides a framework for the comparison. Two examples of interprofessional community-based research projects provide a format to discuss interprofessional research initiatives. Second, the development of principles-based partnerships that link the academic institutions with the community is considered by examining the stages of partnership development between the West Virginia Rural Health Education Program and the University Systems of West Virginia. This is a large, mature, and very successful partnership between a higher education state system and community organization. It is also unique in that it was established through legislative action to provide health services in rural West Virginia. A case is made for how the academic and community partnership can inform community health practice and policy through community-based research. The chapter concludes with a brief discussion of how these activities can be used by faculty as evidence of community-engaged scholarship in their professional portfolio.

CONTEXT OF COMMUNITY ENGAGEMENT

There is no consistently used definition for community engagement associated with the health professions. Community–Campus Partnerships for Health defines community engagement as "the application of intuitional resources to address and solve challenges facing communities through collaboration with these communities"[4] (p. 12). Institutional resources may include, but are not limited to, the expertise and knowledge of students, faculty, and staff; the use of the campus buildings and land; and the institution's political position within their community and influences on local schools, economy, and government. Venues that academic institutions may use for community engagement include, but are not limited to, community service, service learning, community-based research, training and technical assistance, coalition building, capacity building, and economic development.[4]

Service Learning

Service learning is a structured learning experience that meets identified needs in the community "with explicit learning objectives, preparation, and reflection. Students engaged in service learning are expected not only to provide direct community service but also to learn about the context in which the service is provided, the connection between the service and their academic coursework, and their roles as citizens"[5] (p. 274). Also, "unlike practica and internships, the experiential activity in a service-learning course is not necessarily skill-based within the context of professional education"[6] (p. 222). Although service-learning experiences may evolve from discipline-specific academic content, by virtue of working with individuals in the partnering community organization, service learning is innately interprofessional. Professionals staffing community organizations are rarely the same professional discipline as the student.

Service learning differs significantly from volunteerism, community service, traditional practica, clinical rotations, field experiences, and internships.[7] Volunteerism and community service benefit the recipient of the service, not the learner. Traditional practica, clinical rotations, internships, and field experiences include specific course learning objectives and focus on the development of students' skills essential to their profession and education. In contrast, service learning emphasizes an equal balance between the service and the learning components.[7] Academic learning objectives are matched with community-identified needs. Although implementation of service learning into coursework can be discipline specific and skill based, it can also include advocacy and policy-level work on such issues as housing, poverty, the environment, education, and human services.[2] Gelmon and colleagues[8] note that the effect of service-learning experiences on students was much more evident at sites that did not involve an exclusive focus on community-based clinical skill development. Students were strongly influenced when they worked with individuals in nonclinical settings and when they learned about the context of patients' daily lives within the complex and delicate network of support services on which they depended.[8] Although service learning in clinical settings can be valuable, issues of clinical skill development and application usually impede realization and recognition of potential service experience benefits.

Reciprocal learning is the second factor that distinguishes service-learning programs from other community-service programs.[7] The student and the patient are both teachers and learners. Community organizational partners play a crucial role in designing the service-learning experiences in accord with community interests and priorities. Thus both parties help to determine what is learned and provide input on program development.[5–7] It is this element of reciprocity that moves service learning to the level of a philosophy, "an expression of values—service to others, community development and empowerment, reciprocal learning—which determines the purpose, nature and process of *social and educational exchange* between learners (students) and the people they serve"[9] (p. 67). Reciprocity as a philosophy in service learning implies a meticulous effort to "move from charity to justice, from service to elimination of need."[2]

Reflection is another crucial component of service learning. Reflection activities are active learning processes that facilitate students' connection between their service in the community and instructional objectives.[2,10,11] Reflection is the mechanism for moving students toward recognition of achieving specific academic objectives. It is asking the student to step back and be thoughtful about the experience. As students discuss their experience, the facilitator (through questions about what they learned) leads them toward recognition of academic objectives they have met. A common reflection technique is to ask students to define "what," "so what," and "now what" about their experience. *What* happens in this experience? *So what* asks students to consider why things are the way they are and what needs to change. *Now what* empowers students to be agents of social change or at least engaged citizens. Reflection activities can be conducted through oral discussion and structured written essay or journaling.[12,13]

Service-learning experiences facilitate the development of students' professionalism skills and understanding of their social responsibility role as health professionals and citizens within a larger social context.[5,6,10,11] Service-learning objectives can also include educational outcomes in the areas of leadership, ethical or spiritual development, critical thinking, increased understanding of human diversity and commonality, understanding one's professional social responsibility role, and learning to advocate for issues of social justice and social change.[2,11] Studies have reported that when students became cognizant of the many challenges potential patients faced in their everyday lives, their views on their professional roles and citizenship in the community were transformed.[6–8,10] One student working in a remote Appalachian community realized the importance of asking about a patient's home situation during initial physical therapy evaluation, stating, "Many of the homes in this area are built on steep hills, have no access to handicap services, limited resources to perform your suggestions, and no transportation to get to the clinic for adequate intervention"[11] (p. 48). Another student in recognizing her responsibility as a professional stated the following[11] (p. 54):

> This experience had made me aware of the need for more volunteer services, especially with the disabled population. This organization, even though well established, still had staff shortages for several programs. After graduation, I plan to get more involved in volunteering and marketing such programs, so that individuals will take time to help other people who need it so desperately.

Community-Based Research

Community-based research is the most recent iteration of service learning. It involves a collaborative approach to research that equitably involves community members, organizational representatives, and academic researchers in the design and accomplishment of research projects aimed at meeting community-identified needs and objectives. The research is conducted "with" rather than "on" a community partner. Community-based research includes a critical action component such that the knowledge gained is combined with action to enhance the well-being of the community and its constituents.[14,15]

As a form of service learning, community-based research is also intrinsically interdisciplinary. Although it connects well with single discipline-based academic content, again community-based research projects seldom result in strictly involving researchers from one single professional discipline. Students, faculty, and community partners usually bring and apply many different kinds of knowledge and disciplines to their work. Community-based research may also be referred to as community-based participatory research or community action research.[17] *Participatory* is added to the term "community-based research" to honor and indicate that the community partner is an equal participant in research. *Action* is sometimes found in the term because of the aforementioned critical action component associated with community-based research.

Outcomes and products of community-based research are varied and can be divided into three categories: (a) peer-reviewed articles; (b) applied products, such as training materials and resource guides to improve community health, technical assistance, and program development grants; and (c) dissemination products, such as community forums, websites, and presentations or written briefs to legislative bodies and policymakers.[16] Table 11-1 contrasts traditional academic research with community-based research.[14]

Table 11-1. Comparison of Traditional Academic Research and Community-Based Research

	Traditional Academic Research	Community-Based Research
Primary goal of the research	Advance knowledge within the discipline	Contribute to the betterment of a particular community; social change, social justice
Source of research question	Extant theoretical or empirical work in the discipline	Community-identified problem or need for information
Who designs and conducts the research?	Trained researcher, perhaps with help of paid assistants	Trained researchers, students, community members in collaboration
Role of researcher	Outside researcher	Collaborators, partners, and learner
Role of community	Object to be studied ("community as laboratory") or no role at all	Collaborators, partners, and learners
Role of students	None, or as research assistant	Collaborators, partners, and learners
Relationship of the researcher(s) and participants-responders	Short term, task oriented, detached	Long term, multifaceted, connected
Measure of value of the research	Acceptance by academic peers (e.g., publication)	Usefulness for community partners and contribution to social change
Criteria for selecting data collection methods	Conformity to standards of rigor, objectivity, researcher control, preference for quantitative and positivistic approaches	The potential for drawing out useful information, sensitivity to experiential knowledge, conformity to standards of rigor, and accessibility, open to a variety and combination of approaches
Beneficiaries of the research	Academic researcher	Academic researcher, students, community

(Continues)

Table 11-1. Comparison of Traditional Academic Research and Community-Based Research *(Continued)*

	Traditional Academic Research	Community-Based Research
Ownership of the data	Academic researcher	Community
Mode of presentation	Written report	Varies widely and may take multiple and creative forms (e.g., video, theater, written narrative)
Means of dissemination	Presentation at academic conference, submission to journal	Any and all forms where results might have impact: media, public meetings, informal community settings, legislative bodies

Source: Strand K, Marullo S, Cutforth N, Stoecker R, Donohue P. Origins and principles of community based-research. In: *Community-Based Research and Higher Education: Principles and Practices.* San Francisco: Jossey-Bass; 2003:1–15.

An example of a very small scale community-based research projected occurred when Gannon University's Physical Therapy Program was approached by the health care team for two senior citizen high-rise buildings operated by the Housing Authority of Erie, Pennsylvania. The team was concerned about many of their residents' appropriate and safe use of ambulatory assistive devices. Three student physical therapists developed a research project around this community-identified need. They evaluated and made individual written recommendations for over 50 residents about the appropriate adjustment and use of whatever ambulatory equipment they were using. They also collected data about where the resident obtained their assistive device and who adjusted it and trained them how to use the device. This project was approved by all the appropriate institutional review boards for Protection of Human Subjects.

During the study the students saw everything from walking canes to deluxe wheeled walkers and even assessed a shopping cart being used as an ambulation aid. They found that most of the residents never saw a physical therapist or other health care professional for adjustment of or training with their ambulatory devices. Data analysis also demonstrated that a statistically significant number of walkers being used by residents were at inappropriate heights—too high or too low. In two instances, for example, the hand rests were as much as 12 inches too high.

The students disseminated their findings at a national multidisciplinary conference.[18] They also shared their finding in letters to their congressional leaders, making an argument supportive of the proposed Medicare Direct Access legislation for physical therapists. Thus students demonstrated their social accountability and advocated for a health policy change supported by findings of their study. In summary, this community-based research project not only met a community-identified need but also fulfilled the students' educational research requirements for graduation. Subsequently, it has led to the development of more community partnerships and service-learning experience opportunities for our students in the community. Specifically, one student, for an independent study project, developed a brochure on how to select, adjust, and use canes and walkers. She distributed it to local durable medical equipment providers.

Interprofessional Education and Service-Learning Common Teaching Strategies

The primary goal of interprofessional education is to "develop students who have the knowledge, skills and attitudes to become collaborative practitioners who work together in an effective collaborative fashion"[19] (p. 29). The following example of an interdisciplinary service-learning course demonstrates several essential interprofessional education teaching strategies that are also important pedagogical tenets of service learning.

Gupta[20] describes the process of development, challenges, and successes of an interprofessional service-learning experience course, which included the professions of physical therapy, occupational therapy, nursing, social work, and education. The institution partnered with a large urban homeless shelter for families that housed over 350 individuals. The overarching goal of this four credit course focused on students' "understanding the impact of complex social problems on the health and well being of families in poverty and provided an opportunity for collective action to promote social change"[20] (p. 55).

The development of the course involved all stakeholders from the beginning, including community partners, students, faculty, and the academic institution. This unique course evolved over 2 years of laborious hard work and learning from each other the different disciplinary and professional perspectives. The faculty noted that in the early stages their most common barriers to interdisciplinary work were territorial issues, which usually originated from a lack of understanding the other disciplines. For instance, the physical therapy discipline aligned with the biomedical paradigm, which views disease and impairment as an individual deviation from normal biological functioning. Social work and occupational therapy embraced the social paradigm that assumes that factors other than the body influence health and well-being. What united this interprofessional faculty group was "enthusiasm and philosophical alignment around social justice, holistic view of health, interdisciplinary work, service learning and cultural competency"[20] (p. 59).

Similar to this faculty group, a study of academic administrators' attitudes toward interprofessional education found that over two-thirds of the respondents surveyed recognized that faculty attitudes and turf battles were potential barriers to implementing interprofessional learning.[19] It is evident that before students can learn to work collaboratively in practice that faculty need to work through these potential barriers first to realistically model interprofessional practice for the students.

It is evident in both interprofessional education and service learning that the faculty do not function in the traditional role of content expert. There can be a blurring of the line between teacher and student. The faculty role becomes one of a facilitator or coach who works with learner instead of teaching learners. Facilitators need to be mindful of the aspects of facilitation that involve both for team formation and team maintenance.[10,19]

Just as reflection is a crucial element of service learning,[2,5-11] it is also "a key component to interprofessional education teaching strategies"[19] (p. 26). Through reflective exercises, students develop an understanding of each other's professional roles, unique background, and perspectives about clinical decision making distinctive of each profession.[19] The following two reflective comments illustrate these points. They were written by students in Gupta's[20] interdisciplinary service learning course (p. 59):

> There are huge areas of overlap between nursing, education, and occupational therapy, etc. An important aspect of the team work is that all team members understand the other professions involved. This includes listening to and sharing the possibilities of the profession.
>
> It is really important to have a multiprofessional approach to case management to aid in a holistic approach for care. It is really great to have many different perspectives on helping a person/family.

McNair and colleagues[22] developed and evaluated an interprofessional education model in which medical, nursing, physical therapy, and pharmacy students were invited to participate in a 2-week placement of mixed interprofessional team groups in rural community health settings. They were supervised by preceptors for their own disciplines. The teams' central assignment was to design and complete a community-based project. In the end, these projects included a wide range of focal points, including health promotion, health needs analyses and program planning, development of multidisciplinary case conferencing, and raising community awareness of existing health resources. Evaluative outcomes of this brief study supported participating students' belief in the value of interprofessional practice. This finding echoes previous students' comments in Gupta's[20] interdisciplinary service learning course.

In addition, the study[22] also indicated that rural interprofessional educational experiences not only improved participating students interprofessional skills but also influenced employment interest in this area after graduation. Nursing and allied health students' placement in the rural health settings strengthened their intention to work in this setting after graduation.[22] Likewise, in the interdisciplinary service-learning course, one of the students working at the shelter for homeless individuals and families stated that, "It sparked a passion in me to advocate for this population. This course has changed my career path. I do not want to work in a medically based model practice. I want to do community-based practice"[20] (p. 59).

In summary, in both interprofessional education and service learning collaboration with interprofessional practitioners and community partners is essential.[1-3,5-8,21] Reflection is a key component of both.[2,3,5-11,21] The faculty role moves from content expert to facilitator or coach.[10,17] Evidence also suggests that students' experiences in either interprofessional education or service learning can influence their future job placement decisions.[20,22]

DEVELOPMENT OF PRINCIPLES-BASED PARTNERSHIPS

The development of collaborative community partnerships is vital to successful service learning, community-based research projects, and interprofessional education in the community setting. Too often in the past, academic institutions have treated communities as their laboratory. They have gone into the community, provided service to meet academic need or to collect data, and then retreated behind their academic walls without consideration of community needs. Results were neither shared with nor used to benefit the community.[14,23] Thus the community sometimes hesitates or even refuses when approached by an academic institution to "work with" them.

Creating a successful nonthreatening environment for interprofessional education requires a number of conditions, including "institutional support, equal status of participants, positive expectations, a cooperative atmosphere, successful joint work, a concern for and understanding of differences and similarities, [and] a perception that members of the other group"[19] (p. 25). Development of community partnerships in service learning and community-based research requires clear, open, and accessible communications that are built on mutual trust, respect, genuineness, and commitment.[3] Collaborating with a community partner is a two-way street. Understanding the community partner's mission and services needs is important, but the community also needs information about the institution, its culture, policies, procedures, services, and resources.[23] The community's service needs are 24 hours a day, 7 days a week, whereas most academic institution work is by semesters. Information and resource sharing need to be negotiated where the voices of all partners can be heard equally. Community–Campus Partnership for Health identified nine principles for the development of sustainable community partnerships.[24]

1. Agree upon values, goals, and measurable outcomes. The mission and goals are written and agreed upon by all members of the partnership. Measurable outcomes are identified by members on an annual basis. Partners are able to verbally reflect a common mission and goals through interactions with others in the community. The mission, goals, and outcomes should be reviewed on an annual basis.[25]
2. Develop relationships of mutual trust, respect, genuineness, and commitment. Partnering is often challenged by biases and expectations that stakeholders bring to the table on behalf of their respective constituencies. Although these preconceptions have historical precedent, they are not healthy for a developing partnership. A community–campus partnership must grow and mature in such a way as to diminish and eliminate preconceived biases.[26]
3. Build on strengths and assets and also address needs. Reporting problem-oriented data is important, but it only conveys a partial truth in a negative manner. Recognizing the capacity and skills of people and their neighborhoods, however, builds on assets instead of only recognizing deficiencies. In bringing together the community and campus, the gifts and capacities of individuals, citizen associations, and local institutions need to be recognized.[27]

4. Balance power and share resources. Development of collaborative agendas needs to include the interests of all partners. In reality, however, they tend to disproportionately favor the interest of the larger partners with broader scope of services, greater fiscal resources, or better market reputation. The work of achieving a balance of power begins with acknowledging and respecting the importance of each partner's value and unique resources.[28]

5. Have clear, open, and accessible communication. Each partner needs to be aware of each other's viewpoints and diversity in values, beliefs, practices, lifestyles, and problem-solving strategies. Just being aware of differences, however, is not enough. Partners must also learn about what affects each other's worldview, including historical, societal, political, and/or religious influences. Partners must be able to identify their own culture and cultural blind spots, prejudices, and biases. Knowledge bases and resources are shared in successful partnerships. The community is often its own best teacher. It is critical to involve them in the initial planning phase. Whenever possible, recruiting trusted advocates from within the community is the best way to build bridges across distrust and misinformation.[23]

6. Agree on roles, norms, and processes. Like academic institutions, each community organization has its own norms of operation. Working with the community requires a long-term investment, not an episodic one based on when one course is in need of a service dimension. Nurturing the relationship requires frequent meaningful dialogue. The quantity and quality of communication between partners is a sure sign of the health of the relationship.[29] Members of the partnership group create the leadership and together form group norms about the patterns of communication, processes, and decision making.[25]

7. Ensure feedback to, among, and from all stakeholders. All stakeholders should be included in the feedback process, including service users, organizational members, and policymakers. Multiple and diverse approaches to seek and use feedback need to be developed. Differences and conflicts must be managed so they become positive aspects of the communication feedback loop.[30]

8. Share the credit for accomplishments. When sharing the credit for accomplishments, the community partner should be involved in development of the publicity. Often, university public relations offices that are not involved with the partnership publicize programs and accomplishments without sensitivity to the community partner's perspective.[31]

9. Take time to develop and evolve. Partnerships are formed by an ongoing group, and, like most relationships, they develop and mature through a series of continuous stages that broaden and deepen over time. An example of this process is described more fully below.[32] One way that campus and community leaders demonstrate commitment to the progress of the partnership is through attendance at meetings, and by making contributions to support the mission of the partnership.[25]

Hilda Heady[32] is the Executive Director of West Virginia Rural Health Education Partnership and is jointly appointed to the University System of West Virginia. She describes a community–campus partnership model that exemplifies several of the principles already discussed. Heady[32] recounts the development, challenges, and lessons learned through the partnership experience with the West Virginia Rural Health Education Partnership and the seven health profession schools in the state university system. At the time this partnership began there was a critical shortage of primary care providers in the rural underserved areas of the state. The partnership was supported by state legislation that provided $6 million per year to sustain the partnership. During the first stage, partners defined their common ground and common passions. Infrastructure building was the next stage. It is interesting to note that the West Virginia Rural Health Education Partnership with the state university system had no organizational chart, albeit there were attempts to develop one that were abandoned. The partnership is a network rather than a hierarchy.

Performance of mission work defines the third stage. The partnership tests the strength of its foundation. This is where successful and mature partnerships spend most of their time. The West Virginia Board of Trustees for the state universities in accepting the legislative mandate to achieve the West Virginia Rural Health Education Partnership mission made it a degree requirement for students in health professional programs to spend a minimum of 3 months of clinical rotations in rural communities. Partners celebrate and share their successes during the fourth stage, and reflect on their challenges and lessons learned. In the final stage, the partnership recognizes future opportunities that push the partnership to a higher level, applying lessons learned to other social change agendas.[32]

Freyer and O'Toole[26] note that "the sum of a community partnership is far greater than its parts and half the fun is the journey getting there" (p. 24). They offer these suggestions when developing a partnership: (a) get to know each other's strengths and weaknesses; (b) appreciate each stakeholders' priorities and motivations; (c) start small and grow, allowing for space, time, and forgiveness for mistakes; (d) identify and understand areas of mistrust, don't underestimate them; (e) track progress toward goals and priorities; (f) take time to thank your partner; (g) stay flexible; and (h) enjoy the diversity and unique resources of community by moving outside the academic institution.[26] In summary, "When the colleges and communities go beyond common goals and mission to truly believe in each other's dreams, the community-campus partnership can reach a level of depth and strength seldom achieved in joint efforts"[31] (p. 65).

Community-Engaged Scholarship Opportunity for Faculty in Interprofessional Education

Community engagement was defined earlier as the use of institutional resources to address and solve challenging issues facing communities through collaboration with them. Characteristic principles of community engagement are based on "values and norms that involve interactive, collaborative, and respectful community-university partnerships that result in mutually beneficial outcomes and are dedicated to learning with an emphasis on community, responsibility, and stewardship"[33] (p. 81). It is only when these principles of engagement are coupled with standards of scholarship is community-engaged scholarship achieved. Community–Campus Partnerships for Health defines community-engaged scholarship as follows[4] (p. 12):

> *Scholarship that involves the faculty member in a mutually beneficial partnership with the community. Community-engaged scholarship can be transdisciplinary and often integrates some combination of multiple forms of scholarship. For example, service learning can integrate the scholarship of teaching, application and engagement . . . [community-based research] can integrate the scholarship of discovery, integration, application, and engagement.*

Not all community-based activities represent engagement, particularly if they are not done *with* the community. Not all faculty community-engaged activities represent scholarship. The Commission on Community-Engaged Scholarship in the Health Professions gives this example[4] (p. 11):

> *. . . if a faculty member devotes time to developing a community-based health program, it may be important work and it may advance the service mission of the institution, but unless it includes the other components that define scholarship (e.g., clear goals, adequate preparation, appropriate methods, significant results, effective presentation, reflective critique, rigor, and peer review) it would not be considered scholarship.*

Cox[34] describes community-engaged scholarship as having Boyer's original four dimensions of scholarship—discovery, integration, application, and teaching—at its core. The scholarship of engagement evolves within these dimensions through interactive connections with people and places outside the university in the activities of scholarship, including setting goals, appropriate preparation and selection of methods, and reflecting on and dissemination of results.[34] Brukardt et al.[35] remark that "the scholarship of engagement and the idea of community partnerships are not about service. They are about extraordinary forms of teaching and research and what happens when they come together" (p. 2).

Johnson, Maritz, and Lefever[36] offer an example of a community-engaged scholarship outcomes, which began as a pro bono physical therapy clinic in Philadelphia. It started with one physical therapist and a couple of student volunteers offering services one night a week. From this humble beginning it has evolved into the Mercy Circle of Care initiative that brought together a collaboration of citizens, health care providers, social services, the Philadelphia Department of Public Health, and three universities in Philadelphia that provide the core curriculum for three physical therapy programs. Sandmann[33] describes and defines how the Mercy Circle of Care is a community-engaged research and scholarship initiative, having all of the components of traditional research project—purpose, questions, data collection and analysis, and dissemination.[36]

The overall purpose of the Mercy Circle of Care was to address the lack of health insurance, uncoordinated care, and under-resourced health programs in this particular area of Philadelphia. The oversight committee for the Mercy Circle of Care recognized and acknowledged early in its inception that the uninsured use fewer preventative and screening services and were more ill when initially diagnosed. Thus their health issues were more complex, and an interdisciplinary model of care was imperative. Questions raised by this interprofessional collaboration in development of this initiative attended to demographic data and understanding the behaviors of the uninsured or underinsured versus insured patients/clients/service users. Specifically, do they have more chronic condition? Is treatment of musculoskeletal dysfunction more extensive because of delay of care? Do they value the service? [33,36]

The design of a community-engaged research project tends to have greater flexibility. It was chosen because it would be conducted in collaboration with the community partners.[33] The Mercy Circle of Care oversight committee was composed of all collaborating organizations. They also had a data collection subcommittee.[33,36] Community partners assist with the data analysis process, which also had to be understandable for nonacademics.[33] In analyzing their data, the subcommittee collaborated with multidisciplinary faculty to make sense of some of the data, which were unexpected and related to the patterns of participation of the uninsured and underinsured patients. Collaborative discussion with the subcommittee and faculty resulted in new insights. The uninsured patients were more likely to miss visits because of lack of accessible transportation, weather concerns, personal or family illness, and admission to the hospital.[33,36] Community-engaged research uses a variety of dissemination methods and products.[15,33] The Mercy Circle of Care collaboration disseminated their results through the local newspaper and other media outlets. In addition, a couple of the academic faculty are writing scholarly publications and one graduate student completed a master's degree project related to this community–campus collaboration. [33,36]

The Mercy Circle of Care initiative is now a Federally Qualified Health Center. Clinical psychologists and graduate psychology students joined the Mercy Circle of Care program to address the identified need for behavioral and mental health needs of the community. An enrollment specialist was hired to further assist community members with insurance enrollment and to connect them with a variety of other social service agencies that could help address issues that affected their social well-being such as transportation, housing, and employment.

Recognition of Diverse Products and Dissemination Pathways of Community-Engaged Research as Products for Faculty Scholarship

The traditionally accepted product of faculty research for scholarship is the peer-reviewed article. There has been an increase over the past decade of peer-reviewed published articles on service learning. In community-based research, however, a more diverse range of scholarship products or evidence needs to be considered. For instance, the community is a peer and hence potential contributors to the peer review process.[4] The critical assessment of the community-based research product by a representative leader of the community partner should be valued as a peer reviewer.

Applied products are another pathway for dissemination of community-engaged scholarship, which focus on immediate transfer of knowledge into action or application of results. The Mercy Circle of Care example just provided is a case in point of immediate action and application of results. They

hired an insurance enrollment specialist and developed their education activities based on their research results. Other applied products include but
are not limited to innovative intervention program; policies at the community, state, and national level; training materials and resource guides; and
technical assistance. "These products can be evaluated for evidence of scholarship by the extent to which they require a high level of discipline-related
expertise, are innovative, have been implemented or used, and have an impact on the learners (if educational in scope), organizational or community
capacity, or the health of individuals or communities"[4] (p. 16).

Community-engaged scholarship products can be disseminated in community forums, newspaper articles, websites, and in presentations to leaders
and policymakers at the local community, state, and federal levels.[4,16] These
products offer a valuable opportunity for reflective appraisal by peers both
in the community and in the academy.[37]

Although higher education institutions preparing health care professionals have been steadily increasing their community engagement over the past
10 years, faculty review, promotion, and tenure systems have not kept pace.
Faculty frequently site the risks and challenges associated with trying to
achieve promotion and tenure with community-engaged research and scholarship products. Faculty peers tend to classify community-based work as service rather that considering factors that qualify it as scholarship. Standards
for judging quality, productivity, and impact of scholarship tend to exclude
evidence of community-based scholarship.[4] It takes time to develop relationships with the communities, and the process of developing useful products
may take years. It may take even longer to realize and document any community and institutional impact. These factors can present challenges and
barriers to significant and sustained involvement of faculty in the community and can also affect a faculty member's ability to achieve recognition and
document the requirements that most academic institutions require for promotion and tenure.[38] It is beyond the scope of this chapter to detail effective
strategies for faculty to document their community engagement and
community-engaged scholarship. A list of resources, however, has been
placed at the end of this chapter to assist faculty in this process.

In summary, interprofessional education can lead to community-engaged
research and faculty scholarship when interdisciplinary faculty or students
assisted by faculty actively and systematically partner with the community
organizations for the purpose of meeting a community identified need or objective. Opportunities for community-engaged research can include anything

from investigating and recommending an action plan for a large-scale community problem or issue to developing a small-scale community educational program using evidence from best practice. There are measurable outcomes that can be analyzed. Dissemination of the results and/or product, although it may be through a nontraditional pathway, completes the research cycle.

CONCLUSIONS

This chapter defines processes and examples for providing interprofessional education within the community context. Communities, whether they are local, regional, or global, provide a rich framework in which to provide experiential education. Partnerships must be developed and nurtured in a manner that honors and respects the depth of the educational resources that communities offer. In conclusion, these four "pearls" summarize the primary points of this chapter:

1. Community engagement, including service-learning pedagogy and community-based research, connects interprofessional education to the community.
2. Integration of interprofessional education, service learning, and community-based research with the community requires principles-based partnerships.
3. Interprofessional education can lead to community-engaged scholarship when faculty or students assisted by faculty actively and systematically partner with the community organizations for the purpose of meeting a community-identified need, investigating a community problem or issue, or developing evidence-based programs with measurable outcomes that promote community health and wellness objectives.
4. Dissemination of the outcomes and products of community engagement and community-engaged scholarship can inform community-based health care practices and influence advocacy and health policy decisions.

REFERENCES

1. D'Amour D, Oandasan I. Interprofessionality as the field of interprofessional practice and interprofessional education: an emerging concept. *J Interprofess Care.* 2005;(Suppl 1):8–20.
2. Jacoby B. Fundamentals of service-learning partnerships. In: *Building Partnerships for Service-Learning.* San Francisco: Jossey-Bass; 2003:1–19.

3. About Us Page. Community Campus Partnerships for Health website. Available at: http://www.ccph.info. Accessed December 15, 2006.

4. Commission on Community-Engaged Scholarship in the Health Professions. *Linking Scholarship and Communities: The Report of the Commission on Community-Engaged Scholarship in the Health Professions.* Seattle, WA: Community–Campus Partnerships for Health; 2005.

5. Seifer SD. Service-learning: community-campus partnerships for health professions education. *Acad Med.* 1998;73:273–277.

6. Bringle RG, Hatcher JA. Implementing service learning in higher education. *J Higher Educ.* 1996;67:221–239.

7. Furco A. Service-learning: a balanced approach to experiential learning. In: Taylor B, ed. *Expanding Boundaries: Service and Learning.* Vol. 1. Washington, DC: Corporation for National and Community Service; 1996:2–6.

8. Gelmon SB, Holland B, Shinnamon AF. *Health Professions Schools in Service to the Nation: 1996–1998 Final Evaluation Report.* San Francisco: Community–Campus Partnerships for Health; 1999.

9. Stanton T. Service-learning: groping toward a definition. In: Ehrlich T, ed. *Combining Service and Learning: A Resourced Book for Community and Public Service.* Vol. 1. Raleigh, NC: National Society for Experiential Education; 1990.

10. Checkoway B. Combining service and learning on campus and in the community. *Phi Delta Kappan.* 1996;77:600–606.

11. Reynolds PJ. How service learning experiences benefit physical therapist students' professional development: a grounded theory study. *J Phys Ther Edu.* 2005;19:41–51.

12. Eyler J, Giles DE, Schmiede A. *A Practitioner's Guide to Reflection in Service Learning.* Nashville, TN: Vanderbilt University, 1996.

13. Eyler J, Giles DE. *Where's the Learning in Service-Learning?* San Francisco: Jossey-Bass; 1999.

14. Strand K, Marullo S, Cutforth N, Stoecker R, Donohue P. Origins and principles of community based-research. In: *Community-Based Research and Higher Education: Principles and Practices.* San Francisco: Jossey-Bass; 2003:1–15.

15. Israel BA, Schultz AJ, Parker EA, Becker AB. Community-based participatory research: policy recommendations for promoting a partnership approach in health research. *Educ Health.* 2001;14:182–197.

16. Maurana C, Wolff M, Beck BJ, Simpson DE. Working with our communities: moving from service to scholarship in the health professions research. *Educ Health.* 2001;14:207–220.

17. Strand K, Marullo S, Cutforth N, Stoecker R, Donohue P. Teaching community-based research. In: *Community-Based Research and Higher Education: Principles and Practices.* San Francisco: Jossey-Bass; 2003:138–168.

18. Reynolds P, Belczyk E, Dulaney L, Mock B. Investigation of how community dwelling elderly persons obtain and utilize assistive devices for ambulation [poster presentation]. National Community Campus Partnerships for Health 7th Annual Conference, San Diego, April 27–28, 2003.

19. Oandasan I, Reeves S. Key elements for interprofessional education. Part 1: The learner, the educator and the learning context. *J Interprofess Care.* 2005; (Suppl):21–38.

20. Gupta J. A model for interdisciplinary service-learning experience for social change. *J Phys Ther Educ.* 2006;20:55–60.

21. Curran VR, Deacon DR, Fleet L. Academic administrator's attitudes towards interprofessional education in Canadian schools of health professional education. *Journal Interprofess Care.* 2005;19(Suppl 1):76–85.

22. McNair R, Stone N, Simes J, Curtis C. Australian evidence for interprofessional education contributing to effective teamwork preparation and interest in rural practice. *J Interprofess Care.* 2005;19:579–594.

23. Sen Gupta I. There is a clear, open and accessible communication between partners, making it an ongoing priority to listen to each need, develop a common language, and validate/clarify the meaning of terms. *Partnership Perspectives.* 2000;1:41–46.

24. Seifer SD, Maurana CA. Developing and sustaining community-campus partnerships: Putting principles into practice. *Partnership Perspectives.* 2000;1:7–11.

25. Bell-Elkins J. *Assessing the CCPH Principles of a Partnership in a Community–Campus Partnership.* Seattle, WA: Community–Campus Partnerships for Health; 2002.

26. Freyer PJ, O'Toole TP. The relationship between partners is characterized by mutual trust, respect, genuineness and commitment. *Partnership Perspectives.* 2000;1:19–25.

27. Connor K, Prelip M. The partnership builds upon identified strengths and assets, but also addresses areas that need improvement. *Partnership Perspectives.* 2000;1:27–32.

28. Connolly C. The partnership balances the power among partners and enables resources among partners to be shared. *Partnership Perspectives.* 2000;1:33–40.

29. Huppert M. Roles, norms, and processes for the partnership are established with the input and agreement of all partners. *Partnership Perspectives.* 2000;1:47–56.

30. Sebastian JG, Skelton J, West KP. There is feedback to, among and from all stakeholders in the partnership, with the goal of continuously improving the partnership and its outcomes. *Partnership Perspectives.* 2000;1:57–64.

31. Blake JM, Moore E. Partners a\share the credit for the partnership's accomplishments. *Partnership Perspectives.* 2000;1:65–69.

32. Heady HR. Partnerships take time to develop and evolve over time. *Partnership Perspectives.* 2000;1:71–78.

33. Sandmann LR. Scholarship as architecture: framing and enhancing community engagement. *J Phys Ther Educ.* 2006;20:80–84.

34. Cox D. The how and why of the scholarship of engagement. In: Percy SL, Zimpher NL, Brukardt MJ, eds. *Creating a New Kind of University: Institutionalizing Community-University Engagement.* Bolton, MA: Anker Publishing Company; 2006:122–135.

35. Brukardt MJ, Holland B, Percy S, Zimpher N. *Calling the Question: Is Higher Education Ready to Commit to Community Engagement? A Wingspread Statement,* 2004. Proceedings Wingspread Conference, Wisconsin, USA. pg. 9.

36. Johnson M, Maritz C, Lefever G. The Mercy Circle of Care: an interdisciplinary, multi-institutional collaboration to promote community health and professional education. *J Phys Ther Educ.* 2006;20:73–78.
37. Dodds J, Calleson D, Eng G, Margolis L, Moore K. Structure and culture of schools of public health to support public health practice. *J Pub Health Manag Practice.* 2003;9:504–512.
38. Calleson DC, Jordan C, Seifer SD. Community-engaged scholarship: is faculty work in the communities a true academic enterprise? *Acad Med.* 2005;80:317–321.

RESOURCES FOR FACULTY TO DOCUMENT COMMUNITY ENGAGED SCHOLARSHIP

Calleson D, Kauper-Brown J, Seifer SD. *Community-Engaged Scholarship Toolkit.* Seattle, WA: Community–Campus Partnerships for Health; 2005. Available at: http://depts.washington.edu/ccph/toolkit.html. Accessed October 4, 2006.

Glassick CM, Huber MT, Maeroff G. *Scholarship Assessed: Evaluation of the Professoriate.* San Francisco: Jossey-Bass; 1997.

Maurana C, Wolff M, Beck BJ, Simpson DE. Working with our communities: moving from service to scholarship in the health professions research. *Educ Health.* 2001;14:207–220.

Oregon State University Faculty Handbook. Available at: http://oregonstate.edu/facultystaff/handbook/promoten/protenque.htm. Accessed January 31, 2007.

Scholarship of Engagement Online website. Available at: http://www.scholarshipof engagement.org. Accessed October 4, 2006.

Social, Environmental, and Occupational Justice: Too Many High Sounding Words and Not Enough Action

Beth P. Velde, PhD, OT

INTRODUCTION

Social justice compels us to provide health services to residents of rural America. Social justice is more than institutional responsibility for laws and policies that afford equal access and service for all. Social justice goes beyond the belief that governments are responsible for ensuring equal access for all. Social justice occurs when members of a society work together to create a just society. It is too easy to blame the system and not take personal and professional responsibility for social inequities. If rural health disparities exist, as health professionals we have a responsibility to resolve the social injustices related to rural health services. Yet, we continue to pay lip service to the concepts of social justice and health without reducing the disparities.

Disparities in rural health services include higher proportions of poor health conditions when compared with urban areas, lack of access to health providers, and lack of resources to use the providers who are available. Contributors to decreased health care include poor access to medical and mental health practitioners, poor availability of care providers, lack of transportation, poverty, greater exposure to environmental toxins, and loss of family and community.[1–5] These disparities exist at the patient/person, systems, and provider levels.

Why don't more health professionals practice in rural environments? Typical issues raised by health practitioners considering rural practice include social isolation, lack of infrastructure, lack of resources, lack of contact with other health care providers, and a perception that their careers will be limited to generalist practice.[6,7] These issues create a shortage of health services in rural areas.[8]

One way to address rural health issues is to bring rural patients into more urban locations for treatment. This concept may work when rural is defined using the concept of exclusion where urban or metropolitan is defined through population and population density, and rural becomes "everything else." This empirical division based on numbers alone creates a simplistic solution to the rural health disparity problem—just bring those with health needs into the urban health settings when needed. Williams and Cutchin[5] suggest that defining rural only through descriptive categories such as land use (occupation/economic activity), demographic structure (towns, villages, hamlets), nonmetropolitan, environmental characteristics (open countryside), population density, population characteristics (degree of homogeneity), and commuting patterns ignores the sociocultural characteristics (communication patterns, types of human relationships, degree of mobility and change, and the foundation institutions such as the church) and the understanding of the lived experience of the residents. They suggest that rural can best be understood by combining the descriptive categories with the sociocultural characteristics and lived experience. Defining the concept of rural in this holistic manner is congruent with the beliefs of many health professionals. It also suggests that those health professionals serving the residents of rural areas need a different knowledge set and that the place of treatment is important. An urban health setting may not be appropriate. The complexity associated with this type of description of rural highlights how difficult it is for a single professional group to adequately serve the health needs of rural populations.

Because rural areas are inherently linked to the land, an understanding of environmental justice may assist health professionals. Environments include the physical (natural and artificial), social, political–economic, temporal, and cultural. These environments influence health in a variety of ways. For example, in the political economic environment, income frequently defines the type of health care available. Land ownership, a type of financial asset, is a contributer to wealth. Conley[9] argues that land ownership serves as a buffer when difficulties, such as increased economic obligations due to medical expenses, occur. Land ownership has culturally specific meaning. African-Americans living in the south may relate land ownership to control over their lives. Moving from a history of slavery, working someone else's land, to land ownership meant economic benefits and self determination—both contributors to quality of life. Health professionals who understand the role of the environments to health are better prepared to provide holistic services that go beyond "fixing the person."

If rural health practice is complex and practitioners need to understand the unique nature of rural practice and environmental justice issues and work toward social justice, what alternatives exist for changing rural health disparities? Williams and Cutchin[5] suggest interprofessional practice, whereas the National Advisory Committee on Interdisciplinary, Community-Based Linkages[10] suggest a better infrastructure and collaboration among government and private sector agencies who address health issues. Interprofessional collaboration is an active relationship where two or more health or social care professionals work together to solve complex problems or provide services that are related to a specific recipient of care. The service user is placed in the center of the team and contributes to the decisions of the team. Team members collaborate, and roles and functions may overlap. The overlap is negotiated and the desired outcome is to provide the best care possible.

How can health professionals address rural health disparities and implement the concepts of social justice, environmental justice, and a belief in the contextual nature of rural living? The interprofessional work being done in Tillery, North Carolina provides an example.

INTERPROFESSIONAL RURAL HEALTH RESEARCH AND HEALTH SERVICES FRAMED IN JUSTICE: PUTTING THE BIG WORDS INTO ACTION

Tillery, North Carolina has a long history of engagement in issues related to justice. Incorporated in 1889, Tillery was the location of three of the largest slave-holding plantations in North Carolina, the Johnson Plantation, the Tillery Plantation, and the Devereux Plantation. After emancipation, Black sharecroppers and White landowners lived together in Tillery. Reports from descendents of the Black sharecroppers indicate that regardless of their legal status as freedman, their lifestyles did not change. Because of the nature of sharecropping, they remained tied to the land through debt or as subsistence day laborers. In 1934 a third group arrived in Tillery as the result of the New Deal Resettlement program.[11] Approximately 300 families participated in what was known as "40 acres and a mule." Roosevelt's New Deal plan was intended to address "the care of needy persons in rural areas [whose] problem[s are] quite distinct and apart from that of the industrial unemployed. Their security must be identified with agriculture."[12] What opportunities did the New Deal bring to residents of this African-American resettlement community?

> For 100s of African American families, Tillery was a place of hopes and dreams, and possibilities. A beginning for some and a new start for others. Families came from nearby North Carolina towns like Tarboro, Rocky Mount, Enfield, Northampton County and as far away as Virginia, Georgia and Florida. They came by mule and wagon. They came on beat up pick up trucks, the cab filled with small children and the rest of their precious cargo hanging off the sides. To have a new house that no one else had lived in before—a room for the boys and a room for the girls and nobody would come in the cold of the night to threaten us and make us move one more time.[11]

According to Gary Grant, Executive Director of the Concerned Citizens of Tillery, the addition of the resettlement farmers created a triangle of three communities. The White landowning community retained their suspicions about Black residents. The Black community was divided between the share-cropping community and the new landowning Black residents. Many in the sharecropping community were in debt to the White landowners and distrustful of the Black families associated with the resettlement project. Recently, Tillery experienced a fourth group of residents, those who are "goin' home." These new members of the community are individuals who left Tillery to find a job, then returned upon retirement or those who had never lived there but found Tillery a good place to live in retirement.

Since 1996 faculty and students from East Carolina University have been part of interprofessional teams who travel to Tillery to provide services.[13] Although the composition of the teams has varied, over time occupational and physical therapy, nursing, medicine, therapeutic recreation, social work, and exercise science, among others, have participated. The nature of the interprofessional engagement has varied. At times, the university participants met with each other only on the university campus to share ideas and plan for programs. At other times, in addition to the campus meetings, interprofessional teams traveled together to Tillery and met with Tillery residents to collaborate on health issues. Health providers and university researchers who work in Tillery must learn its rich history and an appreciation for the influence of history on its residents. This is the first step in addressing the health issues of its citizens.

These history lessons vary, but one of the most effective strategies has used active learning. In interprofessional groups, students create a three-dimensional model of a community in response to the question, "What do you expect to see when you go to the community of Tillery?" Typical constructions include paved roads, schools, grocery stores, gas stations, churches, parks, movie theaters, and restaurants. The students talk about their constructions and about what community means to them. Next, the students and faculty go to Tillery to meet with Tillery residents in the community center. The residents provide the historical context and talk about customs such as the naming of Black residents who were slaves. Finally, the group tours the area and discovers that Tillery is a cross roads community with few of the buildings they had placed in their models. They see the industrial hog operations, the lack of paved roads, and the high water table. After the tour, the group returns to the community center to compare their observations with their model. This set of active learning experiences provides an understanding of the concept "rural" and of the role of the environments in shaping health. The community helps the university participants understand both social and environmental justice and injustice.

Since the time of the resettlement in the early 1900s, the population has grown to about 3,000 residents, with 98% African-Americans. Within Tillery, 75% of the population is over 65 and 90% are below the federal poverty level. But, even through their struggles, Tillery has a strong sense of community and spirituality. At the geographic center of Tillery lies the community center, a hub of community functions and activities. From Concerned Citizens of Tillery meetings to the Open Minded Seniors' lunches to the Nubian Youth, Tillery has different groups that raise concerns and issues within the community. The "Curin' House," which was originally a potato-curing house, adjoins the community center and has been transformed into a health clinic that offers medical care, therapy, and nutrition education. Current residents speak proudly of their continuing efforts to challenge the system through legislative actions, efforts for health care reform, and solicitation of funding and collaborative relationships with nearby universities.

Like many communities composed of elders, women make up a large proportion of Tillery residents. They are at risk for health impairments such as hypertension, stroke, diabetes, and breast cancer. Residents who experience these health conditions frequently deal with long commutes to see physicians, have difficulty paying for prescription and over-the-counter medicine, and have difficulty accessing rehabilitation services because of lack of availability. Through collaboration between the interprofessional teams, the Tillery People's Health Clinic located in the Curin' House and the Area Wide Health Committee (AWHC) provide services that include health screenings, wellness programs, exercise programs, occupational therapy services, and case management. Recently, an interprofessional team composed of the AWHC director, social work faculty and students, and occupational therapy faculty and students collaborated using the lifestyle performance model.[14] The interprofessional team discussed concepts of lifestyle and occupational justice and agreed that occupations are the way people participate in daily life and are an indicator of health, the foundation for making us human, and that everyone has the right to do activities that are satisfying to self and significant others.

Because of the historical context of Tillery, the team chose to work on environmental issues that impeded residents' health and occupational lifestyles. Solutions included the provision of adapted equipment, home repairs, Medicare and Medicaid educational sessions, home safety assessments, falls prevention programs, and educational programs. Through negotiation among the team members, the professionals involved determined the role of social worker, occupational therapist, and health coordinator. This negotiation included knowledge of the political environment, especially the practice acts for each profession.

My work in Tillery is part of my role as university educator and researcher. Together with my students and colleague, Dr. Peggy Wittman, I have modeled how to integrate health service provision with health research. As a White, female researcher I was acutely aware that too often scientists value removing context and complexity from their studies. They frequently work alone. They believe that objectivity is attained by isolating the scientist from the historical context. Because of these beliefs they fail to attain any attachment to the communities and populations they study.[15]

Values and assumptions shape the way knowledge is acquired[16] and can contribute to injustices when applied to health research. Too often, health research is focused on ways to fix the person, a perception somewhat imbedded in the U.S. value of individualism. Rural communities, like Tillery, survive because of collectivism. The ability of the community to unite and collectively address issues counteracts the geographical distances between people. Because of the community beliefs and values regarding justice, my research has been framed in the critical emancipatory paradigm. Clifford[17] suggests that ethnographic research is a negotiated understanding between researchers where power is explicitly considered in the process. In my case, I was a university researcher who brought some skill in methodology and an interest in understanding the culture of Tillery, including the culture related to health. The other researchers were the community members whose expertise was about their culture. I quickly learned that in Tillery research questions were mutually determined, methodologies negotiated, and research products shared. The outcomes of research had to be more than the making of knowledge, they had to be used to make a difference in residents' lives.

As part of the research process, I had to get the community's permission to engage in research. I had to gain their trust. These processes occurred over time and involved many trips to Tillery, alone, with students, and with university colleagues. Each time I came with questions, not demands. I described my skills and how the community could use them. The harder piece for me as both a researcher and health service provider is figuring out when it is time to leave. While I have been in Tillery, I have seen the community tell other university researchers and providers to leave. The community did this when the university began to dictate research and service—to act paternalistic and authoritarian. I have seen university researchers and service providers leave when the grant money went away. I asked the community, "How I will know when it is time to go?" They indicated that it is time to go when I see the community putting the researcher's needs above their own, when the researcher fails to acknowledge the equal participation of the community, or when the community is able to do its own research and provide its own health services.

With students, colleagues, and community members we have studied community quality of life,[18] the meaning of wellness,[19] the meaning of falls, Tillery as a transformative educational experience,[20] interdisciplinary rural practice,[13] and the meaning of cultural immersion on cultural competence.[21]

CONCLUSIONS

We summarize the value of engagement in rural communities as follows:

An understanding of discrimination, institutional racism and the cultural values of communities engaged in the struggle for human rights and self-determination helps students and faculty understand their own society and prepares them to work in diverse communities in partnership with social change organizations. This promotes the ending of environmental degradation of the poor and people of color, decreases Black land loss, promotes economic development and self-sufficiency, and supports development of occupational lifestyles congruent with the culture.

REFERENCES

1. Andrews GR. Demographic and health issues in rural aging: a global perspective. *J Rural Health*. 2001;17:323–327.
2. Jensen GM, Royeen CB. Improved rural access to care: dimensions of best practice. *J Interprofess Care*. 2002;16:117–128.
3. Lee C. Environmental justice: building a unified vision of health and the environment. *Environ Health Perspect*. 2002;110:141–143.
4. Rogers CC. The older population in 21st century rural America. *Rural America*. 2002;17:2–10.
5. Williams AM, Cutchin MP. The rural context of health care provision. *J Interprofess Care*. 2002;16:107–115.
6. Millsteed J. The contributions of occupational therapy to the fabric of Australian rural and remote communities. *Austral Occup Ther J*. 1997;44:95–106.
7. Peterson C, Ramm K, Ruzicka H. Occupational therapists in rural healthcare: a "jack of all trades." *Occup Ther Healthcare*. 2003;17:55–62.
8. Morris LV, Palmer HT. Rural and urban differences in employment and vacancies in ten allied health professions. *J Allied Health*. 1994;23:143–153.
9. Conley D. *Being Black: Living in the Red*. Berkeley: University of California Press; 1999.
10. National Advisory Committee on Interdisciplinary, Community-Based Linkages. (2001). First annual report to the Secretary, U.S. Department of Health and Human Services, Health Resources and Services Administration. Washington, DC Bureau of Health Professions.
11. Concerned Citizens of Tillery. *Remembering Tillery . . . A New Deal Resettlement*. Tillery, NC: Author; 1996.
12. Foreman C. What hope for the rural Negro? *J Negro Life*. 1934;12:105.
13. Wittman P, Conner-Kerr T, Templeton MS, Velde B. The Tillery project: an experience in an interdisciplinary, rural health care service setting. *Phys Occup Ther Geriatr*. 1999;17:17–28.
14, Velde BP, Fidler GS. *Lifestyle Performance: A Model for Engaging the Power of Occupation*. Thorofare, NJ: Slack; 2002.
15. Wing S. Environmental justice, science, and public health. In National Institute of Environmental Health (Ed.). *Essays on the Future of Environmental Health Research*. Farmington Hills, MI: Gale Group, 2005.
16. Creswell J. *Qualitative Inquiry and Research Design: Choosing Among Five Traditions*, 2nd ed. Thousand Oaks, CA: Sage Publications; 2007.
17. Clifford J. *The Predicament of Culture: Twentieth Century Literature, Ethnography, and Art*. Cambridge, MA: Harvard University Press; 1988.

18. Velde BP, Wittman PP, Lee H, Lee C, Broadhurst E, Caines M. Quality of life of older African American women in rural North Carolina. *J Women Aging.* 2003;15:69–82.
19. Barnard S, Dunn S, Reddic E, et al. Wellness in Tillery: a community-built program. *Fam Commun Health.* 2004;27:151–157.
20. Velde BP, Wittman PP, Mott V. Hands on learning in Tillery. *J Transform Educ.* 2007;5:79–92.
21. Velde BP, Wittman PP. Helping occupational therapy students and faculty develop cultural competence. *Occup Ther Healthcare.* 2001;13:23–32.

SECTION 3

Practice Context

CHAPTER 13

Building a Health Care Workforce That Reflects the People We Serve

Terry K. Crowe, PhD, OT, FAOTA
Patricia Burtner, PhD, OT, FAOTA
Theresa A. Torres, OT

INTRODUCTION

It is well documented that the United States is becoming more culturally diverse.[1] To meet this increasing cultural diversity, we need a health care workforce that looks similar to the people they serve. This chapter covers the current and growing diversity in the U.S. population; the disparities in health care; the limited cultural diversity in health care students, faculty, and providers; strategies for increasing diversity in the health care professions; and an introduction to an occupational therapy educational model that focuses on creating a more diverse workforce.

According to the U.S. 2000 Census,[1] 281.4 million people resided in the United States, with 12.5% of the population identified as Hispanic/Latino (Cuban, Mexican, Puerto Rican, South or Central American, or other Spanish culture or origin regardless of race) and the other 87.5% of the population as non-Hispanic/Latino. The U.S. 2000 Census also stated that 12.3% of the population was Black or African-American; 3.6% was Asian, 0.9% was Native American or Alaska Native, and 0.1% was Native Hawaiian or Other Pacific Islander. In addition, 2.4% (or 6,826,228 respondents) of the people indicated identification with two or more of the five race categories, whereas 410,285 respondents identified with three or more of the five race categories.[1] This most recent census highlights the varied cultural diversity of people living in the United States. The U.S. population is expected to be even more diverse when the next census is taken in 2010.

Disparities in Health Care, Health Providers, and Health Professional Education

Research indicates significant inequalities and disparities in health and health care. For example, the Institute of Medicine reports that individuals who are African-American, Hispanic, or Native American often receive inadequate health care and have morbidity and mortality outcomes that reflect this discrepancy.[2] Health care disparities are consistent and extensive across a multiple range of medical conditions, and health care services are unquestionably associated with worse health outcomes.

With the number of African-American, Hispanic, and Native American population steadily increasing in the United States,[1] the disparities and inequalities in health care will only continue to rise unless there is a conscious effort to significantly change the way health care is delivered and received. Fiscella and colleagues[3] examined the literature and found that people with lower socioeconomic status across racial/ethnic groups have lower overall health care use, even among those with health insurance. Similarly, being a member of a minority group appears to be a risk factor for less intensive, if not lower quality, care. There are complex reasons related to how socioeconomic and race/ethnicity factors influence health care. These factors include health care affordability, less preventive care, geographical access, transportation, education, literacy, health beliefs, racial concordance between physician and patient, consumer attitudes and preferences, and competing life demands including work and child care and provider bias.[3,4] Key indicators of child well-being, including percentage of low-birthweight infants, infant mortality, child death rate, teen death rate, teen birth rate, and percentage of children living in poverty, are poorer for non-Hispanic White groups except for the Asian/Pacific Islander group.[5] For example, infant mortality is 14 per 1,000 births for African-Americans and 5.7 for non-Hispanic Whites. Some statistics are even climbing, raising questions about the impact of cuts of welfare and Medicaid, access to health care, and many physicians stating the growing epidemics of obesity, diabetes, and hypertension creating higher infant mortality.[6]

An added concern is that the U.S. health care team, including physicians, occupational therapists, physical therapists, speech and language pathologists, audiologists, and nurses, are predominantly non-Hispanic White.[7–11] Limited cultural diversity in the workforce may translate into less effective health care, particularly to racial minority consumers. For example, can a White, middle-class, occupational therapist truly comprehend the daily struggles of a Hispanic woman who is a single parent without health insurance? Can a physician who has not interacted with Native American people be sensitive to traditional healing choices of a Native American man? Or what can a Hispanic nurse do when a White, elderly person rejects her advice because her English is spoken with an accent?

Currently, there is a lack of cultural diversity in enrollment in health care professional programs (Table 13-1).[7,8,12,13] For example, in 2005, nationally only 1,043 medical school graduates were African-American, 936 were Hispanic, and only 96 were Native American.[14] This becomes even more challenging as some health professions (e.g., physical therapy, occupational therapy) move to the graduate level when in the past entry level was at the undergraduate level.

There is also a concern that the faculty members who teach future health care providers are limited in cultural diversity.[14,15] Statistics for faculty in occupational therapy, physical therapy, nursing, speech language pathology, and audiology programs could not be found. In medical school and pharmacy educational programs, there is low representation of non-White teachers. Professors who teach medical students are 71.9% White, 12.6% Asian, 4% Hispanic, 3.1 African-American, 1.2% multiple race, and less than 1% Native American/Alaska Native.[14] Professors in pharmacy schools are 74.8% White, 11.8% Asian, 5.6% African-American, 3.2% Hispanic, and less than 1% Native American/Alaska Native.[15]

Table 13-1. Ethnic Diversity of Students in Four Health Care Professions

Health Care Discipline	Students (%)				
	White	African-American	Native American/ Alaska Native	Asian	Hispanic
Medical[7]	62.1	6.5	0.3	18.6	7.0
Occupational therapy[8]	79.5	6.9	0.5	5.2	5.6
Physical therapy[12]	82.1	4.4	0.5	5.8	4.1
Pharmacy[13]	47.2	9.0	0.45	16.0	3.2

Table 13-2. Ethnic/Gender Diversity in Healthcare Providers in Six Healthcare Professions

Health Care Discipline	Male	Female	White	African-American	Native American/ Alaska Native	Asian	Hispanic
					Providers (%)		
Physicians[7]	Not provided	Not provided	36.7	3.3	0.3	5.7	2.8
Occupational therapists[8]	4.3	95.7	86.2	1.7	0.1	5.0	1.6
Physical therapists[9]	34.5	65.5	88.8	1.9	0.5	4.9	2.4
Nurses[10]	5.4	94.6	87	4.9	0.5	3.7	2
Speech/language pathologists[11,*]	4.4	95.6	93	0.02	0.004	0.01	0.03
Audiologists[11,†]	18.4	81.6	93	0.02	0.004	0.02	0.02

*42% did not report race/ethnicity.
†44% did not report race/ethnicity.

Besides a lack of diversity in health care faculty and students, the current workforce is predominantly White (Table 13-2).[7–11] Many of these statistics on providers are pulled from professional associations. Thus statistics often represent only those professionals who are members of the professional associations. We obviously have a major diversity gap in the U.S. health care and higher education systems. This must change if we want to have a health care system that is culturally, socially, and linguistically diverse to better meet the people they serve.

STRATEGIES FOR CREATING A MORE CULTURALLY DIVERSE HEALTH CARE WORKFORCE

New Mexico is a culturally diverse state with poverty levels well above the national average.[5] In 2004, 56% of the children lived in low-income families (compared with 40% nationally). New Mexico, a state with close to 2 million people, was 43.4% Hispanic, 43.1% non-Hispanic White, 10.2% Native American Indian, 2.4% African-American, and 1.3% Asian in 2005.[16] Another descriptor of New Mexico is that it is a predominantly rural state with 35% of residents residing in urban settings and 65% residing in rural areas.[17]

At the University of New Mexico (UNM), the occupational therapy program has made educating a diverse workforce a priority since the program was founded in 1993. We are proud of the numbers of culturally and linguistically diverse undergraduate and graduate students we have educated over the past 13 years who have become practicing professionals. On average, 39% of our graduate students represent minorities, with a range from 25% to 55% across six classes. All of our students have graduated to become occupational therapists, and we have a 100% pass rate on the national certification examination with only a handful of students taking the exam an additional time. We have consciously made several major curriculum adjustments to support all our students, including those who are culturally and linguistically diverse. We have focused on recruitment, retention, graduation, and professional certification with our goal to provide occupational therapists who are competent, ethical, culturally sensitive, and compassionate to practice in the state of New Mexico.[18]

We have graduated eight Native American and 22 Hispanic occupational therapy graduate students in the past six classes (28% of total) (Figure 13-1). Often, these students come from traditional, rural Native American communities in which their life experiences have been very different from other students. Carrie Gashytewa was born and raised in Zuni Pueblo, a community

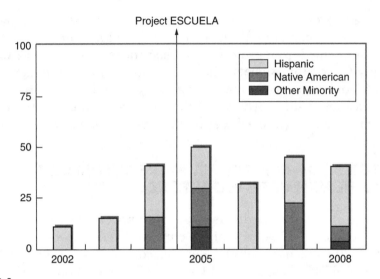

Figure 13-1
Percentage of students recruited for underrepresented cultures. Other = Pacific Islander, Eastern Indian, and those with physical disabilities.

of close to 8,000 (U.S. Census, 2000) people in northwestern New Mexico. As a child she recalls attending religious dances often at night, living closely to family, and being supported by numerous relatives, first speaking her Native language before English, preparing bread in traditional outdoor ovens, and learning the traditional expectations for a Zuni woman. Glennita Haskey grew up on Navajo Nation, the youngest of seven children who was raised by her single mother who is a weaver. She remembers being responsible for much of the household chores while her mother wove rugs, sharing a bedroom with her mother and nieces, and making her own rugs to pay for school clothes and supplies. Matt Sanchez, a Hispanic man, grew up on a ranch homesteaded by his grandparents near a small New Mexican town. He recalls doing ranch chores before and after school, living in a community where residents supported each other and watched over other's children, and having a large extended family.

Glennita Haskey states elegantly why it is critical to educate health care providers who are culturally similar to the people they serve. She was asked why she plans to return to the Navajo Nation to practice as an occupational therapist:

First and foremost, I have a land and a ranch on the reservation. It is a place that I wish to raise my children at and a place that will allow me to practice and

live my Navajo way of life. It is my home where I will not only show my chil-
dren what it means to be Navajo, but also to actually live the ways of life so that
traditional teachings that my mother taught me will be carried on to my chil-
dren. It is a place that I can speak my language, share my knowledge, live my
culture, and to have the opportunity to serve my native people as an occupa-
tional therapist. I would like to take both the Navajo culture and the Western
teachings into my practice and parallel the two so that those who need my ser-
vices will receive the best of both worlds. I will have a better understanding of
the Navajo peoples' environments, families, background, and everyday situa-
tions. I will help individuals and their families to self discover, redesign or de-
velop their priorities despite challenges so that they can have successful lives,
strong self-esteems, and positive outcomes.

INCREASING DIVERSITY BEGINS WITH RECRUITMENT

To create a more diverse workforce, professional programs need to first put resources into recruiting diverse student populations in entry-level professional programs. One strategy that has been helpful at the UNM occupational therapy program is taking a very individualized and consistent approach to recruitment. We have assigned a faculty member and a staff member to communicate with interested students. Although we do occasional group orientations, we make sure that students' questions are individually addressed. In addition, we integrate our enrolled occupational therapy students in public relation activities that draw attention to our profession while recruiting future students. What better way to recruit students than having them hear details from a current professional student? Potential students are invited to sit in on a class or a problem-based learning session. We have also developed an OT Ambassador Program where we link current students, including students with diverse backgrounds, with interested students to talk informally about the program.

McWhirter and colleagues[19] describe a collaborative program between an historically African-American college and a nurse practitioner graduate program that actively recruits and assists African-American students in the application process to be successful. This includes workshops in taking the Graduate Record Examinations, having an ongoing faculty liaison available, and helping students develop their career goal statements on their applications. In Canada, a nursing program has been developed to enhance success for Native Canadian and other nursing students from disenfranchised groups.[20] This program starts with outreach efforts in communities and schools with large populations of Native Canadians and immigrants.

The UNM Medical School received legislative funding to recruit and support medical students from their freshman year until graduation from medical school.[21] Although this program is focused on preparing students to be physicians, during their undergraduate years some students may decide to pursue other health care professions. Besides coursework in the sciences and liberal arts that provide a strong foundation for practicing medicine, students focus on content related to the medical needs of New Mexicans, including six integrated health seminars, and participate in community health projects in rural and medically underserved communities. With obtainment of an undergraduate degree, students are guaranteed entry into the UNM Medical School.

ADJUSTING THE CURRICULUM TO STUDENT LIFESTYLES

Once students from under-represented cultures are enrolled in a professional program, whether an undergraduate, masters, or doctoral program, they may find the intense educational program demanding. For example, our full-time occupational therapy graduate program requires 15 to 17 graduate credits each semester. Like all professional programs, we have many courses that require applied work such as community practice, lab classes necessitating extra hours, and significant outside preparation requirements. We often have students with complex lives (i.e., significant family responsibilities, single parents, living in communities requiring a significant commute, or with significant cultural expectations) or different learning styles that may require pursuing our program part time. However, we recognize that even our part-time option is considered a full-time graduate load at our institution.

Since 2000, 11 graduate students (10%) have opted to pursue the part-time track. Marie Shije, a woman with two children from the small community (less than 700 residents) of Zia Pueblo located 45 minutes from the university, chose this pathway. This option has enabled her to balance her multiple roles as mother, part-time caregiver to her brother who has a disability, student, active tribal community member, and family member. She has been able to successfully graduate but also retains her traditional roots, which include participation in frequent community events such as traditional dances and ceremonies. Although the faculty initially was anxious about creating a part-time option, this has not required a significant amount of extra work. The main responsibility is considering part-time students' class needs related to course time scheduling, tracking students' progress, and informing faculty about class size.

In another flexible approach, McWhirter and colleagues[19] encourage nursing students to take one of the more intensive courses before they actually enroll in the graduate program. This allows students to adjust gradually to the rigors of graduate education and develop technology competencies.

INTEGRATING CULTURAL EXPERIENCES INTO CURRICULA

As all states are becoming more and more diverse socially, culturally, and linguistically, it is important for all professional health care programs to develop applied learning experiences with diverse populations for *all* students. In the New Mexico Occupational Therapy Graduate Program we do this in many ways throughout the curriculum. For example, we build our problem-based learning cases to include the diverse populations represented in New Mexico. We have one paper case, entitled "Baby Ben," that weaves a story of a young boy referred to an interdisciplinary team for assessment and intervention recommendations. He resides on the Navajo Nation and traditional beliefs of the cause of Ben's developmental concerns are revealed by the father during the evaluation. In small groups, the students discuss the differences between Western and traditional Navajo medicine, how the two approaches can be combined for the best outcome for a child with a disability, and what information about cultural rituals and practices the students need to know as practitioners serving this population (including how to access this information).

Another learning opportunity we integrate is for a local expert (Dr. Eliseo Torres) to share with the students his knowledge about traditional Mexican healing practices.[22] Dr. Torres discusses views of health, wellness, and illness from a traditional Mexican perspective and shares some of the details of the practices of traditional healers. For those who wish to explore this area deeper, we offer an interdisciplinary summer course focusing on traditional Mexican medicine in Oaxaca, Mexico each year. Another activity we integrate into our curriculum is a field trip to Jemez Pueblo to observe the traditional feast day. Although many students have grown up in New Mexico, they have not visited one of New Mexico's pueblo communities. We observe the traditional dances and share a meal with a Native American family. Many professional programs strategically build cultural sensitivity and responsiveness and information about health disparities into their curriculums.[23–25]

IDENTIFYING CONFLICTS IN TRADITIONAL CURRICULUM CONTENT WITH CULTURAL BELIEFS

There may be parts of a professional curriculum that contradict or significantly impact cultural beliefs. One activity may be dissecting a human body as part of an anatomy course. Our anatomy course was sequenced the first summer of the professional program. After graduation, one Native American student from a traditional pueblo community shared with us the trauma of taking this course attributed to touching a dead body, which is in conflict with her traditional values. As a new student in the program, she was uncomfortable discussing this subject when she took the course. Curriculums may need to offer alternative ways of learning, such as allowing students to learn anatomy from anatomical models or through online information. This should be openly offered so courses like anatomy do not become a barrier for success. There may be other components of health care curriculums that may culturally impact student learning.

RESPECTING CULTURAL RESPONSIBILITIES AND RITUALS

Often, students have additional expectations and responsibilities that relate to their families and/or cultural communities. Native American students sometimes need to participate in traditional ceremonies. Marie Shije from Zia Pueblo often is involved in dances that occur at least 15 days a year, burials of community members, and community events that sometimes occur with little notice. These events involve elaborate preparation such as cooking special foods. Other students might be expected by family members to remain active with their families even though they are living miles away. Glennita Haskey was not only responsible for her elderly mother's care but at the beginning of her education she and her husband were caring for livestock on the Navajo Nation in Arizona. When floods overwhelmed his family ranch one year, Matthew Sanchez had to return to his home during the semester. For several days he helped his family save cattle, repair fences, and try to prevent further flood damage.

Professional programs need to create an educational environment that supports and is responsive to cultural and community requirements. We need to sensitively open up dialogues with entering and current students about cultural needs and supports. For example, most curriculums are sensitive to Jewish holidays and request faculty to allow students to miss classes that fall on these days. Why not recognize some special days that are important to other cultures?

INCORPORATING FACULTY MENTORSHIP FOR ADDITIONAL EDUCATIONAL SUPPORT

Mentorship is strongly supported in the literature to assist diverse health professional students. McWhirter and colleagues[19] state that "successful mentoring of students often requires a faculty member to go the extra mile to find the instructional strategies by which students with varying backgrounds can achieve academic success" (p. 138). Mentorship includes helping the student with decision making, providing feedback and support, and assisting to keep the student focused.[24]

Amaro et al.[26] introduced the concept of "bridging" teachers. These individuals value cultural diversity and respect cultural differences and integrate this attitude into their daily teaching. Students interviewed described these instructors as mentors who were patient and who made themselves available, open to questions, and provided encouragement.

PROJECT ESCUELA: A PERSONNEL PREPARATION MODEL TO INCREASE DIVERSITY AT UNM

With the call for Personnel Preparation Grant proposals to the U.S. Department of Education Office of Special Education Programs under the Minority of Higher Education competition, UNM Occupational Therapy Graduate Program was awarded a 4-year grant (2004–2008). Project ESCUELA is named for the Spanish word for "school." The letters within the word represent the major content threads of this project—*E*ducating *S*tudents for *C*ultural *U*nderstanding, *E*vidence-Based Practice, *L*eadership and *A*dvocacy.

Project ESCUELA addresses both (a) a specific gap of qualified culturally and linguistically diverse occupational therapy students to work with children of minority groups who are eligible for special education services and (b) the overall shortage of qualified, culturally educated occupational therapists as related services special education personnel available to work with children of cultural groups native to New Mexico in underserved areas. To decrease the shortage of professionally prepared individuals who are culturally and linguistically diverse or who have disabilities, Project ESCUELA is a collaborative project between UNM Occupational Therapy Graduate Program and the Albuquerque Public Schools (APS), one of the largest school systems in the United States. The project is designed specifically to recruit, prepare, and support 25 individuals from underrepresented cultures native to New Mexico (Hispanic, Native American). Over the initial years of the grant, more diversity was noted in the students recruited, as shown in Figure 13-1.

By providing specialized instruction in the school setting as well as individualized mentorship, occupational therapy graduate students are mentored as related service personnel for children receiving special education services throughout the state, including rural school districts. With the addition of newly developed content embedded in the curriculum, specialized instruction is also provided to *all* occupational therapy students enrolled in the occupational therapy graduate program. Students funded by Project ESCUELA begin their specialized mentorship by participating in two semesters of individualized independent study experiences with master therapists in the APS. Each week for 5 hours over the two 16-week semesters, the student works in a school setting planning and administering assessments and intervention to schoolchildren who qualify for occupational therapy services under the Individuals with Disabilities Education Act. As the semesters progress, students not only develop their skills as therapists but also as members of interdisciplinary teams working directly with families. Next, the funded students are placed in early intervention or school districts in rural New Mexico settings for their 3-month fieldwork placement. During these months, the students are full time with an experienced school-based occupational therapist, with intense mentorship in assessment, intervention, and collaboration with families and educational teams.

INCREASED RECRUITMENT OF STUDENTS FROM NEW MEXICO NATIVE CULTURES

Within the UNM structure, several academic support programs were in place to support students from Native American and Hispanic cultures. Although communication about Project ESCUELA was initiated with these programs, the most effective recruitment strategy for students from different cultures was unquestionably personal contact.

The following quote of a student recruited from the Zuni Pueblo reinforces the importance of personal contact when recruiting students from native cultures:

Initially it was very challenging because I was unaware of where to start, being the first family member to attend graduate school. However, acceptance into the UNM Ronald E. McNair Scholars Program opened doors for me. This program prepares first-generation college students for graduate school, entailing application writing, GRE prep, workshops on how to survive in graduate school, and research experience. It was during this time that I met an OT Faculty member, who was my research mentor and a true blessing. With this individual's guidance I was accepted into 5 OT programs in the nation. If it weren't for the

Ronald E. McNair staff and this OT faculty member's patience and big heart to help me, I would have definitely had a harder time with the whole graduate school process.

Carrie Gashytewa MOT, OT, Zuni Pueblo

EVALUATING GRADUATES' IMPACT ON OUTCOMES IN CHILDREN WITH DISABILITIES

Graduates of the UNM occupational therapy program had consistently entered jobs that serve children with disabilities in school districts serving high poverty areas in the state. All graduates had found employment upon completion of the program, approximately 80% to 90% of them within the state of New Mexico depending on the class. Of these graduates, 62% were employed in school districts or education-related settings such as early intervention programs (Figure 13-2).

With the high percentage of graduates seeking employment in educational settings before Project ESCUELA, percentage changes increased only slightly. Changes in rural employment were more noticeable with an increase from 12% in the 1990s to 25% of students returning to or seeking rural employment in 2000 (Figure 13-2).

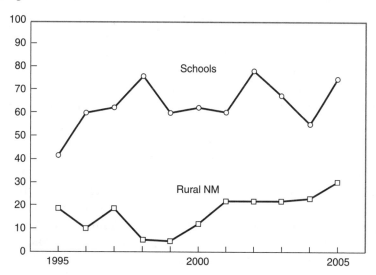

Figure 13-2

Employment of graduates in pediatric (schools and early intervention programs) and rural settings. Schools = school districts and early intervention settings.

HOW DOES FINANCIAL SUPPORT ASSIST INDIVIDUAL STUDENTS?

Bernal and Aragon[27] present critical factors affecting educational success of underrepresented groups. The combination of social, academic, and financial support was emphasized; that is, these multiple barriers need to be addressed rather than providing only financial support. Financial support built into Project ESCUELA includes tuition costs and other direct and indirect costs such as books, photocopy cards, and lab fees. The Project also provides financial assistance to attend state and national conferences for participation and enculturation into the profession. The following quote of an occupational therapy graduate student from the Navajo Nation best describes how financial aid assists students from underrepresented cultural groups:

> *Once you were enrolled in the Occupational Therapy Program, what things supported you to reach your goal?*
>
> *Definitely the UNM financial aid office and funding through Project ESCUELA. Because both my husband and I decided to attend school, our family went from having a paycheck every two weeks to absolutely nothing. The financial aid office certainly helped me find grants and loans to ensure that my housing and child care was covered.*
>
> *Secondly, living at the university's student family housing complex assisted me in graduate school. At the beginning of each semester, the housing office takes a large sum of my financial aid to pay for my rent throughout the semester so I don't have to deal with worry about my housing arrangement throughout the course of the semester. Although I don't receive any disbursement from financial aid because of this arrangement, it is more important to me that my family have a stable living environment. So knowing that my family has a place to call home while attending school helps me to concentrate and focus on studying and to do well in all my classes.*
>
> *Finally, being honest about my situation at home and my personal priorities with the faculty and my advisor was an essential step. The faculty was able to understand my "imbalance" and provided me the guidance I needed. Their counseling and recommendations were not so much directed as "here are answers to your problems or situations" but to help me "to see and find a way out" so that I could explore my options and solve my situations. One example is to transfer from the full-time status to going part time. In this way, I was able to balance my roles as a mother, caregiver, spouse, student, and family member.*

Overall, I think that the continuous reminder from the faculty, advisor, and financial aid staff that I am making progress and that I will be a successful person helps me to keep the picture of what my world will be like when I finish the program refreshed and in my mind. I believe that I am here today because I am moving toward the final phase of my graduate study by concentrating on one day at a time, which leads to one semester at a time, and soon I will be finished.

Glennita Haskey, MOTS, Navajo Nation

CONCLUSIONS

Health care professionals come into contact with people with culturally, socially, and linguistic diverse backgrounds. Preparing health care providers for the future must include locating, encouraging, and supporting capable people from diverse backgrounds and cultures. Multiple strategies to address recruitment, retention, graduation, and certification issues must be used to create a more socially, linguistically, and culturally diverse workforce across health professions. In addition, professional educational schools must provide all students with the opportunity to learn about cultural diversity. We must expect all health care providers to adapt their assessments and interventions to respect the cultural beliefs and practices of the people they serve. Because addressing racial inequalities in health care is a complicated and multifaceted issue, we are not suggesting that by simply increasing the diversity in health care professions this critical problem will be solved. However, health disparities have raised the necessity of creating a health care workforce that is more culturally, socially, and linguistically diverse. Creating a workforce that is responsive to diversity will impact where health professionals deliver health care services, how people participate in the intervention process, and ultimately the health and wellness of all people. Addressing the issue of educating diverse health care providers will ultimately assist to create a health care system that is fairer for all, hopefully helping to eliminate the current significant disparities that exist in health and health care.

REFERENCES

1. Grieco EM, Cassidy RC. Overview of Race and Hispanic Origin: Census 2000 Brief. Washington, DC: U.S. Department of Commerce; 2001.
2. Smedley BD, Stith AY, Nelson AR, eds. *Unequal Treatment: Confronting Racial and Ethnic Disparities in Healthcare.* Washington, DC: National Academies Press; 2002.

3. Fiscella K, Franks P, Gold MR, Clancy CM. Inequality in quality: addressing socioeconomic, racial, and ethnic disparities in healthcare. *JAMA*. 2000;283: 2579–2584.

4. Sampselle CM. Nickel-and-dimed in America: underserved, understudied and underestimated. *Fam Commun Health*. 2007;30 (Suppl 15):S4–S14.

5. Annie E. Casey Foundation. *2006 Kids Count Data Book*. Baltimore, MD: Annie E. Casey Foundation; 2006.

6. Eckhom E. In turnabout, infant deaths climb in south: race disparity persists. *New York Times*, April 22, 2007.

7. Association of American Medical Colleges. *Minorities in Medical Education: Facts and Figures 2005*. Washington, DC; 2005.

8. American Occupational Therapy Association. *2006 Occupational Therapy Workforce Compensation Report*. Bethesda, MD; 2006.

9. American Physical Therapy Association. Race/Ethnic Origin of Members page. Available at: http://www.apta.org/AM/Template.cfm?Section=Demographics &TEMPLATE=/CM/ContentDisplay.cfm&CONTENTID=26307 October 2005. Accessed February 2, 2007.

10. MinoritiyNurse.com. Minority Nursing Statistics page. Available at: http://www.minoritynurse.com/statistics.html March 2000. Accessed May 2, 2007.

11. American Speech-Language-Hearing Association. Summary Membership and Affiliation Counts page. Available at: http://www.asha.org/about/Membership-Certification/member-counts.htm December 2006. Accessed April 2, 2007.

12. Hayward LM, Canali A, Hill A. Case report interdisciplinary peer mentoring: a model for developing culturally competent health care professionals. *J Phys Ther Educ* 2005;19:28–40.

13. American Association of Colleges of Pharmacy. PharmCAS Applications for 2006 Entering Class page. Available at: http://www.aacp.org/site/page.asp?VID =1&CID=614&DID=4397&TrackID September 2006. Accessed February 2, 2007.

14. Association of American Medical Colleges. *Diversity in the Physician Workforce: Facts and Figures 2006*. Washington, DC; 2006.

15. American Association of Colleges of Pharmacy. *Institutional Research Report Series*. Alexandria, VA; 2006.

16. U.S. Census Bureau. State and county quickfacts. http://quickfacts.census.gov/qfd/states/35000.html. Accessed May 10, 2007.

17. U.S. Census Bureau. http://www.census.gov. Accessed February 2, 2007.

18. University of New Mexico Occupational Therapy Graduate Program mission. http://hsc.unm.edu/som/ot/about/mission.shtml. Accessed April 22, 2007.

19. McWhirter G, Courage M, Yearwood-Dixon A. Diversity in graduate nursing education: an experience in collaboration. *J Prof Nurs*. 2003;19:134–141.

20. Labun E. The Red River College model: enhancing success for native Canadian and other nursing students from disenfranchised groups. *J Transcult Nurs*. 2002;13: 311–317.

21. University of New Mexico School of Medicine. Combined BA/MD Degree Program page. Available at: http://hsc.unm.edu/som/combinedbamd. Accessed April 12, 2007.

22. Torres E, Sawyer T. *Curandero: A Life in Mexican Folk Healing.* Albuquerque, NM: UNM Press; 2005.

23. McNeal GJ, Walker D. Enhancing success in advanced practice nursing: a grant-funded project. *J Cultural Divers.* 2006;13:10–19.

24. Thacker K. Academic-community partnerships: opening the doors to a nursing career. *J Transcult Nurs.* 2005;16:57–63.

25. Ford K, Waring L, Boggis T. Living on the edge: the hidden voices of health disparities. *OT Pract.* 2007;17–22.

26. Amaro DJ, Abriam-Yago K, Yoder M. Perceived barriers for ethnically diverse students in nursing programs. *J Nurs Educ.* 2006;45:247–254.

27. Bernal C, Aragon L. Critical factors affecting the success of paraprofessionals in the first two years of career ladder projects in Colorado. *Remed Spec Educ.* 2004;25:205–213.

CHAPTER 14

The AHEC Advantage: Campus–Community Partnerships for Rural Health Education

Robin Ann Harvan, EdD

INTRODUCTION

Area Health Education Centers (AHECs) are campus–community partnerships that train health care providers in sites and programs that are responsive to state and local health and health care delivery needs. As illustrated in Figure 14-1, the only states that currently do not have federally funded AHEC programs or AHEC regional centers are Iowa, Kansas, Michigan, North Dakota, South Dakota, and the Commonwealth of Puerto Rico.

The U.S. Congress created the national AHEC program in 1972. The AHEC program is part of the U.S. Department of Health and Human Services, Health Resources and Services Administration (HRSA), Bureau of Health Professions (BHPr). The mission of the HRSA BHPr is to improve the health status of the population by providing national leadership in the development, distribution, and retention of a diverse, culturally competent health workforce that provides the highest quality care for all.[1] This mission provides direction toward a vision for a nation in which universal access and utilization of quality health care are provided, health workforce shortages are eliminated, health disparities are overcome, prevention is emphasized, and health outcomes are optimal for all.

In 2007, a total of 49 AHEC programs and 211 affiliated AHEC regional centers are ongoing in 45 states and the District of Columbia.[2] As illustrated in Figure 14-2, this network of campus–community partnerships provides multidisciplinary and interdisciplinary educational services to students,

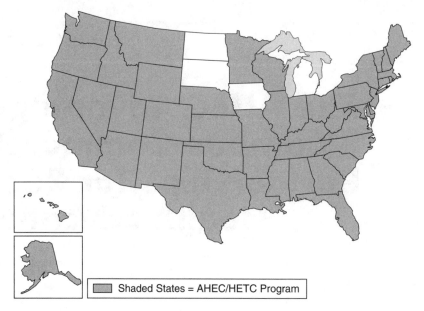

Figure 14-1
States with AHEC programs. (From National AHEC Organization.)

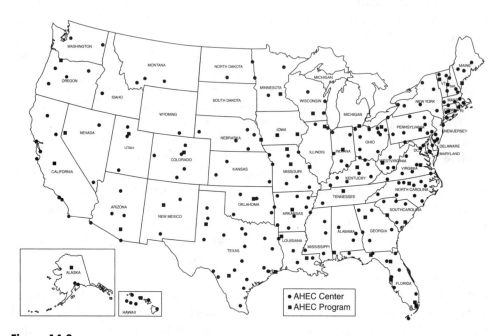

Figure 14-2
Locations of AHEC program offices and AHEC community-based centers. (From National AHEC Organization.)

faculty, and local practitioners, ultimately improving health care delivery in rural and medically underserved areas.[2]

The funding model for the national AHEC program illustrates a federal, state, and local partnership. Legislatively, the U.S. Congress authorizes and allocates federal funding for the national AHEC program. The cooperative agreement between the HRSA BHPr, as the federal agency, and the academic health center receiving funding is that a state and local match of funding be allocated. Figure 14-3 illustrates this funding model.

Nationally, the impact of the AHECs is quite significant. In a typical year, AHECs:

- "Train 32,000 health professions students (17,000 medical students and 15,000 other health professions students) in community-based sites
- Work with approximately 600 federally funded community and migrant health centers, 600 health departments, and 200 National Health Service Corps sites

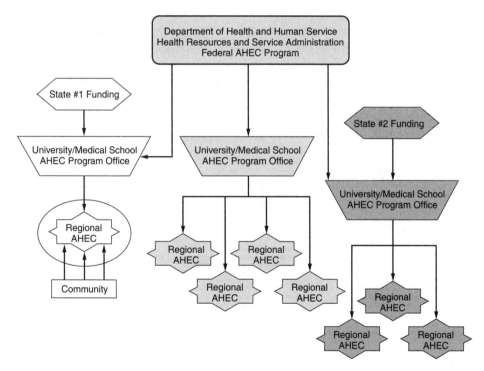

Figure 14-3
AHEC federal–state–local partnership funding model. (From National AHEC Organization.)

- Provide health career enhancement and recruitment activities of 20 hours or more to 25,000 students, grades 9 through 12
- Train 6,000 teachers and counselors in health careers
- Provide continuing education to 330,000 local health care providers."[3]

CAMPUS–COMMUNITY PARTNERSHIPS

The national AHEC program represents a unique network of campus–community partnerships. For each of the 49 AHEC programs nationally, the majority of the AHEC program offices are administratively and programmatically integrated within academic health centers. As illustrated in Figure 14-4, as higher education institutions, academic health centers typically include health professions schools and programs. The AHEC regional centers are community-based partners who have local relationships with community-based academic affiliates, to include the hospitals, community health canters, dental clinics, local pharmacy, and other clinical sites where health professions students practice, learn, and develop their clinical competence. As local community partners, regional AHECs often work with their local public health departments, and they typically have relationships with other organization and agencies affiliated with public health, community health education, and health care delivery. Regional AHECs also typically work with local public schools regarding health education and help promote health careers awareness and development to ensure an adequate future health care workforce. To assist in the recruitment and retention of health care practitioners, particularly in rural and urban medically underserved

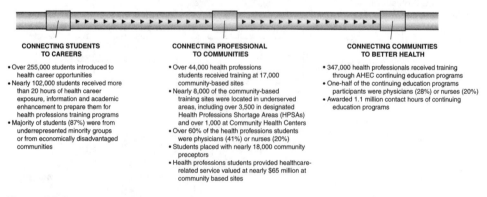

CONNECTING STUDENTS TO CAREERS	CONNECTING PROFESSIONAL TO COMMUNITIES	CONNECTING COMMUNITIES TO BETTER HEALTH
• Over 255,000 students introduced to health career opportunities • Nearly 102,000 students received more than 20 hours of health career exposure, information and academic enhancement to prepare them for health professions training programs • Majority of students (87%) were from underrepresented minority groups or from economically disadvantaged communities	• Over 44,000 health professions students received training at 17,000 community-based sites • Nearly 8,000 of the community-based training sites were located in underserved areas, including over 3,500 in designated Health Professions Shortage Areas (HPSAs) and over 1,000 at Community Health Centers • Over 60% of the health professions students were physicians (41%) or nurses (20%) • Students placed with nearly 18,000 community preceptors • Health professions students provided healthcare-related service valued at nearly $65 million at community based sites	• 347,000 health professionals received training through AHEC continuing education programs • One-half of the continuing education programs participants were physicians (28%) or nurses (20%) • Awarded 1.1 million contact hours of continuing education programs

Figure 14-4
A statewide campus–community partnership for community-based health professions education.

areas, regional AHECs provide local support and continuing professional education opportunities.

The benefits of organizational integration of the AHEC program in academic health centers are as follows:

- AHEC program directors positioned near the top of the organizational hierarchy can translate their greater organizational power into more staff, larger budgets, more in-kind contributions, greater access to information, and more sway in institutional decision making.[4]
- Administrative and programmatic integration raises the profile of the AHEC program within the academic health center and creates opportunities for leveraging activities across related initiatives.[4]
- Organizational integration dampens the potential for turf battles to erupt and decreased the likelihood that related programs will work at cross-purposes.[4]

Campus partnerships with communities are structured whereby the majority of the 211 affiliated community-based AHEC regional centers are separate, legal corporations with 501(c)(3) tax-exempt statuses. Each regional AHEC is an independent, nonprofit organization with its own local board of directors, staff, and advisory committee. The local board of directors for each regional AHEC office consists of members of the communities served by the center and includes both health service providers and consumers. Each regional board of directors determines the AHEC's activities with input from advisory committees, consistent with the needs of its area and its contractual obligations to academic health center. The regional boards are essential to the establishment of partnerships with community-based organizations throughout the state.

The benefits of academic partnerships with community-based nonprofit organizations are as follows:

- Separate, legal status of the local community regional AHECs enhances their perceived independence and credibility in local communities,[4] which in turn increases the instrumental value of the academic health centers as a vehicle for advancing community-based health professions education and other community engagement and service goals.
- Independent status allows the community-based AHECs to seek additional funding from a variety of sources to meet the local needs of local communities.
- The local AHEC board members, who live and work in the communities served by the regional AHEC, can serve as valuable conduits of

information for academic health center leaders regarding local community health needs.[4]

Together, the AHEC program offices and regional community AHECs partner with a wide variety of agencies and organizations. Common partners for statewide AHEC programs include state offices of rural health, state and local health departments, and state health professions societies and organizations. Common clinical and educational partners include local hospitals, physician offices, community health centers, rural health centers, migrant health centers, dental clinics, pharmacies, mental health centers, elementary and secondary schools, community colleges, and local universities. As "interorganizations," regional AHECs serve as vehicles for interorganizational collaborations.[4]

"The AHEC program is a long-term initiative, requiring major changes both in the traditional method of training medical and other health professions students and in the relationship between university health science centers and community health service delivery systems."[5] Since inception, AHECs and community health centers (CHCs) have worked in partnership. Primarily, AHECs have used the CHCs as clinical training sites.[6] The value of services provided by these primary care trainees is estimated to be over $68 million and include primary care residents, medical students, dental and pharmacy students, physician assistant and advanced practice nursing students, and social work students.[6] CHCs have used AHECs for recruiting and retaining health professionals, providing continuing professional education and development, and for technical assistance.

The "scope of collaborative activities between AHECs and CHCs is substantial, and the populations served through these activities are culturally and geographically diverse."[6] The interrelationships between AHECs and CHCs are numerous, and although the outcomes of such contributions may not be well documented, the value added to the community from the unique contributions of each is undeniable in terms of access to quality health care.[6]

AHEC EXPERIENCES IN RURAL AMERICA

Since the inception of the AHEC program in 1972, the mission and core functions have been strategically directed toward enhancing the health workforce pipeline in rural and medically underserved communities. The overall mission of the national AHEC program is to improve the supply, distribution, diversity, and quality of the health workforce, ultimately increasing access to health care in rural and medically underserved areas.

According to the Institute of Medicine (IOM) Committee on the Future of Rural Health Care, the model for achieving greater numbers of rural clinicians is often conceptualized in terms of a pipeline, with each of the following points along the pipeline playing an essential part in achieving the ultimate goal of increasing the size of the rural workforce and its capacity to provide high-quality health care:

1. "Enhanced preparation of rural elementary and high school students to pursue health careers"[7]
2. "Stronger commitment of health professions programs to recruiting students from rural areas, educating and training students in rural areas, and adopting rural-appropriate curricula"[7]
3. "Stronger incentives for health professionals to seek and retain employment in rural areas"[7]

Given the overall mission of the national AHEC program to improve the supply, distribution, diversity, and quality of the health workforce, Figure 14-5 illustrates the three ways AHEC programs work to improve health care

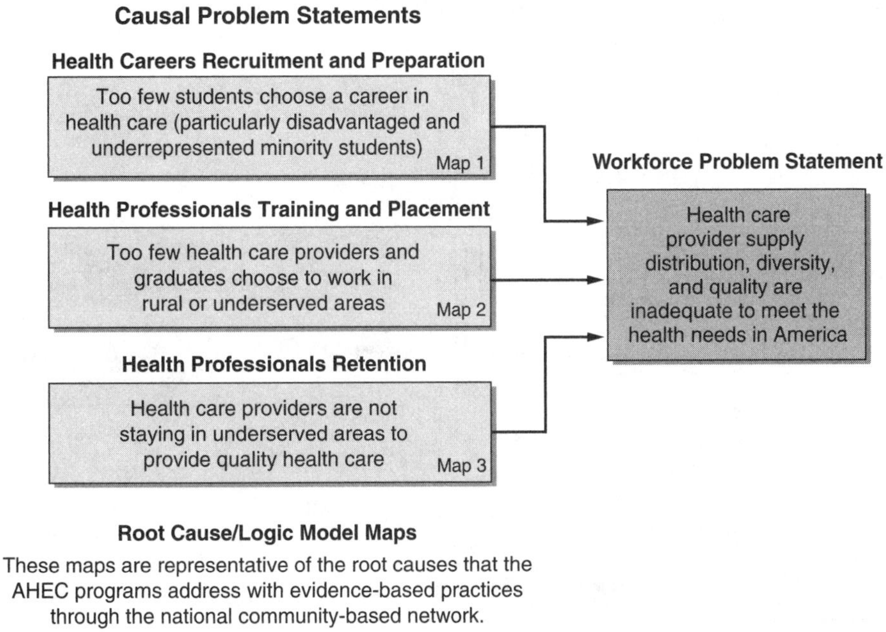

Causal Problem Statements

Health Careers Recruitment and Preparation

Too few students choose a career in health care (particularly disadvantaged and underrepresented minority students)   Map 1

Workforce Problem Statement

Health Professionals Training and Placement

Too few health care providers and graduates choose to work in rural or underserved areas   Map 2

Health care provider supply distribution, diversity, and quality are inadequate to meet the health needs in America

Health Professionals Retention

Health care providers are not staying in underserved areas to provide quality health care   Map 3

Root Cause/Logic Model Maps

These maps are representative of the root causes that the AHEC programs address with evidence-based practices through the national community-based network.

Figure 14-5
Three ways AHECs improve health care workforce resources. (From National AHEC Organization.)

workforce resources. Although the areas of focus and emphasis differ from state to state, AHECs generally perform the following three functions:

1. Health careers recruitment and preparation
2. Health professionals training and placement
3. Health professionals retention

In these three functions, AHECs are (a) connecting students to careers, (b) connecting professionals to communities, and (c) connecting communities to better health.

The following section briefly describes the roles and functions of AHECs in these three areas of focus to improve health care workforce resources.

HEALTH CAREERS RECRUITMENT AND PREPARATION

Figure 14-6 illustrates a map that represents the root cause for this health care workforce problem that the AHEC programs address with evidenced-based practices through the national community-based network.

To address this problem and related causes, AHECs work to connect students from kindergarten through high school to careers in health care.

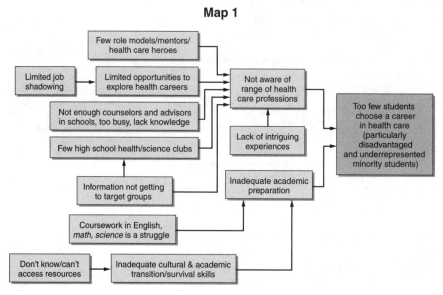

Figure 14-6
Root cause map for health careers recruitment and retention. (From National AHEC Organization.)

"AHECs are committed to expanding the health care workforce, including maximizing diversity and facilitating distribution, especially in underserved communities."[8] To achieve this goal, "AHECs offer the creative, hands-on Summer Health Careers Institute, mathematics and science enrichment programs, and healthy lifestyles programs for elementary, middle school, and high school students. These programs introduce students to a wide assortment of health careers possibilities, guide them in goal setting and educational planning, and offer science courses that strengthen crucial thinking skills. Working with schools, colleges, and community partners, AHECs target students from rural areas, economically disadvantaged students, and those from underrepresented minority groups in school programs and summer institutes."[8]

HEALTH PROFESSIONALS TRAINING AND PLACEMENT

Figure 14-7 illustrates a map that represents the root cause for this health care workforce problem that the AHEC programs address with evidenced-based practices through the national community-based network.

To address these issues, AHECs work to connect health professions students to medically underserved communities. "AHECs, together with health professions schools, departments, and programs, provide community placements,

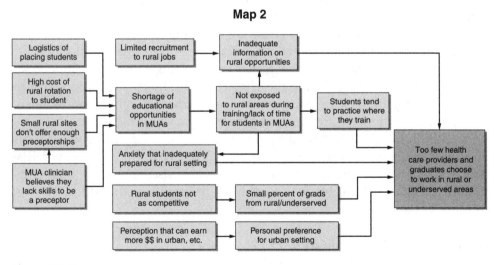

Figure 14-7
Root cause map for health professionals training and placement. MUA = medically underserved area.
(From National AHEC Organization.)

service-learning opportunities, and clinical experiences for medical, dental, physician assistant, nursing, pharmacy, and allied health students in rural and urban underserved communities. AHEC placements give students the opportunity to experience health care in a real-world setting far removed from their health science centers. They get to interact one-on-one with their future patient population in community health centers, county health departments, homeless clinics, local practitioner's offices, and other community primary care sites. Students learn firsthand about economic and cultural barriers to care and the specific needs of underserved and ethnically diverse populations."[8] In 2007, the National AHEC Organization estimated that the added value of services provided by AHEC trainees at the training sites was estimated to be over $64 million dollars:

- $39 million by the primary care residents
- $9.5 million by medical students
- $7 million by dental and pharmacy residents
- $5 million by other health professional students
- $3 million by advanced practice nursing students

AHECs, with their "linkages to local community resources and organizations, are uniquely qualified to facilitate these community placements."[9] Often, students from different health professions disciplines are placed in the same community, at the same clinical site, at the same time, and, sometimes, even sharing the same housing. These are the optimal circumstances that facilitate social and clinical interactions among health professions students.

AHECs use two principal strategies for supporting interprofessional education and training: broadening the physician base by establishing and supporting other primary care practitioners programs (i.e., physician assistant and nurse practitioner students) and developing and promoting training opportunities for team-based models of care delivery.[11] Through both of these efforts, AHECs seek to increase access by improving the supply and distribution of primary care health professions while also improving quality by preparing the health professions workforce to work together effectively on interprofessional teams.[11]

HEALTH PROFESSIONALS RETENTION

Figure 14-8 represents the root cause for this health care workforce problem that the AHEC programs address with evidenced-based practices through the national community-based network.

Map 3

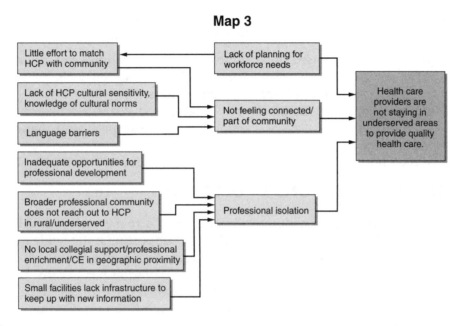

Little effort to match HCP with community

Lack of planning for workforce needs

Lack of HCP cultural sensitivity, knowledge of cultural norms

Language barriers

Not feeling connected/ part of community

Inadequate opportunities for professional development

Broader professional community does not reach out to HCP in rural/underserved

Professional isolation

No local collegial support/professional enrichment/CE in geographic proximity

Small facilities lack infrastructure to keep up with new information

Health care providers are not staying in underserved areas to provide quality health care.

Figure 14-8
Root cause map for health professions placement and retention. CE = continuing education; HCP = health care providers. (From National AHEC Organization.)

To address this health care workforce problem, "AHECs provide accredited, high-quality continuing education offerings and professional support for meeting the needs of health professionals, especially those practicing in rural and medically underserved areas. These programs are designed to enhance clinical skills and help maintain professional certifications. Programs also focus on recruitment, placement, and retention activities to address community and state health care workforce needs."[8] Many of these educational programs are offered to multiprofessional groups of local health practitioners that facilitate interprofessional communication and collaborative health care.

COMMUNITY HEALTH EDUCATION AND DEVELOPMENT

As an expanded component of the overall mission related to the health care workforce, AHECs are also committed to connecting communities to better health. AHECs evaluate and address the health needs of communities within and among the regions and provide innovative, collaborative, and multi-professional responses to those needs. AHECs provide community health education programs on timely topics to promote health literacy, healthy lifestyles, and behaviors and to prevent illness and disease. AHECs facilitate community development through three principal strategies:

1. As a community-based organization, AHECs sometimes serve as fiscal agents for grants and contracts or provide grant writing technical assistance to local community-based organizations.
2. AHECs form, join, and promote broad-based coalitions to improve community health status and strengthen collective problem-solving capacity at the local level.
3. AHECs host, join, and contribute to economic development projects.[10]

AHEC COLLABORATIONS IN COLORADO

The following section provides an illustration of a role a statewide AHEC program can play as a collaborative partner in supporting a statewide initiative to address health care workforce shortages. As a high growth industry, the health care field is projected to increase for Colorado's health care system where the number of available health professionals is not expected to be sufficient to meet the growing need. According to the Colorado Occupational Employment Outlook, significant increases in demand for health professionals are highly likely throughout the state due to an increasing and aging population and a maldistribution of health care providers.[11] Some counties have few or no physicians, dentists, or mental health providers to serve their residents—especially the uninsured and underinsured and those with language or transportation barriers—even in areas where health care providers are available. Of 64 Colorado counties, 51 are designated as health professional shortage areas, 45 are designated as medically underserved areas, and 47 are designated as rural or frontier.

"The Colorado Trust's Health Professions Initiative, a 3-year (2005–2008), $10.2 million effort, provided funding to increase the number of health professionals in Colorado in all disciplines, including primary, mental, and dental health care, as well as pharmacy. Further, the initiative aimed to stimulate partnerships among health professions education schools and programs, community-based organizations, and health professionals to strengthen a community-based clinical training infrastructure and meet the long-term need for health professionals across the state. The Trust made grants to 21 organizations across Colorado—including hospitals, clinics, universities, colleges, and community health care foundations—to support and expand existing programs and to develop new programs that increase education, training, and advancement opportunities, especially for individuals from disadvantaged backgrounds and in rural areas. The grantees received training and technical assistance from the Colorado AHEC system (program office and regional centers) and participated in networking opportunities to share strategies and identify opportunities for collaboration. In addition, the Trust awarded funds to the Colorado Rural Health Center to support a variety of rural health career programs."[12] An independent evaluation of the initiative was conducted by the Center for Research Strategies "to help the Trust understand the impact of the collective work of the grantees as well as to inform the health professions education field."[12]

"An examination of grantee activities and lessons from the wider health professions education field provided a sense of the complex infrastructure required to recruit, train, and place an adequate number of health professionals. Collectively, the 22 grantees demonstrated that increasing the community-based clinical training capacity in Colorado requires multiple strategies as well as cooperation with stakeholders that traditionally have not been part of health professions training. Grantees provided examples of promising strategies aimed at strengthening three components of the health professions community-based clinical training infrastructure: health professions students, health professions education programs, and community partners engaged to train, recruit, and retain health professions students."[12]

These components of the health professions community-based clinical training infrastructure "are interconnected, and any intervention aimed at one component alone is insufficient to create a long-term solution to health professional shortages. Because communities are beginning to recognize this interdependence, communities that are experiencing shortages are proactively stimulating the training cycle by promoting health care career awareness programs among local residents, subsidizing students who have an interest in health careers, offering locally based training and clinical rotation experiences, and developing active recruitment and retention programs for health professionals."[12]

The framework illustrated in Figure 14-9 shows the three components of the health professions community-based clinical training infrastructure and six broad strategies derived from the lessons learned in this initiative.[12] These strategies show promise for strengthening the components of the health professions community-based clinical training infrastructure.

The grantees' work illustrates the importance of early health career exposure and student assistance programs that enable diverse students from underserved urban and rural areas to pursue health careers. Local community-based faculty development and support, expanded clinical training sites,

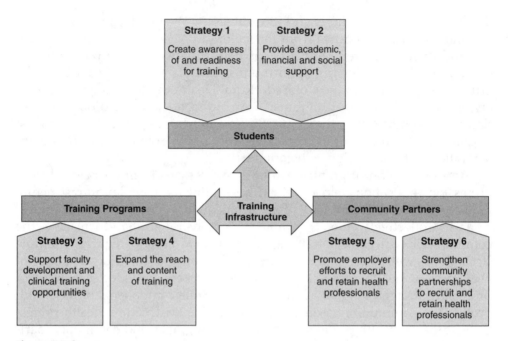

Figure 14-9
Strategies for strengthening the health professions training infrastructure. (From The Colorado Trust:
Solving Colorado's Health Professions Shortage, 2007.)

distance learning with advanced curricula, and clinical training opportunities are strategies that help to ensure that optimal education is accessible and available in rural and medically underserved areas.

Several grantees used creative program approaches that address more than one strategy and, in some cases, more than one infrastructure component. For example, training programs are addressing student needs through flexible program formatting, while simultaneously working with community partners to create clinical rotation experiences. Community partners are financing "grow-your-own" programs to stimulate interest in health careers among local students as well as hosting distance learning sites for health professions education schools.

Overall, the evaluation of the Colorado Trust's Health Professions Initiative shows that a key strategy for addressing health care workforce shortages is the development of an infrastructure that can support enough students at all stages in the health care workforce training pipeline. Figure 14-10 illustrates both the *supply* and *demand* sides of health care workforce development pipeline.

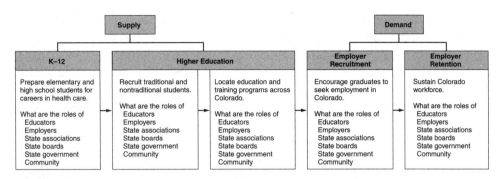

Figure 14-10
Health care workforce development pipeline.

To strengthen the supply of health professionals, students from kindergarten through secondary school need to participate in health careers exposure and awareness programs, and higher education needs to recruit, retain, and train diverse health professions students, with part of their clinical training located in medically underserved sites. Partnerships are imperative and AHECs know this imperative well.

Close partnerships between health professions education schools and programs and community partners are imperative to:

- Support local students and health professionals serving as clinical preceptors and instructors
- Provide community-based clinical sites and learning experiences
- Offer leadership in the recruitment and retention of health professionals

Given health care workforce shortages, demand for health professionals can be improved with community engagement and employer involvement in the recruitment and retention of health professionals.

LEADERSHIP TO LEVERAGE THE BENEFITS

The IOM Committee on the Future of Rural Health Care offered several guiding principles for reforming rural health care applicable to the role of the national AHEC program:

- "Rural communities should focus greater attention on improving population health in addition to meeting personal health care needs. . . . . Collaborative efforts are needed at the community level to create environments that minimize the likelihood of illness or disease (for example, through immunization campaigns) and to provide incentives for residents to pursue healthy lifestyles (for example, encouraging regular exercise)."[7]

- "A core set of health care services (primary care, dental care, basic mental health, and emergency medical services) should be available within rural communities."[7]
- "When care cannot be delivered locally, links should be established to services in other locales."[7]
- "The spectrum of services available in rural communities should be based on the population health needs of the local community."[7]
- "The provision of rural health care services should be shaped and guided by local community and rural organizations and institutions. . . . Solutions to rural health care issues should be shaped by the structured input of rural residents. . . . Health literacy must be fostered in ways that acknowledge the culture of the rural population."[7]
- "Rural health care requires a team of well-trained health care clinicians, managers, and leaders working together. These teams must provide continuous services, maintain adequate coverage, and establish and foster seamless linkages with other elements of the health care system both locally and at a distance." Educational institutions have "the responsibility to select, train, and support health professionals for rural practice."[7]

In redesigned health systems, rural teams must have effective methods of providing supervision, expert consultation, and emergency backup to offer patients seamless care regardless of the setting or team member engaged with the patient at any given time. All team members must have strong communication skills and a clear understanding of each other's roles and responsibilities. In rural settings, it is not uncommon for health care workers to know each other and to have worked together for years, a situation intensified by the markedly smaller number of clinicians and managers involved. Yet competency in team care requires much more than familiarity. It involves learning approaches to maximize collaborative work; ensuring that timely information reaches those who need it; and managing patient transitions across settings and over time, even when team members are in different physical locations.[7] (pp. 83–84)

Clearly, collaboration is key to quality reform in rural health care. With the focus on building partnerships between education and community-based practice by building coalitions and campus/community partnerships, AHECs are in an excellent position to offer a national educational network focused on solutions for these challenges.

AHEC collaborations exist with a variety of academic institutions, including academic health centers, public and private colleges/universities, community colleges, and public school systems. Collaborations also exist with a variety of public health and health care organizations and institutions, including hospitals, community health centers, and public health departments. AHECs focus across the health care workforce development pipeline and the continuum of health professions education, including health career awareness and recruitment. They support student and resident community-based clinical training, including multidisciplinary and interdisciplinary training. AHECs provide local practitioner support and continuing education to reduce professional isolation, increase retention, and enhance the practice environment. They promote improved health and increased disease prevention that is responsive to local community needs. AHECs also have developed technical assistance expertise that could prove extremely valuable in achieving systemwide educational reform.[13]

Legislative reauthorization and adequate federal funding appropriations are critical for sustaining and strengthening the national AHEC network. The National AHEC Organization provides the following justifications:

1. "Many geographical areas, communities, and populations lack adequate access to high-quality preventive, primary, and specialty health care, a lack that contributes to significant health disparities that impair America's public health and economic productivity.

2. These health disparities have many causes, including shortages and inadequate distribution of culturally and linguistically competent health care providers at all levels. These workforce issues most acutely affect community-based health care safety-net providers, including but not limited to CHCs, Native American health centers, rural health clinics, critical access hospitals, public health departments, and their patients.

3. Developing and maintaining a health care workforce of optimum size, distribution, quality, and effectiveness requires community-based assessments and solutions, designed and implemented in partnership with a broad range of academic institutions and programs.

4. AHECs provide a national network of community-based and governed entities that, in partnership with community resources and academic centers, provide an infrastructure effectively serving as the workforce development arm of America's health care safety net.

5. The community-based AHEC network has demonstrated flexibility and capacity to respond to changing national, regional, and local health care workforce needs and priorities."[6]

CONCLUSIONS

Strong leadership is called for to sustain and leverage the benefits of the national AHEC program. This national network of campus–community partnerships is strong but needs the strength of leadership to maximize the advantages and opportunities for addressing health workforce shortages, for improving access to quality health care services, and for eliminating health disparities in rural and underserved communities.

REFERENCES

1. U.S. Department of Health and Human Services. *Health Resources and Services Administration.* Available at http://www.hrsa.gov/about/default.htm. Accessed September 17, 2008.
2. Coe D. *My Health Career.* Northern Arizona Area Health Education Center. Available at http://www.myhealthcareer.net/nahec/. Accessed September 17, 2008.
3. Bureau of Health Professions. *Area Health Education Centers.* Available at: http://bhpr.hrsa.gov/ahec/. Accessed February 14, 2008.
4. Weiner BJ, Ricketts TC, Fraher EP, Hanny D, Coccodrilli LD. Area health education centers strengths, challenges, and implications for academic health science center leaders. *Health Care Manag Rev.* 2005;30:194–202.
5. The Rhode Island Area Health Education Center Program (AHEC). Mission Statement. Available at *http://biomed.brown.edu/ahec/.* Accessed September 17, 2008.
6. National Area Health Education Centers Organization. *Area Health Education Center and Community Health Center Collaboration: Effective Partnerships for the Recruitment of Health Professionals.* Kansas City, MO: National Rural Health Association; 2006.
7. Institute of Medicine. Committee on the Future of Rural Health Care. *Quality Through Collaboration: The Future of Rural Health Care.* Washington, DC: National Academy of Sciences; 2005.
8. Colorado Area Health Education Center. *Health Careers and Workforce Diversity.* The University of Colorado Denver. Available at http://www2.uchsc.edu/ahec/ healthCareers.asp?cat=healthCareers. Accessed September 17, 2008.
9. National Area Health Education Centers Organization. *Training Health Professions Students.* Wexford, PA: National AHEC Organization.
10. Cecil G. Sheps Center for Health Services Research. *An Evaluative Study of the Area Health Education Centers Program.* Final Report to the Area Health Education Centers Branch, Division of State, Community and Public Health, Bureau of Health Professions, Health Services and Resources Administration; 2002.
11. Henry S. *Expanded Role for AHECs: Providing Technical Assistance for a Health Professions Workforce Initiative.* The National AHEC Bulletin, 23(2), Spring/Summer 2007.
12. Gallagher K, Beer T. *Solving Colorado's Health Professionals Shortage: Initial Lessons Learned from the Health Professions Initiative Evaluation.* The Colorado Trust; 2007.
13. Harvan, RA. *The Role of AHECs and HETCs in Bridging the Gap to Quality in Health Professions Education.* The National AHEC Bulletin, 21(1) Autumn/Winter 2004.

Professionalization and the Ethic of Care: From Silos to Interprofessional Moral Community

Laura Lee (Dolly) Swisher, PT, MDiv, PhD

INTRODUCTION

Within the last two decades there has been increasing interest in interprofessional education.[1–3] Supporters of interprofessional education note that traditional educational experiences produce health care practitioners who practice in professional "silos," lacking the knowledge and ability to collaborate with other professionals. The silo is often used as a metaphor for noncollaborative education because the structure of the silo is characterized by high walls without connection to other structures or organizations. Moreover, the silo has few doors or areas of access. Although the silo may continue to be filled higher and higher with good quality materials, neither the silo nor its contents have any interaction with the surrounding environment. In spite of this interest in interprofessional education, there remain many barriers to true interprofessional education.[1,2] Two important barriers to interprofessional education are resistance from faculty and students and issues of perceived status and power between professions.[1,2] As Irvine et al.[1] describe it, "Interprofessional relationships continue to be characterized by conflict rather than co-operation and are frequently distorted by mutual suspicion, hostility and disparities between the way that a particular profession views itself and how it is viewed by other occupations" (p. 199). Little attention has been given to the manner in which the dominant underlying Western ethic of justice may reinforce the barriers to interprofessional education and collaboration, nor to the possibilities that the ethics of care may offer to overcome these barriers.

This chapter uses the underlying ethics of care and justice to analyze forces that may contribute to a culture of interprofessional conflict versus cooperation and suggests educational strategies to address these forces. The argument is developed that the goal of interprofessional ethics education should be the creation of an interprofessional moral community, and accomplishment of this goal requires insights from the ethics of care.

The chapter begins by contrasting the ethics of justice and the ethics of care. In contrast to early care literature, which may have viewed justice and care as contradictory viewpoints (justice vs. care),[4] this analysis follows the thinking of more recent feminist ethicists (such as Virginia Held[5]) in suggesting that these two ethical perspectives are complementary lenses with which to view moral life. Each lens brings important issues and information into view, and it is therefore important to use each lens in considering ethical issues rather than focusing on one lens or the other. After this description, we provide a delineation of the sociological process of professionalization. The two ethical lenses are used to analyze the process of professionalization, producing insights from the perspectives of justice and care regarding barriers and resources for educating for interprofessional collaboration rather than competition. The importance of the notion of mutual autonomy within the ethics of care has particular significance for interprofessional education in overcoming the barrier of competitive market-based understandings of professional autonomy. The chapter concludes with a discussion of the possibilities of the ethic of care as a foundation building an interprofessional moral community and associated educational strategies to accomplish this goal.

JUSTICE AND CARE

Carol Gilligan[4] is generally credited with the ground-breaking insights that became the basis for the ethic of care. Working as a research assistant for Lawrence Kohlberg,[6] Gilligan observed that Kohlberg's moral developmental framework may not have captured the experience of females. Gilligan was critical of the emphasis of Kohlberg's theory on abstract universal rules of conduct and impartial moral judgments that appeared to Gilligan to ignore contextual judgments and relationships. Her work gave rise to the development of what has come to be known as the ethics of care. In contrast to the dominant Western ethical tradition that emphasizes rational decision making, abstract universal principles, and impartial judgments, the ethic of care emphasizes relationships, emotion, narrative-contextual detail, and "particular" judgments within relationships.[5] Benner[7] describes the ethic of care succinctly: "A care ethic is relational and focuses on meeting the other with respect, characterized by recognition, support for growth or self-acceptance, and/or allowing the other 'to be'" (p. 48). Although the earliest formulations of the ethic of care portrayed this ethic as contradictory and antithetical to the ethic of justice, more recent literature has viewed these as more complementary. As Held[5] and others note, however, it is not the case that the two perspectives can serve as simple addenda to the other because they represent separate ethical paradigms, and it is therefore important to use both perspectives.[8,9] In this chapter, we view these as separate lenses for analysis to attend to both perspectives. Table 15-1 provides a comparison of features of the two perspectives.

Table 15-1. Comparison of the Ethics of Care and the Ethics of Justice

	Ethic of Justice	*Ethic of Care*
Focus	Consistent application of principles governing fairness, quality, and rights for the individual	Cultivation of attentiveness, responsiveness, trust, and caring relationships
Ethics and moral understanding	Abstract, universal rules achieve impartiality successful in balancing competing individual interests	Responding to particular others through interrelatedness and responsiveness
Human nature	Independent, self-sufficient rational individuals who act out of self-interest	Relational and interdependent beings who seek well-being cooperatively
Autonomy	Autonomy as rational control and self-sufficiency	Shared understanding, mutual empowerment, and cooperation in pursuit of community
Values	Impartiality, justice, fair distribution	Trust, solidarity, mutual concern empathy
Moral practices	Protection of individual rights, impartial judgments, fair punishment, equal treatment	Cultivation of relationships, responding to needs, demonstration of sensitivity, moral discourse to understand the perspective of others

(Continues)

Table 15-1. Comparison of the Ethics of Care and the Ethics of Justice *(Continued)*

	Ethic of Justice	Ethic of Care
Society and individuals	Free and equal individuals constrained by law, focused on economic interests working cooperatively when it benefits self-interest; public and private clearly delineated	Society composed of interdependent people in relationship with varying degrees of dependence and ability to act freely out of self-interests
Emotion	Values "impartial" judgments	Values emotions
Aims for	Moral minimum	Going beyond the moral minimum
Best suited tools and contexts for specific ethical theories	The marketplace and universal contexts: Kantian = legal, contractual disputes Utilitarian = public policy	Particularistic contexts: family, friends, and personal relationships
Analogy	Moral practice as science	Moral practice as art

Source: Based largely on the model of ethics of care described by Virginia Held.[5] *The Ethics of Care: Personal, Political, and Global.* New York: Oxford University Press, 2006.

Subsequent discussion emphasizes the following limitations of the dominant Western justice-based ethic as a foundation for interprofessional collaboration in health care:

- An individualistic focus of the ethics of justice may reinforce market competitive hierarchical concepts between health care providers that maintain professional silos and inhibit moral discourse.
- Emphasis on individual decision choices may hinder efforts to look at broken or hierarchical structures and relationships that may support provision of care or effective implementation of the ethical decisions. (In spite of the emphasis on individual decision making, implementation often requires organizational, political, or social action.)
- The underlying concept of both personal and professional autonomy is inadequate to understanding the complex interactions between patients/clients, health care providers, and administrators.

- A minimalist analytic emphasis does not adequately inform the constructive processes of caring interrelationship and collaboration. The result is what Benner[7] describes as an emphasis on health care as production versus practice.

In spite of these possible limitations of the ethic of justice, there are clearly also strengths of the justice perspective. For example, the ethics of justice provides relatively clear principles for making ethical decisions and a significant literature addressing the problem of competing duties or principles. Likewise, the care perspective also has strengths and limitations as an ethical model and as an educational focus. Table 15-2 delineates the strengths and weakness of the two perspectives. In light of the strengths and weaknesses of both perspectives, it is tempting to view the two ethical models as

Table 15-2. Strengths and Limitations of Two Ethical Approaches

	Ethics of Justice	Ethics of Care
Strengths of ethical model	Clear principles for decision making Extensive literature describes applications Rational and logical	Narrative and context-rich moral discourse Creating and valuing inter-relationships Critique of structures
Possible limitations of ethical model	Individualistic focus Difficulty in critiquing social structural deficiencies Abstract and impartial bias may not attend to contextual and narrative details that are ethically important Flawed notion of professionalism and autonomy undercuts interprofessionalism and teamwork Minimalist ethic—what should be done in reaction to a problem—provides a poor foundation for link to constructive collaborative efforts	Does not produce clear indicators of "what should be done" May not protect rights

(Continues)

Table 15-2. Strengths and Limitations of Two Ethical Approaches (Continued)

	Ethics of Justice	Ethics of Care
Opportunities for interprofessional education	The decision-making framework applied to "paradigmatic" cases relatively easy to implement Group discussion focused on cases provides valuable opportunity for interprofessional collaboration	Student-generated narrative ethics Interprofessional dialogue about individual and professional perspective Team perspectives on ethical situations Development of shared or mutual autonomy in interprofessional teams Professional life in teams as an interprofessional moral community
Pitfalls for interprofessional education	Power and status difference between professions may undercut interprofessional oral dialogue (i.e., structure affects communication) If not written to accomplish interprofessional goals, cases may actually inhibit interprofessional collaboration and reinforce professional barriers	Succumbing to a superficial view of care as an attitude or value rather than a "practice"

complementary. It is not simply the case that the two views are complementary, however, so that one might use one viewpoint to augment the other.[5] It is more accurate to believe that the two viewpoints provide a different focus on the ethical issues. Therefore it is important to use both lenses. Consider how the ethics of justice and the ethics of care might deal with a commonly used type of scenario in end-of-life health care as presented next.

SAMPLE VIGNETTE

Let us suppose that a young college student has been involved in a tragic automobile accident, suffering a traumatic brain injury. In spite of prompt medical intervention, it appears that the student has suffered brain death and will not recover from the coma that ensued from the accident. Like many young people, the young student did not have an advance directive. Because it is clear that the patient's prospects for recovery are limited, family and friends now disagree in what to do in the face of medical recommendations to discontinue life support. Analysis of the situation from the standpoint of the ethics of justice might focus on the criteria for determination of brain death and legal and ethical guidelines that delineate who has the "right" to serve as surrogate decision making. One difficulty that arises in this analysis is that the legally designated decision may not have personal knowledge of the person for whom they are making judgments. An ethic of care, on the other hand, would begin from the standpoint of relationship and the rich contextual detail of the family context.

PROFESSIONALIZATION

Professionals have been an important part of life in America since the birth of the country.[10,11] One important line of sociological scholarship explores the process of professionalization,[12,13] delineating the steps that must be navigated and the characteristics that an occupation must possess to be regarded as a profession. For example, Ritzer[11] described three different perspectives on professionalization: structural, processual, and power. From this perspective an occupation must not only possess the right characteristics or traits (such as a body of knowledge, a code of ethics, and autonomy in decision making) and go through an appropriate process of gaining political protection through licensure, but must also gain status and recognition within society to be considered a profession.

In recent years, there has been increasing emphasis on the power approach to describing professionalization from both positive and negative perspectives. From the positive side, Forsyth and Danisiewicz[14] delineated the processes that a profession might navigate in attaining professional status through the use of power. To achieve this status, the profession must demonstrate that the service it performs is important to clients, exclusivity or monopoly of the task, and complexity in applying its body of knowledge (p. 62). The power approach has also been developed from a negative perspective, however, as an increasing number of scholars and members of the public expressed dissatisfaction with the monopolistic practices, examples of unethical behavior, and lack of accountability of professionals. As a result of public dissatisfaction and decreased trust in professional behavior, some observe that institutions have sought to limit the power of professionals through "deprofessionalization."[15]

Mutual Autonomy and Interprofessional Collaboration: Paradox of Autonomy

There is widespread agreement that autonomy is a critical feature of professions. Whether it is viewed as an intrinsic attribute, or part of the process of gaining acceptance, or as the exercise of political power, autonomy is considered a critical feature of professional status. Concepts about professionalism and professional autonomy present barriers and opportunities in interprofessional education.

Our beliefs about professional autonomy are heavily influenced by the underlying ethic of justice. Professional autonomy is construed as "right" gained by a profession through strategic action for its collective self-interest within the social and political arena. It is both assumed and permitted within this ethical framework that rational individuals (both individually and collectively) act in self-interest. Perceptions of professional status, autonomy, and power, however, may prove to be barriers to interprofessional collaboration and teamwork. The paradox of professional autonomy is that although every occupation strives to achieve and possess professional autonomy, it is often turf wars over autonomy that most undercut interprofessional collaboration.

As previously discussed, the ethic of care has observed that many of the assumptions about autonomy are incorrect. Moreover, there are many cultures in which autonomy and autonomous action are not valued as positive attributes. We are not, individually or collectively, simply independent rational actors. As professionals we are interdependent with and dependent on other professionals and patients, clients, and families in providing care. Effective interprofessional teams intrinsically recognize this interdependence, and they learn that autonomy is not statically invested with the physicians or other members of the team.

Held[5] described a concept of "mutual autonomy" that she proposes more closely represents the human condition (p. 55):

> *Mutual autonomy is very different from traditional autonomy would be, if there were such a thing. Traditionally, autonomy has been understood in terms of self-sufficiency, self-direction, noninterference, rational control and the like. . . .*

Mutual autonomy is different from individual autonomy. It includes mutual understanding and acceptances of how much sharing of time, space, daily decisions, and so on there will be, and how much independently arrived at activity.

This concept of mutual autonomy is an important concept for interprofessional education, collaboration, and practice. It is an important antidote to individualized market concepts inherent in the justice-based concepts of autonomy.

CREATING AN INTERPROFESSIONAL MORAL COMMUNITY GROUNDED IN CARE AND JUSTICE

Professionals often view relationships with those in their own profession as a moral community. Special obligations are owed to members of one's own profession: the obligation to mentor others, to support the professional organization, to provide care to family members, to provide peer review, to share the work of caring for the disenfranchised within society, or even to provide help in a time of need. The argument for turning away from competitive marketplace notions of interprofessionalism and toward a care-based notion of professional autonomy is also an argument for an interprofessional moral community. As Benner[7] notes, "The ethos of the buyer-seller relationship does not adequately capture the moral demands of caring for the disenfranchised, the vulnerable, and the suffering" (p. 58). Where interprofessional teams function most effectively, they indeed seem to understand themselves as a kind of caring moral community—defined more by interrelationships and caring practices than by the rights and duties of the ethics of justice. The abilities and skills to develop these types of caring moral communities, however, are seldom taught during professional education. This suggests that an appropriate goal for interprofessional ethics educational efforts should be directed toward developing interprofessional moral community in preparation to work in interprofessional teams. Educational efforts directed toward this goal would include practice in negotiating mutual autonomy, attentiveness to the unique narrative professional perspectives, and developing shared practices, behaviors, and attitudes rooted in both care and justice. Figure 15-1 contrasts sample interprofessional educational activities that might be associated with the ethics of care and ethics of justice.

Educational Content and Activities Associated With the Ethics of Justice	Educational Content and Activities Associated With the Ethics of Care

• Focus on individual decision-making
• Purpose is for the individual to reach a "right" decision using rational tools
• Ethical case dilemmas focused on universal impartial principles for decision-making
• Health care relationships are hierarchical
• Perspective is that of the health care provider with emphasis on the physician
• Adjudication of competing rights, duties, and principles
• Individual rights–the "separated self"
• Content
  – What it means to be a professional, especially from the standpoint of your own profession with regard to autonomy
  – Code of Ethics of your profession
  – Ethical theories–Kant
  – Decision frameworks
  – Professional issues sensitivity
  – Individual values clarification
  – Cultural sensitivity
  – Implementation skills–such as, communication and negotiation skill
  – Interprofessionalism as overcoming competing professional interests
	• Focus on cultivation of caring practices and relationships[5]
	• Moral discourse and dialogue
	• Attentiveness to context[5]
	• Responsiveness to needs[5]
	• Appreciating narrative nuance
	• Shared relationships and responsibility to meet needs
	• Teams focused on moral community
	• Content
	  – Human interdependency
	  – Interest are interwined, not independent
	  – Mutual autonomy of professionals
	  – Interprofessionalism as developing trust to support moral community
	  – Limitations of market perspectives for caring relationships
	  – Emotion is helpful in understanding narrative and context
	  – Motives

Figure 15-1
Contrasting educational content for care and justice.

CONCLUSIONS

Professionalization and socialization during professional education may exacerbate barriers to interprofessionalism. Overcoming the barriers of professional rivalry and competition for status depends in part on a paradigm shift that focuses on the creation of an interprofessional moral community grounded, at least in part, in the ethic of care. This chapter explored conceptual barriers to interprofessional practice within the ethical foundations for interprofessional education. The argument was developed that the ethical foundation in the Western ethic of justice reinforces barriers to interprofessional practice. Features of the ethic of justice that work against interprofessional practice are the focus on individual rights, an inadequate notion of autonomy, the minimalist analytic ethic that attends to principled decision making at the expense of constructive interrelationship and caring practices, and difficulty in critiquing structures of domination. These features are exacerbated by the current tendency to reduce social interactions to market relationships. An alternative to the ethic of justice construed within market assumptions is a care-based model of professionalism based on care, mutual autonomy, and relationship. Overcoming the barriers of professional rivalry and competition for status depends in part on a paradigm shift that focuses on the creation of an interprofessional moral community grounded, at least in part, in the ethic of care. Development of an interprofessional moral community has the potential to transform education, practice, students, health care practitioners, and health care organizations.

REFERENCES

1. Irvine R, Kerridge I, McPhee J, Freeman S. Interprofessionalism and ethics: consensus or class of cultures? *J Interprofess Care*. 2002;16:199–210.
2. Yarborough M, Jones T, Cyr TA, Phillips S, Stelzner D. Interprofessional education in ethics at an academic health sciences center. *Acad Med*. 2000;75:793–800.
3. Kelley M, MacLean M. Interdisciplinary continuing education in a rural and remote area—the approach of the Northern Educational Centre for Aging and Health. *Educat Geront*. 1997;23:631–649.
4. Gilligan C. *In a Different Voice: Psychological Theory and Women's Development*. Cambridge, MA: Harvard University Press; 1982.
5. Held V. *The Ethics of Care: Personal, Political, and Global*. New York: Oxford University Press; 2006.
6. Kohlberg L. Stage and sequence: the cognitive-developmental approach to socialization. In: Goslin D, ed. *Handbook of Socialization Theory and Research*. Chicago: Rand McNally; 1969.
7. Benner P. A dialogue between virtue ethics and care ethics. *Theoret Med*. 1997;18:47–61.
8. Botes A. An integrated approach to ethical decision-making in the health team. *J Adv Nurs*. 2000;32:1076–1082.
9. Smeyers P. "Care" and wider ethical issues. *J Philos Educ*. 1999;33:233–251.
10. Sullivan WM. *Work and Integrity: The Crisis and Promise of Professionalism in America*, 2nd ed. Chicago: University of Chicago Press; 2005.
11. Ritzer G. Professionalization, bureaucratization and rationalization: the views of Max Weber. *Social Forces*. 1975;53:627–634.
12. Carr-Saunders AM. Professionalization in historical perspective. In: Vollmer HM, Mills DL, eds. *Professionalization*. Englewood Cliffs, NJ: Prentice-Hall; 1966.
13. Pavalko RM. *Sociology of Occupations and Professions*. Itaska, IL: F.E. Peacock Publishers; 1971.
14. Forsyth BF, Danisiewicz TJ. Toward a theory of professionalization. *Work Occup*. 1985;12:59–76.
15. Reed RR, Evans D. The deprofessionalization of medicine. *JAMA*. 1987;258: 3279–3282.

"Against the Current": Strategies for Success in Health Care—A Case Example of a Rural, Native American Community

Joy D. Doll, OTD, OT
Wehnona Stabler, MPH

INTRODUCTION

According to tribal leaders, in the English languge "Omaha" translates to "those going against the current." This chapter presents the story of the Omaha people who constantly face momentous health issues, including chronic disease and substance abuse. The Omaha people struggle to address barriers to access in care such as poverty, geographical isolation, and the culture of reservation life. The life and community of the Omaha Tribe provides insight into how a community facing significant barriers has gone "against the current" to meet their most basic health needs. This chapter also reflects on the unique needs of the Omaha Tribe as a rural population with specific examples of the importance of interprofessional practice in promoting social change and improving health status.

As is the case with many Native American reservations, the Omaha reservation is located in a rural area. According to the National Rural Health Association, rural populations face significant challenges in addressing health issues, including lack of transportation, lack of technology, low literacy levels, and health professions shortages.[1] Due to these issues, a health disparity exists in rural health care. Compared with urban or suburban populations, residents living in rural areas are also more likely to partake in risky behaviors, are at increased risk for developing chronic diseases, and are more likely to be uninsured.[2,3] Regarding risky behaviors, rural residents are more likely to smoke, less likely to exercise, and have higher rates of obesity. Rural health care settings offer less specialty care services and preventative medicine to adequately meet the health needs of rural residents. The culture of rural life has changed as well with increasing diversity and decreasing employment related to farming. Because of lack of employment opportunities, poverty levels are high with as many as one-fifth of rural residents in the United States living below the poverty level.[1-3]

Not only is rural health care unique, but the needs and issues of a Native American community require different strategies to battle chronic disease, address historical trauma, and honor the culture that is intimately bound to health and wellness.[4-7] Compared with the general population, Native Americans face significant health disparities, with Native Americans being twice as likely to live in poverty, be unemployed, and lack an education. According to the Centers for Disease Control and Prevention, the rate of diabetes among Native Americans doubled from 1994 to 2004, posing a significant threat to the wellness of Native people.[8] Mortality rates for Native Americans are significantly higher than the general population for heart disease, accidents, diabetes, alcoholism, suicide, and tuberculosis and are the highest of any minority group.[4-7]

The health disparities of rural, Native American populations can leave any health care professional feeling overwhelmed and helpless to influence the wellness of individuals, much less the community as a whole. With limited resources, rural Native American communities are forced to be creative in their efforts to meet needs. With the complications of the underinsured, clients may not get health needs adequately addressed or even addressed at all, leading to poor chronic disease management along with acute problems. The Omaha Tribe is one example of a rural, Native American community that has created processes to help address community health needs. According to Tribal leaders, partnerships with organizations and entities are a must to bring in resources to meet needs and encourage interprofessional health care practices promoting improved patient care. Simpson et al. state[9] that underserved communities need interprofessional practice models to approach chronic disease models efficiently and to address both health professional shortages in rural areas and increasing health disparities.[9] Simpson et al.[9] define inter-professional health care as "a partnership among professionals involving individuals and communities based on (1) a shared mission, (2) a shared bio-psychosocial paradigm, and (3) a shared responsibility for decision-making and problem solving, with leadership based on the expertise that is needed for improving health outcome in a shared relationship with individuals, families, and communities."[9] The combination of the recommendations of national professional organizations and the recognition by communities needing to maximize resources calls for partnership and teamwork across health professionals and community members.

OVERVIEW OF OMAHA TRIBE

The Omaha Tribe of Nebraska resides on a reservation located in northeast Nebraska, 70 miles from Omaha, Nebraska on a portion of the Tribe's original land base. Macy, Nebraska is the Tribal Headquarters of the Omaha Tribe, who have an enrolled population of about 6,000 and a reservation population of a little over 4,200. The economy of the Tribe is tied closely to tribal government with the largest employers including the Tribe, the tribal casino, and the Carl T. Curtis Health Education Center, the tribally run health facility.[10]

The Omaha Tribe maintains a rich culture, including traditional health practices that are still used to promote health and wellness. Common practices, like Native American Church services, sweat lodges, sundance, smoking sacred tobacco, and burning cedar, are all methods for purification of the mind, body, and soul. These practices are relevant today because Omaha Tribal members may choose to use them for healing in collaboration with traditional Western medicine. Health care professionals should be aware of these practices not only because of their effect on health status but also in an effort to attain cultural awareness, as most of the health care professionals working on the reservation are non-Native. Many of these practices are spiritual in nature, calling on health care professionals to respect and acknowledge their relevance in health care to the Omaha people. Because of the richness of the Omaha culture, this chapter briefly mentions traditional practices and their relevance to health care today.[11,12]

In traditional Omaha ways, connections with the Great Spirits or Wakonda (God) were very important. Ceremonies and rituals existed to promote cleansing of the body, mind, and soul to reconnect with Wakonda. Today, cedar, or sometimes sage, is burned and the sacred smoke is rubbed on the body to promote healing. The smoke from burning these plants is seen as a healing force and a messenger to Wakonda. The ritual of burning cedar can be both formal, where the smoke is waved and people are offered to accept it, or informal, when it may be burned during a meeting to cleanse the room. Tobacco is also sacred, and when prayers are spoken in the presence of the tobacco, the words transfer into the tobacco, allowing thoughts to go to the spirits via the smoke. Even though tobacco is still used in this manner by Omaha people, it is also abused in the form of cigarettes, which are not viewed as sacred.[11,12]

Sweat lodges are also used for cleansing and purification and can be associated with the Native American Church and other ceremonies. Traditionally, women did not participate in sweats because they already have a natural cleansing process in their monthly cycle. Today, both women and men can participate in sweat lodges and frequency of participation in sweats varies from daily to not at all. On the reservation, the Native American Church is the predominant religion, but Omaha families move easily between traditional native beliefs and modern Christian denominations, including Catholic, Mormon, Baptist, and Presbyterian. Omaha people believe that the main objective is to know God and that all religions provide ways to get to know God. In Native American Church ceremonies, the use of peyote is common and a sacrament, providing a sense of transcendence and connection with the spirits.[11,12]

Historically, the Tribe used a clan system with each clan holding a significant role within the community, and many members still recognize the clan system today. The clan system is based on the sacred circle or the Huthuga, which divided the 10 original clans into the Earth and Sky. Traditionally, the Huthuga provided a way to maintain order and provided each Omaha with their place in the circle. Each clan had duties, roles, and responsibilities along with taboos. One example would be not marrying within one's own clan. Today, Omahas still identify with their clanship, which follows their father.[13]

Although this section is a brief introduction into Omaha culture, these descriptions demonstrate the importance and relevance to the Omaha culture in regard to health and health care. Many successful health programs integrate cultural elements into modern approaches. Omaha practices define much of the community-based health outreach with projects geared toward relevant cultural events. One program that exemplifies this point is the Last Buffalo Hunt Walking Program, which incorporates a valued cultural traditional practice with modern physical activity practices.

Project Exemplar—The Last Buffalo Hunt Walking Program
The Last Buffalo Hunt Walking Program is a healthy walking program integrating the cultural dimension of the buffalo hunt, which dictated much of the Omaha's life throughout their existence. The route of the last buffalo hunt to take place was mapped by children at the Omaha Nation School and then used as a basis for developing a comprehensive walking program encouraging participants of all ages to walk the distances of their ancestors who participated in buffalo hunts. Participants are grouped into quartets and required to walk about ten miles per day among the group walking a total of 342 miles over one month in the summer prior to the Omaha powwow celebration. Pre- and post-screenings are done to assess changes including blood pressure, glucose testing, body composition and weight. This program is offered at the Four Hills of Life Wellness Center to all members of the Omaha Tribe. Teams are tracked and awarded prizes if completing the distance of the last buffalo hunt. Furthermore, the project provided a powerful method for teaching and reinforcing the rich history and cultural values of the Omaha people.[14]

Besides community-based health care services, Omaha tribal members have access to a tribally run health system called the Carl T. Curtis Health Education Center, which includes an outpatient clinic, dentistry, pharmacy, podiatry, a 10-chair dialysis unit currently running two shifts, a 24-bed nursing home, an alcohol program, a behavioral health program, and a diabetes program. In 2005 the Carl T. Curtis Health Education Center received 37,000 outpatient visits and currently holds 8,000 patient charts. Under the auspices of the Omaha Tribe Diabetes Program, adult tribal members have access to a comprehensive wellness center, the Four Hills of Life Wellness Center, and youth have access to daily programs at the Valentine Parker Jr. Youth Prevention Center.

DEMOGRAPHIC DATA FROM OMAHA TRIBE

The Omaha Tribe is located 30 miles from Sioux City, the closest metropolitan area, in Thurston County. The median age of Omaha tribal members is 18 years of age, with a high school graduation rate of 69%, 11% less than the national average. Only 9% of tribal members receive education beyond high school, and 49% of individuals are living below poverty level with the average income of $19,500. Thurston County has the lowest per capita income in the state of Nebraska. A state health survey by the Nebraska Health and Human Services revealed that 39.2% of Omaha tribal members are unemployed, 58.9% make $19,999 or less in annual income, and 49% of individuals are living below poverty level. According to a state survey, approximately 40% of tribal members are unemployed, with 50% having been out of work for more than a year. Thirty percent of Omaha tribal members report never having graduated from high school or receiving a GED, whereas 7% report being a college graduate.[10]

Among Native American households in Thurston County, 42.4% consist of single-parent families compared with a national average where 27% of households are single-parent families.[15] Many residents on the reservation do not have access to a vehicle, and transportation services are limited, making accessibility an important aspect of providing care and meeting community need. Health services are also limited due to funding, the income level of residents, and the shortage of available health care providers. Although the Omaha Tribe faces many challenges, leaders within the community have been innovative in seeking ways to meet needs. Later in this chapter, lessons and recommendations are discussed on maximizing resources in an underserved community.[10]

OVERVIEW OF TRIBAL HEALTH CARE DELIVERY SYSTEM

The Omaha Tribe health care system has been designed based on the needs of the community and includes programs relevant to major health issues. All services including long-term care, a dialysis unit, wellness programming, youth wellness programming, alcohol treatment, primary care services, and the tribal diabetes program have been designed to be patient centered and to attempt to address chronic disease prevention and management.

Long-Term Care Services

When the Carl T. Curtis Health Education Center was being designed in the mid-1970s, the tribal council was very forward thinking and added a nursing home onto the facility. At that time, there were hardly any nursing homes in Native communities. The Omaha Tribe believed that the current system of sending elders who could no longer live independently off the reservation to receive services was inadequate and culturally destructive. The separation of the elder from the rest of the community negatively influenced the quality of life of the entire community. Omaha elders were dying alone separated from family and culture. In Omaha culture, elders are the teachers of culture and honored for their knowledge and experience. Their removal from the community did not allow for elders to educate younger tribal members on traditional practices, not to mention the psychological effects on the individual elders. The tribal council added the nursing home to the Carl T. Curtis Health Education Center to ensure that elders could continue to educate others and be a part of the community even if assistance was needed for daily living.

Today, the nursing home is home for elders and individuals who have had a traumatic injury needing constant care or for those in need of hospice care. Services at the nursing home include dietetics, physical therapy, occupational therapy, podiatry, and optometry. The facility is only Medicaid certified so does not function as a traditional nursing home typically associated with Medicare. Many of the aforementioned services, therefore, are offered to the residents on a consultative or as-needed basis. Restorative aides work full time to carry out treatment plans created annually by the physical therapist and occupational therapist. If treatment is beyond the aide's capabilities, then physical and occupational therapy services are provided. Also available to the residents are diagnostic services through the Carl T. Curtis Health Center, including laboratory and x-ray services, and dental services. Another benefit of having the nursing home attached to the facility ensures that elders and nursing home residents receive necessary primary care. A full-time activity director organizes both individual and group events. Outings are planned at least monthly when the weather permits, and a variety of events are provided in-house as well.[16]

Dialysis Unit

With type 2 diabetes rampant among the Omaha people, many individuals progress to the point of requiring dialysis. Issues of transportation along with distance to services and the drain on funding helped the Omaha Tribe decide to open a 10-bed dialysis unit in 2005. Having these services on-site allows Omaha community members to receive services on-site instead of traveling nearly 60 miles three times a week. The Tribal Dialysis Center receives no funding from Indian Health Services and is solely a tribal enterprise. These services are also innovative and unique in tribal communities and demonstrate a commitment to ensure quality care for patients managing chronic disease.

Community Services

Four Hills of Life Wellness Center

The Four Hills of Life Wellness Center offers a comprehensive list of services to members of the community, including exercise facilities, community health education, substance abuse counseling, physical therapy, and occupational therapy. The Wellness Center is open and free to all members of the Omaha Tribe over the age of 16. Exercise classes and a personal trainer are on-site to provide support for those wanting to work toward healthy living. Many of the programs carried out at the Wellness Center integrate cultural dimensions, which promotes community buy-in and the success of the program. One such program is the Sobriety Powwow, which takes place every New Year's Eve, providing an opportunity to engage in a cultural activity and prevent alcohol and drug use.

A community health educator is on-site to organize health promotion events regarding smoking cessation, seatbelt safety, and sexually transmitted diseases. A substance abuse counselor is also available to organize substance-free activities such as the Sobriety Powwow, tailgating before athletic events, and other such activities. The counselor also provides both individual and group counseling to community members struggling with substance abuse.[17]

In 2005, physical and occupational therapy services were moved from the Carl T. Curtis Health Education Center to the Wellness Center providing therapy with more space and access to more equipment. Both services are currently provided 1 day a week on an outpatient basis. Rehabilitation services have proved pivotal and demonstrated a savings to the Tribe by sending patients to therapy rather than an expensive specialist off-site for musculoskeletal and neurological problems. This has saved contract health dollars, which are used to send patients out to receive specialty services not available in the tribal health system. Contract health services are any services not included in the basic primary care services, including any specialty care. A case management team prioritizes individuals based on the health issue, and patients only qualify if the specialty care is "life or limb," meaning the issue threatens the patient's life or could cause them to lose a limb if not managed. Furthermore, contract health services are not provided on-site and require additional transportation and time to receive care. Contract health services are not only costly but require transportation between 30 and 80 miles to attend appointments. For a community struggling to meet the basic needs of its members, having as many services within the community is of utmost importance, including occupational and physical therapy.

Alcohol Program

The Omaha Alcohol Program provides early intervention, youth prevention programs, an intensive outpatient treatment program for both adolescents and adults, court-ordered driving under the influence classes, and weekly support groups (Alcoholics Anonymous, sweats, and Talking Circles). The mission of the Omaha Alcohol Program is "to provide community based intervention activities, services that enhance individual and community lifestyles through a holistic approach, including immersion of cultural, physical, mental and emotional environment" (ehealth.creighton.edu). The Omaha Alcohol Program is based on the belief that cultural beliefs and practices along with traditional substance abuse treatment are the keys to a substance-free lifestyle. All staff in the Omaha Alcohol Program are certified or provisionally licensed dependency counselors following the guidelines laid forth by the American Society of Addiction Medicines criteria and the state of Nebraska. An emerging issue is methamphetamine abuse, and current programming is ill prepared to deal with this problem.

Valentine Parker Jr. Youth Prevention Center

The Valentine Parker Jr. Youth Prevention Center opened in 2005 as a place focused specifically on the needs of the youth of the Omaha Tribe. The Prevention Center offers daily activities and special events. Family night occurs every Wednesday, which includes both youth and family members in a variety of activities. In the summer months, the Center also operates the swimming pool. All programs held at the Prevention Center focus on culture, physical activity, and healthy living. Junk food and soda are banned, and only healthy snacks are served, including fruits, crackers, and sugar-free juice. Each year key leaders in the community meet to organize and brainstorm the youth activities to take place. The Valentine Parker Center has proved invaluable on the health and wellness of Omaha youth, keeping them not only physically active but socially involved. The Center has a sophisticated tracking system where children log in when they arrive and log out after activities to record numbers and the length of time of participation. This tracking system helps the Omaha Tribe recognize the program value on the overall wellness of youth by promoting physical, spiritual, and mental health.

Outpatient Primary Care Services

The Carl T. Curtis Health Education Center provides basic primary care services to members of the Omaha Tribe. The facility is staffed by a medical director and supported by a contracted endocrinologist, nurse practitioner, and two physician's assistants. The pharmacy, with a staff of two pharmacists, provides all the prescriptions for the community as no other pharmacy exists in the community. Community members receive basic primary care services by an interprofessional team as other health care team members are called upon for their expertise because physician specialists are not within close reach. Fridays at the clinic are designated solely for individuals with diabetes to ensure that individuals with diabetes receive continual disease management.[16] The clinic also operates a small acute care room as an emergency room when medical providers are on-site.

Omaha Tribe Diabetes Program

The Omaha Tribe Diabetes Program develops programs and services specifically catering to the needs of community members with diabetes. Basic education is provided to any tribal nember diagnosed with diabetes across the life span regarding the use of a glucometer and diabetes management along with comprehensive prevention programs in collaboration with the Four Hills of Life Wellness Center and the Valentine Parker Jr. Youth Prevention Center. In addition, the diabetes program holds yearly school screenings that assesses every student on weight, height, vision, blood pressure, and acanthosis nigricans, seeing about 500 children per year. These school screenings help target which youth need additional education to promote diabetes prevention.[18] In the most recent screenings, 20% of children were identified to have the acanthosis marker.

HISTORY OF CARL T. CURTIS HEALTH EDUCATION SYSTEM

In 1976 Carl T. Curtis, a senator from Nebraska, came to visit the Omaha Tribe. He was appalled at their health care and the lack of access to address basic needs. At the time the Tribe shared a Public Health Service hospital with the Winnebago Tribe, which was located 9 miles away in Winnebago, Nebraska. The distance proved difficult for many tribal members because many did not have vehicles or even phones to call if health care was needed. Twice a month a nurse and pharmacist would travel from the Winnebago Public Health Service hospital to Macy to address the health needs of the

Omaha people. The nurse and pharmacist visited with patients in a trailer trying to meet basic health needs. A station wagon acted as the emergency vehicle, but with only one gas pump in Macy, which had limited hours, even fueling the vehicle was difficult. Witnessing all these problems, Senator Curtis told the Tribe there were economic development funds and upon his election helped the Omaha Tribe write a grant to receive funding to build a tribal health facility that would specifically serve the needs of the Omaha Tribe.

LESSONS LEARNED

The Omaha Tribe is a community that faces many barriers from chronic disease to the challenges of rural health care, including being a health professions shortage area.[19] Yet, the health system developed by the Tribe is helping to meet needs. How does an underserved community meet high levels of needs with few resources? The Omaha Tribe serves as an example of a community trying to answer that question. Based on reflections by Wehnona St. Cyr, MPH, Tribal Health Director, the following are a summary of lessons learned:

1. All decisions should be made for patient welfare. According to community leaders, if health care systems decisions are made with the patient in mind at all times, then the health care system will meet community needs. This requires that health care administrators are in touch with community needs and get out of the clinic to fully understand the health needs of the community.
2. Cultural awareness must occur. Health care professionals must not only be willing to work in a rural setting but also have a desire to gain cultural awareness of the individual community. Participating in cultural activities and practices may help fulfill this knowledge or simply asking questions to explore the cultural nature of patients. All in all, to work in a Native American community, health care professionals must be open and accepting of traditional practices and how culture affects health care choices.
3. Culture is integral in prevention and treatment. The Omaha culture holds meaning for community members and aids in coping with historical trauma. Culture must be integrated into all health care and community-based programming not only to provide meaning but to demonstrate the integration of culture and health. Health care profes-

sionals must cater both individual and community activities to promote
and recognize the cultural beliefs and rituals of community members.

4. Partnerships are essential. Partnerships with agencies and organizations help meet needs by combining resources.[20] For example, the Omaha Tribe has had an active partnership with Creighton University for 14 years, which has led to assistance with grant writing, health professions recruitment, and program development.

5. Do not underestimate students. Students from academic institutions can prove to be a valuable resource, displaying a willingness to learn about the culture and truly spending the time to understand the communities' needs. Students can also assist with gathering research, conducting focus groups, performing community needs assessments, and helping to run community-based programming. Furthermore, students may lead to the recruitment and retention of caring and qualified health care professionals to serve the community by role modeling to high school students within the community.

6. Interprofessional practice happens naturally. In underserved communities, health care professionals have to work together to combine resources to meet health needs. Health care professionals must have a team-oriented approach to care and be willing creatively and openly. Although interprofessional health care comes with many challenges, it proves to be the most efficient manner in underserved communities to meet needs.

7. Community capacity building is the best approach. Despite all the needs with the community, many strengths exist. Taking an approach that builds on these strengths to address massive health care problems promotes community buy-in and ensures a community-driven approach to tackling health care issues. To bridge the gaps in health care services, the Omaha Tribe is always looking at ways to maximize resources. Community capacity building calls on the entire community to mobilize for social change and is especially relevant when dealing with major health issues. Using this approach proves to be successful in addressing the environmental barriers that exist to healthy living.[21]

8. Tribal communities must be willing to take risks. Although Native American tribes can never live fully as they originally did, each tribe can promote health and wellness by combining culture with science to promote innovative methods for addressing individual and community health issues.

CONCLUSIONS

Despite being a rural, underserved, Native American community, the Omaha Tribe of Nebraska exists as an example of a community maximizing all its resources to face health care challenges. This chapter provides a glimpse into the current system and strategies used by community health leaders to impact community-wide health issues. The picture painted here in this case provides insight for health care professionals and community health leaders working in rural areas on how to face health care problems that almost overwhelm communities and how to strategize to facilitate individual and social change for overall well-being.

REFERENCES

1. National Rural Health Association. Rural health disparities collaboratives: benefits, barriers and adaptations for the future. NRHA website. 2005. Available at: http://www.nrharural.org/pubs/pdf/HDCfocus-call.pdf. Accessed February 9, 2007.
2. Hartley D. Rural health disparities, population health and rural culture. *Am J Public Health*. 2004;94:1675–1677.
3. Galambos CM. Health care disparities among rural populations: a neglected frontier. *Health Social Work*. 2005;30:179–181.
4. Castor ML, Smyser MS, Taualii MM, Park AN, Lawson SA, Forquera RA. A nationwide population-based study identifying health disparities between American Indians/Alaska Natives and the general populations living in select urban counties. *Am J Public Health*. 2006;96:1478–1484.
5. Doshi SR, Jiles R. Health behaviors among American Indian/Alaska Native women, 1998–2000 BRFSS. *J Women's Health*. 2006;8:919–927.
6. Jones DS. The persistence of American Indian health disparities. *Am J Public Health*. 2006;12:2122–2134.
7. Dapice A. The medicine wheel. *J Transcultural Nurs*. 2006;17:251–260.
8. Centers for Disease Control and Prevention. Diagnosed diabetes among American Indians and Alaska Natives aged <35. United States, 1994–2004. CDC website, 2006. Available at: http://www.cdc.gov/mmwr/preview/mmwrhtml/mm5544a4.htm. Accessed February 9, 2007.
9. Simpson G, Rabin D, Schmitt M, Taylor P, Urban S, Ball J. Interprofessional health care practice: recommendations of the National Academies of Practice expert panel on health care in the 21st century. *Issues in Interdisciplinary Care: National Academies of Practice Forum*. 2001;3:5–19.
10. Nebraska Department of Health and Human Services Office of Minority Health. *Health survey: Omaha Tribe of Nebraska in Thurston County, Nebraska*. Lincoln, NE: Health and Human Services, 2004.

11. Fletcher A, LaFlesche F. *The Omaha Tribe*, Vol. 1. Lincoln, NE: University of Nebraska Press; 1992.
12. Fletcher A, LaFlesche F. *The Omaha Tribe*, Vol. 2. Lincoln, NE: University of Nebraska Press; 1992.
13. Tyndall W, Wolfe M, Coffey M. Huthuga diagram. ULCC website. 2007. Available at: http://teacherweb.esu1.org/vstabler/stories/StoryReader$15. Accessed August 1, 2008.
14. Ekstrum J. Last Buffalo Hunt Walking Program. 2006.
15. U.S. Census Bureau. Statistics on single parent families. 2000.
16. Cross P, Champ-Blackwell S. Carl T. Curtis Health Education Center. Omaha Tribe eHealth website. 2007. Available at: http://ehealth.creighton.edu/commres_OmahaAlcohol.htm. Accessed February 9, 2007.
17. Cross P, Champ-Blackwell S. Four Hills of Life Wellness Center. Omaha Tribe eHealth website. 2007. Available at: http://ehealth.creighton.edu/commres_OmahaAlcohol.htm. Accessed February 9, 2007.
18. Cross P, Champ-Blackwell S. Omaha Alcohol Program. Omaha Tribe eHealth website. 2007. Available at: http://ehealth.creighton.edu/commres_OmahaAlcohol.htm. Accessed February 9, 2007.
19. Health Resources and Services Administration. Health Professions Shortage Areas search. HRSA website. 2007. Available at: http://hpsafind.hrsa.gov/HPSASearch.aspx. Accessed February 9, 2007.
20. Warne D. Research and educational approaches to reducing health disparities among American Indians and Alaska Natives. *J Transcult Nurs*. 2006;17:266–271.
21. Chino M, DeBruyn L. Building true capacity: indigenious models for indigenous communities. *Am J Public Health*. 2006;96:596–599.

SECTION 4

Educational Context

Improving Diabetes Outcomes in Rural Practices: Power of Collaborative Care

Doyle M. Cummings, PharmD, BCPS, FCP, FCCP
Paul Bray, MA, LMFT
Maria C. Clay, PhD

INTRODUCTION

The number of adults with diagnosed diabetes mellitus in the United States has increased 61% since 1991 and is projected to double by 2050,[1] with similar trends being seen around the world.[2] Diabetes is the sixth most common cause of death and is associated with serious complications, including cardiovascular disease, renal failure, blindness, neuropathy, and limb amputation. Data from the UKPDS (UK Prospectus Diabetes Study Group)[3] clearly showed that improving glycemic and blood pressure control in patients with diabetes can result in significant reductions in both morbidity and mortality.[3] The American Diabetes Association and other entities published guidelines for diabetes care based on this and other evidence.[4] Many patients, however, particularly rural patients, do not receive these recommended levels of care, demonstrating the need for redesigning systems of care to improve the use of these evidence-based guidelines to minimize long-term morbidity/mortality.

The major risk factor for type 2 diabetes, obesity, is also reaching epidemic proportions in both adults and children, suggesting that this disease will continue to impact both patients and our health care system for many years to come.[5] Of great concern is that the disease preferentially impacts persons of color with prevalence ratios in African-Americans, Latinos, and Native Americans of 1.5 to 2 times that in Whites. Substantial literature also describes both racial and socioeconomic disparities in care delivery and in the prevalence of complications.[6–8] This growth in the prevalence of diabetes and its complications has led to the development of focused diabetes care programs, particularly in urban centers, designed to provide comprehensive care for patients with diabetes mellitus.

DIABETES IN RURAL AMERICA

Rural patients with type 2 diabetes represent a very at-risk population. As reported by the National Rural Health Association, rural areas are more likely to be underserved with 25% of the nation's population living there but only 10% of the nation's physicians practicing there. There are 2,157 health professions shortage areas in rural areas compared with 910 in urban areas. On average, per capita income is $7,417 less in rural areas than urban areas, rural residents are less likely to be covered by employer-based health insurance, and the rural poor are less likely to be covered by Medicaid benefits than their urban counterparts. To maintain hospital services in many of these rural communities, the federal government has established critical access hospitals, which receive cost-based reimbursement for services delivered. The primary care practices associated with rural hospitals, however, usually do not receive higher reimbursement and represent the fragile environment for care delivery in rural communities.

In a study by Dansky and Dirani,[9] the health services use patterns of Medicare beneficiaries with diabetes mellitus were compared in rural and urban areas. Patients with diabetes in sparsely populated rural communities reported fewer physician office visits than their urban counterparts. Further, it has been shown that low income, rural patients with type 2 diabetes are more likely to receive care from a primary care physician and less likely to receive care from a specialist than their urban counterparts.[10,11] Extremely busy primary care providers in rural communities have had to shoulder the burden of providing comprehensive chronic care for patients with diabetes mellitus, often without sufficient resources.[12] Because of migration of young people from rural communities, such communities are often left with an aging populace, especially minority patients, who may contribute disproportionately to premature morbidity/mortality and increased health care costs. The Institute of Medicine's recent report details the fragile nature of health care in rural communities and calls for major changes in government policy and support.[13] The report also encourages rural communities to implement a population health focus in their delivery of health services. It suggests that many interventions are available that might improve the delivery of care for chronic disease such as diabetes mellitus but these interventions need to be tested and prioritized in such settings.

Diabetes Outcomes

Patients in rural primary care practices have diabetes outcomes that are inadequate relative to published guidelines. In studies in both the United States and Canada, it has been shown that diabetes care in rural areas, delivered by primary care providers, is inadequate relative to the standards described by the American Diabetes Association (ADA) and often is of lower quality than that in urban settings.[10,14-16] Zoorob and Mainous[15] reviewed a random sample of 100 charts from patients with type 2 diabetes mellitus seen by rural family physicians in Ohio. They found that family physicians did not consistently follow the ADA standards of care. HbA_{1c} tests were performed in only 15% of patients, and annual lipids were measured in less than half of patients. In a study by Andrus et al.[14] glycemic control, blood pressure control, and low-density-lipoprotein cholesterol goals were compared in a representative sample of rural and urban patients with diabetes mellitus in Alabama. The percentage of patients in this study meeting ADA-recommended standards are shown in Table 17-1. Rural patients had lower quality outcomes in every category studied.

In a study by Coon and Zulkowski,[17] diabetes care was examined in 399 patients in rural Montana. Although glycemic control was better than the national average, it still was worse than that recommended in ADA guidelines.

Table 17-1. Comparison of Diabetes Outcomes* in Rural and Urban Patients

Parameter	Urban	Rural
Mean HbA_{1c}, %	7.4	8.5
Percent with HbA_{1c} < 7.0%	49	33
Percent with BP < 130/80	22	8
Percent with LDL < 100 mg/dl	37	11

*Outcomes were glycemic, blood pressure (BP), and low-density-lipoprotein (LDL) cholesterol control.
Source: Andrus MR, Kelley KW, Murphey LM, Herndon KC. A comparison of diabetes care in rural and urban medical clinics in Alabama. *J Commun Health.* 2004;29:29–44.

Further, blood pressure and lipids were not well controlled. In additional studies by Porterfield and Kinsinger[18] and Bell et al.,[19] hyperglycemia among rural patients was also less well controlled relative to published guidelines. Based on data from UKPDS and other sources, we would anticipate that inadequate control of blood sugar, blood pressure, and lipids would place rural diabetic patients at greater risk for end-organ complications. This is also borne out in 5-year mortality trends from the late 1990s. In rural eastern North Carolina the adjusted mortality rate from diabetes is 29 per 100,000, whereas the rate in the more urban Piedmont region of North Carolina is 25 per 100,000. Further, Massing and colleagues[20] describe a "diabetes belt" in the eastern coastal plain of North Carolina and report that recommended testing in the region was only performed at about half the rate recommended by current guidelines. These findings do not necessarily imply that providers practice bad medicine but may more reflect an ineffectual delivery system in need of redesign.

REDESIGNING SYSTEMS OF CARE

Redesigned systems of care have demonstrated efficacy in urban and managed care settings. It is clear from large-scale studies, including the UKPDS, that intensive medical care designed to achieve tighter glycemic and blood pressure control as well as other treatment endpoints in patients with diabetes mellitus is associated with improved morbidity and mortality. The extent to which findings have been translated from these well-controlled clinical trials into the reality of primary care office practice where most of routine diabetes care occurs in this and other countries is not well understood. This is especially true in rural settings where health care resources are already insufficient. To address this need, a variety of interventions have been developed to improve the quality and consistency of medical care delivered to patients with diabetes mellitus in an effort to replicate the improved outcomes obtained in these highly controlled clinical trials. Most of these studies have involved redesigning or reengineering the delivery of health care in the primary care setting. Most have been undertaken in urban or managed care settings, however, and not in rural communities. Such redesign is necessary because the current health care delivery system is geared toward acute rather than chronic care as described by Bodenheimer.[21] Visits are designed to identify a specific cause of symptoms and to provide acute treatment—a system that works well for infections and other acute illnesses but is ill designed to address chronic diseases. The origins of the traditional acute care model have been prevalent in Western medicine for more than a century. Even the traditional medical note, which begins with a "chief complaint," demonstrates that the system is geared toward addressing acute problems. System redesign is necessary to close the gap between the current acute care model of practice and the optimal care needed for chronic diseases evidenced in highly controlled trials. Further, most innovative models involve the expanded use of nonphysician personnel to take more responsibility in chronic care management.

Some of the individual components of interventions to improve the care management process have been recently reviewed by Norris et al.[22] In this systematic review, Norris et al. evaluated the effectiveness of various disease management interventions in 27 studies of varying design quality. The authors reported that evidence supports the effectiveness of disease management on glycemic control; on screening for diabetic retinopathy, foot lesions and peripheral neuropathy, and proteinuria; and on the monitoring of lipid concentrations. Care management was effective in improving both glycemic control and provider monitoring of glycemic control, although this was only well studied in managed care settings. Care management was effective both when delivered as a single intervention and when delivered with one or more additional educational, reminder, or support interventions. Likewise, in a systematic review of 41 studies involving 48,000 patients by the Cochrane Collaboration, the authors describe the effectiveness of interventions directed at health professionals, organizational change interventions, as well as patient-focused interventions in improving diabetes-specific outcomes.[23] In a recent publication by Shojania et al.,[24] the effects of various quality improvement strategies for type 2 diabetes mellitus on glycemic control were compared using a meta-regression analysis. These authors demonstrated the importance of team-based care with nonphysicians assuming expanded roles in patient management.

REDESIGNED SYSTEMS OF CARE IN RURAL PRACTICES

Redesigned systems of care have not been studied in rural practices. Although these studies provide evidence that redesigning care delivery can result in improved outcomes and efficiency of care, most of these studies are limited by the fact that they have nearly all been conducted in urban and/or managed care settings. By contrast, the delivery of health care services for patients with diabetes mellitus in fee-for-service practices in underserved rural communities differs substantially. System redesign techniques have not been carefully evaluated in these settings. Similarly, many system redesign efforts have not focused on the unique needs of minority patients to minimize disparate health outcomes and reduce associated costs. In particular, more work in this setting is needed because this is where a substantial burden of disease exists—among underserved minority patients with limited access to contemporary diabetes services.

NEW MODEL OF CARE DELIVERY

The above information demonstrates that diabetes care in rural communities is not adequate and is in need of new systems for improving the process of care delivery. The goal of any new model for care delivery is to improve the quality of the care process and ultimately patient outcomes in a way that is well received by patients. Although some new patient care strategies have been explored, few provide comprehensive change. To date, most of the more comprehensive efforts to improve diabetes care have been informed by the chronic care model originally described by Wagner.[25] There are six fundamental areas identified by the chronic care model forming a system that encourages high-quality chronic disease management and one that is clearly distinct from the traditional acute care model so prevalent in medical practice:

1. Self-management support. Patients have a central role in determining their care, one that fosters a sense of responsibility for their own health. To achieve this role patients must have basic information about diabetes, understanding of and assistance with self-management skill building, and ongoing support from members of the practice team, family, friends, and community members. Better patient outcomes are achieved through use of evidence-based techniques that emphasize patient activation or empowerment, collaborative goal setting, and problem-solving skills—all important skills in self-management.

2. Delivery system design. Effective management of chronic illness requires more than simply adding interventions to an existing system focused on acute care. Rather, it necessitates basic changes in delivery system design. These changes require (a) a shift in emphasis to "planned" rather than acute visits, (b) expansion of roles and responsibilities for all professionals (e.g., nurses, health educators, pharmacists) to augment involvement in managing complex chronic conditions, (c) timely access to key clinical data, (d) enough time to interact with patients and one another (i.e., interprofessional collaboration), and (e) reg-

ular, planned follow-up with patients. Meeting these needs often requires innovation in the scheduling and organization of care, such as planned group or individual visits.

3. Decision support. Treatment decisions are based on explicit, proven guidelines that are creatively integrated into the day-to-day practice of all providers in an accessible and easy-to-use manner. In particular, this information is most needed at the point of care when decisions regarding management are often made within a limited time frame. Although clinical guidelines are often available on government or association web pages, the sheer volume of information can be overwhelming. Guidelines for the most common conditions encountered, such as diabetes mellitus, are best used in the busy office practice and are now available for downloading onto personal digital assistants.

4. Clinical information system. Because most providers in rural areas do not have electronic health records, a system that records all relevant patient care information, known as a "registry," can be used. Providers can use the registry to record critical elements of the care plan, produce quick care summaries at the time of a visit, and enter data to alter the care plan as needed. A patient registry is most useful when patient data are available to the provider(s) and can remind providers of needed services, represent feedback on performance of both the clinic and the provider(s), and serve as a source of up-to-date information and decision support for encounters. Health care teams can also use the registry to contact groups of patients with similar care needs and deliver planned care and educational sessions.

5. Organization of health care. Health care systems, even small practices working together, can create an environment in which organized efforts to improve the care of people with chronic illness take hold and flourish. Critical elements include a coherent approach to system improvement, leadership committed to and responsible for improving clinical outcomes, and incentives to providers and patients to improve care and adhere to guidelines.

6. Community. Linkages between health clinics and community resources such as health departments, churches, and senior centers are crucial to the success of comprehensive chronic illness care programs. Practices can form partnerships with community organizations to develop evidence-based programs, resources, and health policies that support patients in their efforts to manage chronic disease. Although community

resources are limited in rural communities, effective linkages can be made in most communities to facilitate lifestyle changes in patients.

This chronic care model has been extensively used to facilitate organizational change for chronic disease care for diabetes and other chronic diseases.[24] Organizations need to focus on the six areas defined above, encourage patients to take an active part in their care, and support providers with the necessary resources and expertise. In the most recent assessment of system redesign for diabetes care using the chronic care model, HbA_{1c} fell significantly in the redesigned practice but not in the usual care settings.[26] A key element in redesigned systems of care such as the chronic care model is the facilitation of interprofessional collaboration.

INTERPROFESSIONAL COLLABORATION

The Institute of Medicine's Committee on Quality of Health Care in America has advocated for increased use of interprofessional teams as a strategy to improve health care.[27] The traditional acute care model has not generally encouraged collaborative, interprofessional care. Market forces are now forcing us to reexamine current care strategies. Insurers and consumers alike are looking at the outcomes of care for populations of patients, including the care of patients with specific diseases such as diabetes mellitus, with a goal of providing the highest quality of care for the least cost. Insurers are now beginning to pay providers for specific performance outcomes in diabetes and other targeted conditions. Driven by these market forces as well as by changes in information systems and medical technology, the process of health care delivery is beginning to undergo substantial transformation.

Moreover, one can no longer make the assumption that improving the health of a population, such as a rural population of diabetic patients, is simply a function of the number of physician providers per population. Instead, today's best integrated health delivery systems are evolving toward a model of care in which interdisciplinary teams of providers manage the care of the sickest patients. Resources are used in the most efficient way, mistakes or duplication of services is avoided, and the expertise of a number of nonphysician health practitioners, including nurses, pharmacists, dietitians, health educators, social workers, physical therapists, occupational therapists, and others, is brought to bear in an environment that values collaboration. As described in the Institute of Medicine report, to ensure effective and efficient coordination of care, health professionals must work interdependently in carrying out their roles and responsibilities, conveying mutual respect, trust, support, and appreciation of each discipline's unique contributions to health care. The challenge for most rural communities is assembling the health care professionals needed and building a redesigned care delivery process when resources are limited.

New models of care delivery must be built on new relationships between health professionals. The emphasis is away from traditional hierarchical structures that place physicians as responsible for delivering most aspects of the care delivery process and toward more interprofessional, collaborative care. Although most providers are already practicing in a multidisciplinary fashion, referring patients to other providers when appropriate, the focus here is on developing a patient care plan that is the product of the inter-disciplinary interaction of different health professionals working as a well-coordinated team. The emphasis is on collaborative care planning and the assumption is that no one professional has all the required knowledge and skills necessary for optimal care to be achieved.

Interprofessional collaboration has already been shown to result in im-proved care outcomes. A recent meta-analysis[24] demonstrates that team-based care that uses nonphysician providers such as nurses or pharmacists results in greater improvement in glycemic control in patients with chronic diabetes mellitus. It is clear from this study that the expanded use of non-physician health professionals collaborating as a team can improve diabetes outcomes and suggests great potential for various collaborative care models in the care of patients with diabetes mellitus.

From the health care delivery system perspective, patient-centered care in-cludes providing care that is respectful of and responsive to individual pa-tient preferences, needs, and values and ensures that patient values guide all clinical decisions. Although we often think of the health care team as limited to the practitioners themselves, it is clear that involving the patient more di-rectly in their care is an important component of high-quality care. In a sur-vey of physician's attitudes and practices regarding patient-centered care, only 36% of physician providers reported getting feedback from their pa-tients about care plans.[28] Despite progress to date, considerable change must occur before the patient will be routinely embraced as a member of the pa-tient care team. This should remain our goal for diabetes care—to educate and encourage patients to take a more active role in the day-to-day decisions for their care. The additional challenge in rural communities is that many of the patients with diabetes mellitus come from diverse cultures, each of which has unique values and norms regarding food, physical activity, medical care, and medications. Each unique culture presents a different set of challenges for the interprofessional diabetes care management team. For each culture, the appropriate care strategies relating to diet and exercise changes, medication use, and the role of the provider team in care must be translated, modified, or adapted to be both acceptable and effective. Diabetes care team members in rural areas must be trained in culturally sensitive care practices and may require language training as well. As described below, culturally accepted alternative care providers may also play important roles in patient management and can be incorporated into the patient care team. The redesigned care delivery process must accommodate and utilize all these cultural influences to promote improved care outcomes.

Another relatively new member of the health care team is the lay health advisor or promotora. Their specific activities include patient and community education, patient counseling, monitoring patient health status, linking people with health and human services, and enhancing provider patient communication and adherence to care. The value of these individuals has been previously documented.[29,30] Lay health advisors have been successfully used in the management of patients with type 2 diabetes mellitus and have tremendous potential to assist the health care team in improving care outcomes.[29] With adequate training, these individuals have the potential to improve access to and use of needed health care services as well as the adoption and continuation of patient-specific behaviors necessary for disease management. Unfortunately, precious little is known about the nature and content of communications between lay health advisors and an interprofessional health care team.

EASTERN NORTH CAROLINA CHRONIC CARE PILOT PROJECT

Because of the higher prevalence of diabetes mellitus and its complications and the relative lack of published experience with redesigning care delivery for diabetes mellitus in rural communities with traditional fee-for-service practices, the authors piloted a new care delivery process in this rural region of North Carolina. The care delivery outcomes for the project and its feasibility have been previously published.[31,32] In short, the project recruited a rural fee-for-service primary care practice serving predominantly minority patients to act as a feasibility site for improved diabetes care delivery, whereas another similar rural practice served as a control site. Over the period of 6 to 12 months the care delivery processes in the "intervention" rural practice were progressively redesigned as informed by the chronic care model. Staff members were retrained in new roles, and new nonphysician providers were recruited and used to provide innovative care delivery. Stronger linkages were built with churches and other community entities to encourage self-management support. A patient registry was built using disease management software available in the public domain, and data on diabetic patients were entered and utilized to develop and monitor practice changes. From the registry, a cohort of 112 diabetic patients who were at increased risk for complications due to elevations in either blood glucose, blood pressure, or blood lipids was identified to serve as an outcome measure in this pilot project. A similar cohort was also assembled at the control rural practice.

In the pilot project, in addition to the family physician provider, the following team members were recruited: a nurse, a pharmacist, and a dietitian. Although additional team members, including patients and lay health advisors, might be desirable, this was not feasible for this initial pilot project. Most of these additional nonphysician providers were not readily available in this small rural community; thus the project used a "circuit rider" model in which the team members came to the practice from other communities on an identified day each week. One aspect of the practice's redesigned care delivery process was to proactively schedule the diabetic patients to return for care on these preidentified dates when the team was assembled. On these dates, the interprofessional team members would initially review the diabetes registry and the medical records of patients to be seen and would proactively plan what care was needed for each diabetic patient before the visit. This change alone allowed for tremendous interprofessional collaboration and brought greatly expanded resources to the patient care process, and it was this live synchronous communication among providers that served as the primary activity of the project's interprofessional collaboration. Additional interprofessional collaboration occurred subsequent to the visit in an asynchronous fashion using e-mail and telephone. The team also provided extensive self-management training to patients using a mixture of group visit and individual session structures. The nonphysician providers, particularly the nurse, became efficient chronic care managers and independently saw patients for follow-up once a plan of care had been established by the interprofessional team.

The outcomes of these patients were compared with those from the control practice in which care was unchanged. As detailed by Bray et al.,[31] in the intervention practice, median HbA_{1c} at baseline was $8.2 \pm 2.6\%$ and median

HbA$_{1c}$ at an average follow-up of 11.3 months was 7.1 ± 2.3% (difference 1.1; $p < 0.0001$). In the control practice, median HbA$_{1c}$ increased slightly from 8.3 ± 2.0% to 8.6 ± 2.4% over the same time period. In the intervention practice, 61% of diabetic patients had a reduction in HbA$_{1c}$, whereas the percentage of patients with an HbA$_{1c}$ of less than 7% improved from 32% to 45% ($p < 0.05$). These preliminary findings support the prior work of Litaker et al.,[33] who demonstrated improved clinical outcomes in diabetic patients managed by an interprofessional team consisting of a physician and a nurse practitioner compared with that of a physician alone. The above pilot study extends this work in that it involved four different professions collaborating in an inter-disciplinary fashion and it took place in a rural community without substantial resources. More details on the feasibility of this chronic care model application are available.[32]

The transition from the traditional acute care model for diabetes mellitus to a new model of care delivery such as that described in the chronic care model involves substantial change. This transition to a more shared and interactive interprofessional model of care often requires changes in power, structure, and professional culture.

Power

Interactive models require new definitions of power. First, power must be shared with other professionals and with the patient. This necessitates trust in the patient's role and the professional competency of the other providers. Trust often comes only after a significant amount of time is invested to develop a working relationship. Second, power must be distributed such that staff members assume new and expanded roles/responsibilities depending on patient needs. This requires nurses, physician's assistants, pharmacists, and other nonphysician providers to assume greater responsibility for direct patient care—both collaboratively as a team and independently once a plan of care has been developed. For example, in diabetes care, point of care testing of glycemic control (i.e., HbA$_{1c}$) is becoming more commonplace and is something that office staff can routinely perform under a standing order policy from providers. Likewise, adjustment of medication dosages once the therapy plan has been developed by the team can be independently managed by the pharmacist or nurse care manager. This distributed power allows for the development of a more efficient care model that effectively utilizes the knowledge and skills of multiple providers.

Structure

As demonstrated by Bower et al.,[34] the organizational structure of the practice can influence the processes of care delivery, and the combination of organizational structure and care processes can influence patient outcomes. Team work, designed to replace the traditionally independent nature of health care delivery, is preferred as a more efficient and effective process of care. Composition of the team becomes less a function of traditional professional roles and more a function of patient needs, competency levels of existing personnel, and availability of resources. Models such as the chronic care model that allow for group visits, team interactions, and greater utilization of professional resources is one example of innovative team structure in practice.

Professional Culture

To be effective, transitions must also alter the professional cultures of practice. Interprofessional care processes may be difficult for some rural providers, many of whom may have been trained and acculturated in a more hierarchical model and may have practiced independently for many years. Nevertheless, to achieve transitions in practice, changes in professional culture must be made. The patient must become the focus of the cultural change. A good team has as its first priority meeting the patient's needs. This naturally leads to a greater reliance on evidence-based care. Mutual respect brought about by changes in power and new working relationships achieved through new models of health delivery will gradually shift the culture to one that values interprofessional collaboration.

CONCLUSIONS

Interprofessional patterns of care delivery are effective and are increasingly becoming the norm for the management of patients with diabetes mellitus and other chronic conditions. Their inclusion in redesigned systems of care represents an innovative model that requires a sharing of power, new structures or practice patterns, and a cultural shift away from traditional hierarchical models of care delivery. The authors demonstrated that redesigned systems of care for diabetes mellitus can be successfully established even in underserved rural communities and have great potential to improve outcomes and diminish health disparities.

CHAPTER 17: IMPROVING DIABETES OUTCOMES IN RURAL PRACTICES

REFERENCES

1. Narayan KM, Boyle JP, Thompson TJ, Sorensen SW, Williamson DF. Lifetime risk for diabetes mellitus in the United States. *JAMA.* 2003;290:1884–1890.
2. Wild S, Roglic G, Green A, Sicree R, King H. Global prevalence of diabetes: estimates for the year 2000 and projections for 2030. *Diabetes Care.* 2004;27:1047–1053.
3. UK Prospective Diabetes Study (UKPDS) Group. Intensive blood-glucose control with sulphonylureas or insulin compared with conventional treatment and risk of complications in patients with type 2 diabetes (UKPDS 33). *Lancet.* 1998;352: 837–853.
4. American Diabetes Association. Clinical practice recommendations 2006. *Diabetes Care.* 2006;29(Suppl 1):S4–S42.
5. Ogden CL, Carroll MD, Curtin LR, McDowell MA, Tabak CJ, Flegal KM. Prevalence of overweight and obesity in the United States, 1999–2004. *JAMA.* 2006;295: 1549–1555.
6. Rostand SG, Kirk KA, Rutsky EA, Pate BA. Racial differences in the incidence of treatment for end-stage renal disease. *N Engl J Med.* 1982;306:1276–1279.
7. Lavery LA, Ashry HR, Van Houtum W, Pugh JA, Harkless LB, Basu S. Variation in the incidence and proportion of diabetes-related amputations in minorities. *Diabetes Care.* 1996;19:48–52.
8. Dagogo-Jack S. Ethnic disparities in type 2 diabetes: pathophysiology and implications for prevention and management. *JAMA.* 2003;95:9.
9. Dansky KH, Dirani R. The use of health care services by people with diabetes in rural areas. *J Rural Health.* 1998;14:129–137.
10. McCall DT, Sauaia A, Hamman RF, Reusch JE, Barton P. Are low-income elderly patients at risk for poor diabetes care? *Diabetes Care.* 2004;27:1060–1065.
11. Woodwell DA, Cherry DK. National Ambulatory Medical Care Survey: 2002 summary. *Advance Data.* 2004;346:1–44.
12. Rothman AA, Wagner EH. Chronic illness management: what is the role of primary care? *Ann Intern Med.* 2003;138:256–261.
13. Committee on the Future of Health Care, Institute of Medicine. *Quality Through Collaboration: The Future of Rural Health.* Washington, DC: National Academies Press; 2005. Available at: www.iom.edu. Accessed December 2006.
14. Andrus MR, Kelley KW, Murphey LM, Herndon KC. A comparison of diabetes care in rural and urban medical clinics in Alabama. *J Commun Health.* 2004;29:29–44.
15. Zoorob RJ, Mainous AG. Practice patterns of rural family physicians based on the American Diabetes Association standards of care. *J Commun Health.* 1996;21: 175–182.
16. Toth EL, Majumdar SR, Guirguis LM, Lewanczuk RZ, Lee TK, Johnson JA. Compliance with clinical practice guidelines for type 2 diabetes in rural patients: treatment gaps and opportunities for improvement. *Pharmacotherapy.* 2003;23: 659–665.

17. Coon P, Zulkowski K. Adherence to American Diabetes Association standards of care by rural health care providers. *Diabetes Care.* 2002;25:2224–2229.
18. Porterfield DS, Kinsinger L. Quality of care for uninsured patients with diabetes in a rural area. *Diabetes Care.* 2002;25:319–323.
19. Bell RA, Camacho F, Goonan K, et al. Quality of diabetes care among low-income patients in North Carolina. *Am J Prevent Med.* 2001;21:124–131.
20. Massing MW, Henley N, Biggs D, Schenck A, Simpson RJ Jr. Prevalence and care of diabetes mellitus in the Medicare population of North Carolina. Baseline findings from the Medicare Healthcare Quality Improvement Program. *NC Med J.* 2003;64: 51–57.
21. Bodenheimer T. Interventions to improve chronic illness care: evaluating their effectiveness. *Dis Manage.* 2003;6:63–71.
22. Norris SL, Nichols PJ, Caspersen CJ, et al. The effectiveness of disease and case management for people with diabetes. A systematic review. *Am J Prevent Med.* 2002; 22:15–38.
23. Renders CM, Valk GD, Griffin S, Wagner EH, Eijk JtM van, Assendelft WJJ. Interventions to improve the management of diabetes mellitus in primary care, outpatient and community settings. *Cochrane Database of Systematic Reviews.* 2003; 1:1–25.
24. Shojania KG, Ranji SR, McDonald KM, et al. Effects of quality improvement strategies for type 2 diabetes on glycemic control: a meta-regression analysis. *JAMA.* 2006;296:427–440.
25. Wagner EH. Chronic disease management: what will it take to improve care for chronic illness? *Eff Clin Pract.* 1998;1:2–4.
26. Piatt GA, Orchard TJ, Emerson S, et al. Translating the chronic care model into the community. *Diabetes Care.* 2006;29:811–817.
27. Institute of Medicine. *Crossing the Quality Chasm: A New Health System for the 21st Century.* Washington, DC: National Academies Press; 2001.
28. Audet AM, Davis K, Schoenbaum SC. Adoption of patient-centered care practices by physicians: results from a national survey. *Arch Intern Med.* 2006;166:754–759.
29. Fedder DO, Chang RJ, Curry S, Nichols G. The effectiveness of a community health worker outreach program on healthcare utilization of west Baltimore City Medicaid patients with diabetes, with or without hypertension. *Ethnicity Dis.* 2003; 13:22–27.
30. Earp JA, Eng E, O'Malley MS, et al. Increasing use of mammography among older, rural African American women: results from a community trial. *Am J Public Health.* 2002;92:646–654.
31. Bray P, Thompson D, Wynn J, Cummings DM, Whetstone L. Confronting disparities in diabetes care: the clinical effectiveness of redesigning care management for minority patients in rural primary care practices. *J Rural Health.* 2005;21:317–321.
32. Bray P, Roupe M, Young S, Harrell J, Cummings DM, Whetstone LM. Feasibility and effectiveness of system redesign for diabetes care management in rural areas: the eastern North Carolina experience. *Diabetes Educ.* 2005;31:712–718.

33. Litaker D, Mion L, Planavsky L, Kippes C, Mehta N, Frolkis J. Physician–nurse practitioner teams in chronic disease management: the impact on costs, clinical effectiveness, and patients' perception of care. *J Interprofess Care*. 2003;17:223–237.
34. Bower P, Campbell S, Bojke C, Sibbald B. Team structure, team climate and the quality of care in primary care: an observational study. *Qual Saf Health Care*. 2003; 12:273–279.

CHAPTER 18

Developing Health Professional Students into Rural Health Care Leaders of the Future Through Best Practices

Patrick S. Cross, PT, DPT
Joy D. Doll, OTD, OT

INTRODUCTION

People who live in the rural areas are more likely to live in poverty; have higher rates of suicide, mortality, chronic illness, and smoking among those over 12 years old; report fair or poor health status; and have higher self-reported rate of obesity than suburban residents.[1,2] Although people who live in rural areas have increased medical needs, they are less likely to receive recommended preventive services and have fewer number of average visits to a health care provider. Lack of transportation, distance from health care services, shortage of health care professionals, and individuals being less likely to have employer health insurance or obtain Medicaid, if eligible, contribute to why individuals in rural areas do not receive needed services.[2] Community health promotion and interprofessional collaboration may be effective strategies to extend scarce resources and meet the needs of rural communities.

Sociomedical Versus Biomedical Models

To adequately address the prevalence of chronic disease and substantial health issues, a community-based approach, exploring all the factors influencing the health of the community members, may be effective. Gahimer and Morris[3] support this notion (p. 440):

> *Changes in population characteristics, lifestyles, environmental factors, and health disorders have altered the leading causes of death and illness. Concerns of government policy makers about growing cost of health care have prompted restructuring and reorientation of the system toward one that focuses on community and health promotion.*

A community-based approach to health care requires professionals to think outside the traditional biomedical model and consider a social approach to provision of health care. In the social model, focus moves away from the authority of health care professionals and concentrates on health promotion and holistic care of the person and community. To maximize outcomes, care is comprehensive and the client or community representatives may be a crucial member of the team. A multitude of factors, including socioeconomic status, biological factors, health habits, lifestyles, social relationships, psychological traits, safety, availability of transportation, culture, access to medical care, and the physical and social environments, may influence the health status of an individual or a community. Through prevention and promotion of health, wellness, and fitness, risk factors that lead to disablement may be modified.[4] In a community facing high levels of poverty, community members' most immediate needs, such as acquiring food and shelter, may take priority over traditional health care. If this is the case, then the health care team may consider that immediate issues take precedence to chronic disease management and overall wellness.

The fourth report of the PEW Health Professions Commission[5] identified 21 competencies for health professionals for the 21st century, with eight areas that focus on community-based and interprofessional care (Table 18-1). Goal one of Healthy People 2010 calls health care professionals to "help individuals of all ages increase life expectancy and improve their quality of life."[6] The U.S. Department of Health and Human Services[6] acknowledges that health disparities exist based on geographical location, which includes rural populations, and that the health care systems should set a goal to eliminate such disparities. In areas that are underserved, such as rural communities, quality of care has become an issue based on the barriers to receiving care. The Institute of Medicine[7] identified core competencies for increasing patient care, including providing patient-centered care and health care professionals providing care through interdisciplinary teams.

Table 18-1. Community-Based and Interprofessional Related Health Professional Competencies[5]

- Improving access to health care for those with unmet health needs

- Relationship-centered care with individuals and families

- Partnering with communities in health care decisions

- Working in interdisciplinary teams

- Practicing preventive care

- Integrating population-based care and services into practice

- Ensuring care balances individual, professional, system, and societal needs

- Being advocates for public policy that promotes and protects the public's health

Adapted from O'Neil EH. *Recreating Health Professional Practice for a New Century.* San Francisco: PEW Health Professions Commission; 1988.

Community-based work often calls care professionals to a higher level of duty and a commitment to bettering the community. This call is not only rooted in professional duty but also a sense of social justice[8] and moral action in response to injustice. To address the broad influences on the community health status, the health care team must work and communicate together and promote patient-centered care. The term *interdisciplinary*, or *interprofessional*, denotes more than just multiple disciplines—"the different disciplines strive for some form of mutual understanding, knowledge, and awareness in pursuit of common goals or objectives"[9] (p. 13). Traditionally, interprofessional models of health care delivery function under the following assumptions: (a) community capacity building is a basic need, (b) community capacity building requires a social approach to health care and an interprofessional team of health care providers, (c) community solutions should be both need based and asset based recognizing the community's health issues holistically, and (d) heightened interprofessional competence comes from working at relationships over time.[8] According to Charles and associates,[10] "The consequences of not working well together are often more severe in rural centers" (p. 41).

Any community trying to address widespread health issues must recognize that it takes a significant commitment, and interprofessional models of health care delivery develop over time through considerable planning and sustained efforts. For this type of model to be successful, each member of the team must first commit to self-awareness, which includes knowledge of the extent of their practice areas and how they work with others on the team.[8] Communication also needs to be open and honest for the health care team to function successfully.

EDUCATIONAL DESIGN

Cleary and Howell[11] surveyed academic institutions in the United States with both entry-level physical therapy and occupational therapy programs. Of the surveys returned, it was noted that 67% of physical and occupational therapy students who attend the same university take classes together, but most of the interdisciplinary education occurs in the basic science courses, with few contacts taking place during clinical experiences.[11] Hamilton, Smith, and Butters[12] did a survey of medical schools in the United States. The researchers found that 87.2% of medical schools had some type of rural training or public service, but only 21.2% of medical schools had an interdisciplinary student team experience.[12]

To prepare students to practice in rural settings, curriculums should be designed that integrate interprofessional student learning experiences into multiple aspects of the curriculum. Success depends on consistent collaboration across involved health disciplines as well as administrative support. Beyond the basic science courses, an interprofessional curriculum could include the development of community-based and interprofessional practice skills,[13–15] rural health issues,[13] cultural considerations,[13] as well as journaling[10] or reflective exercises, which aid students in developing a profound understanding of their personal beliefs, culture, and discipline,[16] before community integration. An instrument like the Readiness for Interprofessional Learning Scale is an appropriate tool for assessing both professional and student readiness to engage in interprofessional education.[17]

Class discussions, small group discussions, team assignments, presentations, learning modules, case studies, and grand rounds that illustrate the integration of clinical, interdisciplinary, and rural contexts in patient care are modes that may be used to promote interprofessional development.[13] An example of the use of case studies to promote the initial stages of collaboration and increase knowledge about other disciplines is described below.

Exemplar

According to a letter from Joy Karges, PT, EdD, MS, in January 2007, at the University of South Dakota, an interdisciplinary workshop, consisting of students from 12 medical and health science departments (audiology, alcohol and drug abuse studies, dental hygiene, dietetics, health care administration, medicine, nursing, occupational therapy, physical therapy, physician assistant studies, social work, and speech-language pathology) has been conducted annually since 1999. During the workshop, students are divided into interprofessional teams. Each member of the team fills out a preworkshop questionnaire that determines how much knowledge each student has about the services each of the different disciplines represented provides, as well as how comfortable each student is in representing his or her own discipline. The teams are given medial charts, with past medical history and laboratory values, for two patients. Faculty members simulate each clinical case within these small group settings. For each case, the team has 45 minutes to review the chart and conduct an interview of the client. This is followed by a 30-minute care planning meeting. Then the team meets again with the client, provides recommendations, and develops a patient-centered plan of care. Feedback related to the process and discipline specific recommendations is provided by the faculty member following each case. The workshop concludes with students completing a postworkshop questionnaire, similar to the initial survey, and a form assessing the workshop.

Once basic skills are established and students have an understanding of their values, beliefs, and profession, as well as background knowledge of other disciplines, community-based engagement experiences can occur. It has been suggested that an effective strategy for training students is to conduct educational activities in a variety of settings using various strategies.[18] Although various settings and strategies may be used, Slack and colleagues[19] examined five interdisciplinary rural health training programs, in various parts of the country, participating in the Quentin N. Burdick Grant Program. Despite the differences in populations served, locations, and represented disciplines, similarities existed among the programs, including student assessment of community needs, interaction with community professionals and residents, educational support for students, and inclusion of both clinical and community-based activities.[19] One successful academic–community partnership that was supported by interdisciplinary rural health training grants is highlighted in the Exemplar section at the end of the chapter.

Obstacles

Multiple obstacles must be overcome to provide meaningful experiences. Because of multiple disciplines being involved, barriers related to establishing a common goal,[20] differences in program structures and philosophies,[9,11] scheduling conflicts,[9,10,13,21] teaching loads,[9] student learning needs,[9] and department expectations[10,11] may exist and need to be addressed. Academic institutions need to develop and support infrastructure for interprofessional education that can address the potential barriers.[10,22] This may include an office or a committee that specifically addresses the complexities of interprofessional education. At first, the initiation of planning meetings and development of infrastructure may be costly but is critical to the success of a program.[10]

It is also essential that educational experiences and projects are molded around community-identified needs.[13,14,19] The academic institution and community must concur on the essential factors, including goals, responsibilities, and funding. Once an agreement is established, site, faculty, and preceptor preparation, as well as on-site coordination, must occur. Housing in the community is important because it allows team bonding and informal discussion between students[10] and allows students to feel part of and gain a better understanding of the community. Expectations and roles of all individuals involved is essential.[13] Preceptor training may better prepare individuals for students.[10] Modeling is especially important for students as "medical students contemplating practice location, real world clinical experiences and role models facilitate decision-making"[23] (p. 113).

There also needs to be faculty incentives and recognition, especially in relation to promotion and tenure, for community-based work.[16,18,22] The recognition should not only be made by educational institutions but also by professional associations and educational accrediting bodies.[24] Some academic institutions have begun to recognize the value of scholarship of engagement, identified by Ernest Boyer,[25] which has been defined by the National Review Board as "academically relevant work that simultaneously meets campus mission and goals as well as community needs."[26] Typically, developing an academic–community partnership needed to implement scholarship of engagement is demanding, taking time to develop relationships and understand community needs.[27–29] This process is only further complicated when student learning is involved.

Funding can also be an issue but is imperative because institutions may not prioritize monies for service learning and without allocating resources needed to conduct activities, including transportation and supplies, the project may not be able to prosper. Obtaining external funding not only aids in accomplishing objectives and assisting the community, but also serves as a means for faculty scholarship. Recently, Congress has cut funding for interprofessional student training grants. Students, faculty, professional organizations, and members of communities need to inform policymakers in private foundations, government, and academic institutions about budgetary limitations associated with implementing community-based programming.[24]

Benefits

Effective campus–community partnerships and interprofessional experiences can benefit the community, clients, practitioners, students, and academic institutions. Communities benefit through the extension of cost-effective delivery of professional services and health promotion activities that address the health concerns of the community.[15,21,30] Parallel to this, clients benefit from having increased services by having previously unmet needs fulfilled and optimizing their care. In addition, the relationship aids in the recruitment of health professionals in the area,[10,19,23] and provides educational opportunities for professionals, staff, and community members.[15] The increased opportunity for contact with faculty at academic institutions reduces the isolation of rural practitioners, which ultimately benefits the clients.[19] A partnership can also help a community receive external funding for projects through using the skills and resources of academic institutions and their faculty.

Students also benefit from the relationship, much more than just adding an activity to a resume. Through a comprehensive interprofessional curriculum, with both didactic and community integration components, students have the ability to enhance cognitive and affective skills and develop a unique skill set that will improve patient care (Table 18-2).

The university or higher education institution benefits from campus–community partnerships. Often, this is through positive publicity and increased relations with the community. Individuals are seen as members of their respective institutes and professions. This may serve as a recruitment tool for individuals from that area and even individuals from outside the area whose family or friends may live in the community where the partnership exists. Dissemination of information from the partnership, through scholarly publications and presentations, as well as funding of grants, brings prestige to an academic institution. The availability of unique experiences and research is an attractive tool for recruiting students. Finally, interprofessional learning may be a cost-effective mechanism for a higher education institute. Faculty resources and classrooms may be shared, instead of paying multiple instructors to teach essentially the same information but within various departments.

Table 18-2. Health Care Skills Enhanced Through Community-Engagement Experiences

Cognitive	Affective
• Knowledge of the roles of other professions[10,11,30] and interprofessional collaboration[8,13,31]	• Appreciation for own and other professions[10]
• Generalist and primary care skills, including advanced clinical reasoning and differential diagnosis skills[10,21,23,31]	• Flexibility with time management[31]
	• Cultural sensitivity[13,31]
• Understanding of the disablement process[31]	• Verbal and nonverbal communication skills with patients[13,31] and other professionals[11]
• Ability to analyze and assess community needs, organizations, and skills[13,31]	• Ethical foundation of social and distributive justice,[21] patient advocacy,[21,31] and moral agency[14,21]
• Program development based on community needs[14]	• Self-reflection
• Ability to identify and apply ways to work with scarce resources[13,14]	
• Patient education, behavior change, and adherence facilitation[14]	
• Disease prevention and health promotion[10,14]	
• Understanding of public health focus[11]	
• Knowledge about various cultures	

Exemplar

In 1994 a representative from the Omaha Tribe sought assistance for the provision of rehabilitation services to Native Americans being served at the Winnebago Public Service Hospital in Winnebago, Nebraska, which serves both the Omaha and Winnebago Tribes. Creighton University was approached and agreed to provide physical therapy services twice a month. With the need and demand for physical therapy services, twice a month was not sufficient. To increase services a Health Resources and Services Administration (HRSA) grant was written to fund a full-time position and incorporate student learning in the rural and culturally rich Native American communities. At this time, student groups of physical and occupational therapy students began participating in service-learning activities in the communities.

Since that time, the partnership between the tribes and Creighton University has grown and faced many accomplishments and challenges. Today, both physical therapy and occupational therapy services are sustained by the communities themselves, including two physical therapists and one occupational therapist. Three additional HRSA grants were written to sustain the projects and added the inclusion of pharmacy, nursing, and medicine into the student learning experiences. In 2001, the Office of Interprofessional Scholarship, Service and Education (OISSE) was formed, within the Creighton University School of Pharmacy and Health Professions, and established an infrastructure for maintaining the partnership, organizing the expanded student training, and promoting collaboration in scholarship.

Directed by a group of core faculty from the disciplines of physical therapy, occupational therapy, pharmacy, and nursing, the OISSE coordinates all outreach and student training in the rural communities. Students are offered multiple levels of opportunities to allow them a multitude of opportunities to learn about both the rural and cultural aspects of health in these communities (Table 18-3). These levels of opportunities allow students to continue to be involved with the communities and grow in their involvement throughout their professional academic careers.

Table 18-3. Student Opportunities Through the Office of Interprofessional Scholarship, Service and Education

Student Opportunity	Disciplines	Description
Service learning	• OT • PT • Pharmacy • Nursing	Students across the health sciences can choose a variety of activities in the Native communities to meet service learning requirements • Leading exercise courses • Educational presentations • Health screenings • Health promotion projects • Physical activity with youth • Health careers education

(Continues)

Table 18-3. Student Opportunities Through the Office of Interprofessional Scholarship, Service and Education *(Continued)*

Student Opportunity	Disciplines	Description
Classroom activities	• OT • PT • Pharmacy • Nursing • Medicine	Faculty wanting to include the Native American communities in course projects can do so. Examples include • Educational presentations • Health care training • Community assessments • Data analysis • Health promotion planning and implementation
Community-based participatory research projects	• OT • PT • Pharmacy • Nursing • Medicine	Include a variety of activities • School health screenings • Quality assurance projects
Native American immersions	• OT • PT • Pharmacy • Nursing	Three-day immersions into the health and culture of the Omaha and Winnebago Tribes. Activities include • Interprofessional case studies • Clinical observation • Health care team discussion • Cultural activities • Community health outreach projects
Native American special interest group	• OT • PT • Pharmacy • Nursing	Service activities organized by an interprofessional group of students interested in outreach to Native American communities. Students must have done prior activities with the community to participate in group.
Culturally driven courses	• Pharmacy • PT • OT	Two courses have been developed and implemented focused on Native American culture both including community immersions.
Clinical experiences	• OT • PT • Pharmacy • Nursing	Ranging from 1 to 12 weeks Students are encouraged to live in the community to fully experience the culture and health care issues

OT, occupational therapy; PT, physical therapy.

Through reflection and journaling, students who completed activities through the OISSE valued the experience and noted development in the cognitive, affective, and psychomotor domains of learning. Since 2000, over 930 students from across the disciplines of medicine, nursing, pharmacy, physical therapy, and occupational therapy have participated in community experiences in the Native American communities. Students complete online pre- and postreflections regarding culture, interprofessionalism, and their overall experience with the underserved communities. The mixture of quantitative and qualitative surveys used by the OISSE demonstrate an impact from these experiences, including a significant impact on students' thoughts on culture and a future career with an underserved population (Table 18-4).

The Omaha and Winnebago Tribes of Nebraska have recruited Creighton University graduates to work at their facilities, including occupational therapists, physical therapists, pharmacists, and a nurse practitioner. Many of these individuals completed service-learning experiences, research, and/or clinical affiliations on the tribal lands through OISSE. In addition, one-third of surveyed graduates who completed a service-learning activity sponsored by OISSE- and/or HRSA-funded projects have practiced or are currently practicing in a rural setting or with an underserved population.

The professional and paraprofessional staff have also benefited from in-services and services provided by Creighton University students, including transfer training for nursing assistants, athletic taping in-services, presentations to wellness staff on exercising with various populations safely and effectively, assistance with youth health screenings, workstation ergonomic assessments, and community-based participatory research projects. In addition, professionals and administrators have had the opportunity to collaborate with individuals in the academic setting to disseminated scholarship through publications and presentations at regional, national, and international conferences.

Most importantly, the community has benefited through patient care being optimized through a more comprehensive approach to client care, with the client as a member of the team, through interventions initiated, such as the Omaha Tribe's Diabetes Program's interprofessional diabetes management critical pathway which was designed by tribal employees in collaboration with students and faculty from Creighton University. In addition, the community has benefited from assistance in applying for grants and from collaborative interventions that meet the needs and desires of the community,

Table 18-4. Student Reflections from Rural, Interdisciplinary Training

Discipline	Reflection
Nursing	"I enjoyed this experience and learned many amazing things about the Native American culture that I was not aware of. I feel that this is an experience that every health care professional should complete before moving into the real world of working. It is an opportunity that I feel honored to have had this year." "I definitely loved this experience. I was able to do a lot of hands-on activities with patients and was able to get to know them, even for only 3 weeks, very well. I was able to connect with many of them at a deeper level and really feel as if I were doing more than just 'fixing their problem.'"
Pharmacy	"I really enjoyed this experience and learned a lot. I liked it because I got a better understanding of not only my profession, but also the professions of nursing, PT [physical therapy], and OT [occupational therapy]. It showed me how important communication between all of the disciplines is in the well-being of the patient. I also got to see one area that I could possibly go into after graduation (the IHS [Indian Health Service]), which was nice to start to see my options as a pharmacist." "Wow. This experience was absolutely amazing. Seeing interdisciplinary care in person, in practice was wonderful. It was so refreshing to see that this is practiced, not just something I read about in my textbooks."
Physical therapy	"I felt that the experience was worthwhile; it was challenging, rewarding, inter-professional, and an immersion experience. The 'Case Studies' component offered the several disparate professions an opportunity to see what each profession had to offer the 'client.' The exercise gave us the opportunity to exchange ideas, question practices, and form good peer relationships." "I felt that this experience was incredibly beneficial. I learned a great deal about the Native American community including their rituals, lifestyle, and challenges/barriers individuals of this culture face on a day-to-day basis. I truly believe that this experience has helped me become a more culturally sensitive healthcare professional. I am much more aware of the cultural biases that I may have previously held and my eyes have been opened to a culture with which I had very little previous experience."

Table 18-4. Student Reflections from Rural, Interdisciplinary Training *(Continued)*

Discipline	Reflection
Occupational therapy	"These experiences offer students an opportunity to interact in a substantive manner with other medical professionals. Partnering with the rehab staff to conduct patient evaluations, organizing and running community events around health issues respective to the cultural health issues, and reading the pre-experience materials to gain valuable information, all culminated into an exceptional educational experience for me." "I felt that this experience was great! It allowed me to interact with other disciplines and learn how we are different and similar. This in turn will lead to future team development to ensure that the patients' best interest and safety is at hand."

such as weight management and exercise programs, on-the-field sport injury management, exercise videos, health professions education, substance abuse prevention activities, and assistance with health care delivery, including school screenings and physicals.

CONCLUSIONS

A strong academic–community partnership that incorporates best practices, including immersion of students into rural communities, interprofessional collaboration, and community health promotion activities that are driven by community need, can extend scarce resources, improve care of patients, facilitate higher levels of cognitive and affective skills in students, encourage collaboration of professionals, and promote future practice in underserved, rural settings.

REFERENCES

1. Blumenthal S, Kagen J. The effects of socioeconomic status on health in rural and urban America. *JAMA*. 2002;287:109.
2. National Rural Health Association. Health disparities in rural populations: an introduction. National Rural Health Association website. Available at: http://www.nrharural.org/advocacy/sub/policybriefs/HlthDisparity.pdf. Accessed June 13, 2006.

 3. Gahimer J, Morris DM. Community health education: evolving opportunities for physical therapists. In: Shepard KF, Jensen GM, eds. *Handbook of Teaching for Physical Therapists*, 2nd ed. Boston: Butterworth-Heinemann; 2002:440.
 4. American Physical Therapy Association. On what concepts is the guide based? *Guide to Physical Therapist Practice*, 2nd ed. Alexandria, VA: American Physical Therapy Association; 2003:15–25.
 5. O'Neil EH. *Recreating Health Professional Practice for a New Century*. San Francisco: PEW Health Professions Commission; 1988.
 6. U.S. Department of Health and Human Services. What are its goals. Healthy People 2010 website. Available at: http://www.healthypeople.gov/About/goals. htm. Accessed June 10, 2006.
 7. Institute of Medicine. *Health Professions Education: A Bridge to Quality*. Washington, DC: National Academy Press; 2003.
 8. Jensen GM, Royeen CB. Improved rural access to care: dimensions of best practice. *J Interprof Care*. 2002;16:117–128.
 9. Cloonan P, Davis F, Burnett C. Interdisciplinary education in clinical ethics: a work in progress. *Holist Nurs Pract*. 1999;13:12–19.
10. Charles G, Bainbridge L, Copeman-Stewart K, Art S, Kassam R. The Interprofessional Rural Program of British Columbia (IRPbc). *J Interprof Care*. 2006;20:40–50.
11. Cleary KK, Howell DM. The educational interaction between physical therapy and occupational therapy students. *J Allied Health*. 2003;32:71–77.
12. Hamilton C, Smith C, Butters J. Interdisciplinary student health teams: combining medical education and service in a rural community-based experience. *J Rural Health*. 1997;13:320–328.
13. Lilley SH, Clay M, Greer A, Harris J, Cummings HD. Interdisciplinary rural health training for health professional students: strategies for curriculum design. *J Allied Health*. 1998;27:208–212.
14. Cochran TM, Jensen GM, Gale JR, et al. Practice and educational innovation: revision of rehabilitation roles to extend scarce resources in a rural community. Poster presented at the National Rural Health Conference, Reno, Nev., May 19–21, 2006.
15. Cross P, Voltz JD, Parker D, et al. Community-collaboration: defeating diabetes and transforming students into caring professionals. Poster presented at the Center for Disease Control Diabetes and Obesity Conference, Denver, Colo., May 17–18, 2006.
16. Harris DL, Henry RC, Bland CJ, Starnaman SM, Voytek KL. Lessons learned from implementing multidisciplinary health professions education models in community settings. *J Interprof Care*. 2003;17:7–20.
17. Reid R, Bruce D, Allstaff K, McLernon D. Validating the Readiness for Interprofessional Learning Scale (RIPLS) in the postgraduate context: are health care professionals ready for IPL? *Med Educ*. 2006;40:415–422.
18. Miller BK, Ishler KJ. The rural elderly assessment project: a model for interdisciplinary team training. *Interprof Collab Occup Ther*. 2001;15:13–34.
19. Slack M, Cummings D, Borrego M, Fuller K, Cook S. Strategies used by interdisciplinary rural health training programs to assure community responsiveness and recruit practitioners. *J Interprof Care*. 2002;16:129–138.

20. Lowry L, Burns C, Smith A, Jacobson H. Compete or complement? An interdisciplinary approach to training health professionals. *Nurs Health Care Perspect.* 2000; 21:76-80.

21. Gale J, Cochran T, Wilken M, Cross P, Parker D, Voltz J. Community-based primary care: a model for practice. Poster presented at All Together Better III, London, England, April 10–12, 2006.

22. Cochran TM, Jensen GM, VanLeit B, Daniels Z, Cummings D, Voltz JD. Educating health professionals for the 21st century. Presented at the National Rural Health Conference, Reno, Nev., 2006.

23. Rabinowitz HK, Paynter N. The rural vs. urban practice decision. *JAMA.* 2002; 287:113.

24. Brashers VL, Curry CE, Harper DC, McDaniel SH, Pawlson G, Ball JW. Interprofessional health care education. *Iss Interdisc Care.* 2001;3:21–31.

25. Boyer, EL. *Scholarship Reconsidered: Priorities of the Professoriate.* New York: Jossey-Bass; 1990.

26. Clearinghouse and National Review Board for Scholarship of Engagement. Frequently asked questions. Available at: http://schoe.coe.uga.edu/about/FAQs.html. Accessed February 8, 2007.

27. Fogel SJ, Cook JR. Consideration on the scholarship of engagement as an area of specialization for faculty. *J Social Work Educ.* 2006;42:595–606.

28. O'Meara KA. Encouraging multiple forms of scholarship in faculty reward systems: does it make a difference? *Res Higher Educ.* 2005;45:479–510.

29. Huyser MA. Faculty perceptions of institutional commitment to the scholarship of engagement. *J Res Christian Educ.* 2005;13:251–285.

30. Lough MA, Schmidt K, Leshan L. An interdisciplinary service learning program promotes collaborative health care. *Nat Acad Pract Forum.* 1999;1:255–261.

31. Cross PS, Cochran TM, Lohman M. Therapy roles in a Native American culture—a qualitative study. Platform presentation at the American Physical Therapy Association Combined Sections Meeting, Nashville, Tenn., January 4–8, 2004.

CHAPTER 19

Interprofessional Education and Multicultural and Community Affairs

Omofolasade "Sade" Kosoko-Lasaki, MD, MSPH, MBA

INTRODUCTION

Traditionally, interprofessional education and collaboration of health workers is challenging and difficult to achieve. The highly sophisticated but seemingly fragmented health care system in the United States today is unlikely to address future needs for the country. New health care systems require paradigms of collaboration and partnership within and outside the "normal" confines of health care. The integration of multiple professional competencies and the lessons learned from developing countries, with very scarce resources, can be transposed to the health care needs of rural and poor communities in the United States. In this chapter, discussion focuses on some of the lessons learned in interprofessional collaboration in a Jesuit University and how this, together with personal skills and experience in the practice of rural medicine in developing countries, has inspired the development of an interprofessional curriculum that, hopefully, will help the students in the health professions schools to appreciate and provide care for the less fortunate in rural and poor diverse communities.[1]

BACKGROUND

Creighton University (CU), founded in 1878, is a private, Jesuit, comprehensive university located in Omaha, Nebraska. CU's mission is guided by the fundamental philosophy of education through service, caring, and community. CU is dedicated to the pursuit of truth in all its forms and is guided by the living tradition of the Catholic Church. As Jesuit, CU participates in the tradition of the Society of Jesus which provides an integrating vision of the world that arises out of a knowledge and love of Jesus Christ. This mission guides CU in preparing students for lives of service, professional distinction, and personal fulfillment. Further, CU is committed to providing an environment that recognizes and appreciates the value of cultural diversity and promotes the well-being and success of all persons.

In celebrating CU's 125th anniversary, the University established strategic objectives[2] that include fostering an inclusive and diverse human community of students, faculty, and staff. Embracing service, caring, and community has allowed CU to cultivate a culture of success as a regionally dominant and nationally prominent institution.

Creighton's Health Sciences is made up of the Schools of Medicine, Dentistry, Pharmacy and Health Professions (Occupational Therapy and Physical Therapy), and Nursing. Each school is unique in characteristics with its own mission statement and governance. The leadership for each school is under the auspices of a dean. The Dean of the School of Medicine also serves as the Vice President of Health Sciences.

The School of Medicine's mission is "To improve the human condition through excellence in educating students, physicians and the public, advancing knowledge and providing comprehensive patient care." The School of Dentistry's mission is "To educate students who can demonstrate the attainment of competence and the progression toward proficiency in providing for the oral health needs of society." Creighton's School of Pharmacy and Health Professions (Occupational Therapy and Physical Therapy) focuses on preparation of practitioners who perform patient-centered care while advancing knowledge, promoting justice, and embracing change. Finally, CU School of Nursing offers value-centered educational programs that provide opportunities and guidance for students to develop their intellectual, spiritual, and physical potential and to master the knowledge and skills necessary to practice professional nursing.

In 2000 the Office of Health Sciences Multicultural and Community Affairs (HS-MACA; www.creighton.edu/hsmaca/) was created at CU under the direct supervision of an Associate Vice President for Health Sciences. This Office has a mission to empower CU in the training and development of future leaders for an increasingly multicultural society. HS-MACA provides support and retention services to students by providing diversity awareness to the entire campus community. HS-MACA serves as the critical structure that facilitates collaboration across the independent and complex health professions schools. The office promotes minority affairs through recruiting and retaining disadvantaged students in the CU Health Sciences Schools. HS-MACA also promotes local involvement in multicultural communities, civic functions, and community service organizations. HS-MACA coordinates multicultural activities with other areas of the University and works to enhance cultural awareness of Health Sciences faculty, students, and staff. HS-MACA also ensures that all students matriculating in the health profession schools at CU achieve a satisfactory level of academic performance and graduate with the goal of better serving the needs of an increasingly diverse U.S. population.

Success of HS-MACA

The successful implementation of HS-MACA, an office that serves as a bridge for all the health professions schools, is centered around its mission statement that evolves from that of the university that it serves. In addition, leadership is provided by the Associate Vice President, an African-American physician who has practiced in rural and poor countries in West Africa, the Caribbean, and Asia and, who is compassionate about reducing disparities in health care and facilitates discussions with faculty, students, and staff in all the schools. Finally, the culturally diverse staff in HS-MACA promotes the desired networking with all the health science schools and the rest of the university and builds linkages with the community that Creighton serves.

Need for Health Care Professionals in Nebraska

The City of Omaha has a population of 390,007 and ranks as the nation's 44th largest city. Within a 50-mile radius of Omaha are more than 1 million people, five designated health professional shortage areas, and 35 census tracts that are designated medically underserved areas. The total minority population base in Omaha is approximately 83,930 individuals. Revised 2000 Census estimates show the demographics of Douglas County, of which Omaha provides the population base, to be close to that of the United States as a whole: 78.4% White, 13.3% Black, 7.5% Hispanic, 1.7% Asian, and 0.7% Native American. Whereas the Black, Hispanic, and Native American populations represent 22.5% of the population, the ratio of underrepresented minority health care providers is dramatically lower. The need for underrepresented minority health care providers in Douglas County, of which Omaha is the largest city, is critical (Table 19-1). Black, Native American, and Hispanic physicians represent less than 4% of the

Table 19-1. Health Care Professionals in Omaha/Douglas County

Job Title	Douglas County	State of Nebraska
Primary care physicians	1,086	1,948
Registered nurses	5,889	18,680
Physical therapists	378	1,017
Occupational therapists	223	557
Dentists	392	1,110
Pharmacists	747	1,882

Source: The Nebraska Department of HHS, Nebraska Health Information Project, 2005 Data Book.

total (Table 19-2). Similarly, Black, Native American, and Hispanic nurses represent less than 3% of the total. Underrepresented minorities are dramatically absent from health care professions in the Omaha metropolitan area.

HS-MACA's Programs Addressing Health Disparities

HS-MACA's programs have demonstrated that different health professional perspectives enhance the learning environment for everyone and benefit students, staff, and faculty by advancing a variety of educational outcomes. The programs promote cross-cultural understanding and expose the interprofessional students to common goals and values critical to the health professions, particularly those based on team work and mentoring in the K–12 programs. We realize that interprofessional health education is not a result but a means of achieving a concrete set of educational objectives and ideology. HS-MACA's programs are periodically reviewed and evaluated. The success of these programs is due to the strong and effective collaborative approach with all the health science schools. Some of the successful collaborative efforts are well detailed in the literature.[3-5] The health science faculty and students continue to work very closely with the "pipeline" students from the 4th grade to the undergraduate schools to develop and encourage interest in the health science professions. In addition, the health professions students' exposure and interactions with the diverse and underserved schools and communities in rural and urban Nebraska will prepare them for

Table 19-2. Ethnicity Breakout of Health Professionals in Nebraska

Health Profession	Asian	African-American	Native American	Hispanic	White	Other/Unknown	Total
Physicians	161	35	4	40	2,508	480	3,228
Physician assistants	4	2	1	2	391	114	514
Dentists	17	4	1	10	823	116	971
Pharmacists	19	3	3	12	1,155	343	1,535
Nurse practitioners	2	2	2	3	298	125	432
Registered nurses	90	103	25	126	11,421	87	11,852
Licensed practical nurses	21	128	24	117	4,529	81	4,900
Total	314	277	60	310	21,125	1,346	23,432

Source: The Nebraska Department of Health and Human Services System, 2006.

clinical practice in the future. Examples of programs that provide this exposure are detailed below.

Health Careers Opportunity Program (HCOP)

Starting with financially and/or educationally disadvantaged students in the seventh grade and proceeding through the high school and college years, "Pipeline to Success at Creighton University" (the HCOP program) shepherds young people through educational activities so they are prepared to handle health professions programs. Seventh and eighth grade students take part in a Health Careers Exploration Club. High school students attend monthly meetings and a 6-week summer program. College students attend a 6-week summer session for three summers. Postbaccalaureate students attend an 8-week diagnostic summer session. CU's Health Professions Schools are partnering on this project with the College of Arts and Sciences and community partners such as the Omaha Public Schools, Boys and Girls Club, and Charles Drew and Indian-Chicano Health Centers. The health professions students lecture the precollegiate students in their science classes, help with science projects, and serve as after school mentors. In addition to encouraging students to pursue health careers, HCOP addresses the health care needs in rural and urban poor areas by educating the students about diseases that may be prevalent in their families. Students who understand this may be able to educate their own families about the prevalence and the prevention of that disease. Every Friday during the summer the academy is devoted to health professions guest speakers that focus on diseases particular to certain ethnic groups. Diabetes, cancer, hypertension, sexually transmitted diseases/acquired immunodeficiency syndrome/human immunodeficiency virus/sudden infant death syndrome, alcoholism, and asthma are topics of discussion with health experts.

Focus on Health Professions

CU and the Omaha Public Schools Office of Gifted Education cosponsor this activity. This program is for students in 7th through 12th grades and is designed to give disadvantaged students information about and opportunities to experience health science careers. Seventh grade minority students are nominated for the program if they show academic aptitude by having a California Achievement Test score at the 85% level or above and express an interest in a health professional career. The health professions students volunteer in the classrooms in both rural and urban poor areas. This experience is very enriching and rewarding for both parties.

Center of Excellence

CU School of Medicine, Center of Excellence is a federally funded program through the U.S. Department of Health and Human Services, Bureau of Health Professions, and Health Resources and Services Administration. The program is a comprehensive approach to solving the problem of underrepresented and disadvantaged persons in the nation's health care workforce. As a result, the number of new underrepresented and disadvantaged students entering CU School of Medicine has steadily grown, and the percentage of minority faculty has also been augmented. Underrepresented and disadvantaged student performance is continually improving due to the Pre-Matriculation Program, a preview of the first year curriculum to increase passing rates, and the Retention and Success Program, personal and academic development courses throughout all 4 years of medical school. Additionally, Center of Excellence objectives include increased faculty development, faculty/student research, and student clinical experience as well as a Minority Health Information Resource Center. The Pre-Matriculation Program has been expanded to include students in the Schools of Dentistry, Pharmacy, and Health Professions. The increase in qualified health professions students will help to address the health disparities that are experienced in rural and urban poor areas in the United States.

HEALTH PROFESSIONS PARTNERSHIP INITIATIVE

CU's four health science schools and undergraduate college, along with other community partners, have collaborated to increase the communication, coordination, and effectiveness. These interprofessional educational collaborations have succeeded in implementing initiatives and programs that increase the academic achievement and the health career preparation of the students to provide much needed health care service in rural and urban poor areas of the country (Table 19-3).

HS-MACA's Experience in Cultural Proficiency Training

The goal of the cultural competency training in all HS-MACA programs is to increase students' understanding of and appreciation and respect for cultural differences and similarities. Specifically, HS-MACA provides students the tools to (a) appreciate their own cultural values and assumptions, (b) recognize their own cultural biases, (c) improve their understanding of

Table 19-3. Summary of HS-MACA Pipeline Activities in Rural and Urban Poor Nebraska

Grades 6–8 Exposure/Investigation	Grades 9–12 Cultivation	Grades 13–16 Motivation	Grade 17 Post-bac	Grades 16–20 Retention
HCOP Health Careers Information activities	HCOP Summer Institute	HCOP Summer Institute	Diagnostic summer session	Professional development seminars
Academic monitoring	HCOP academic year monthly meetings	Summer Research Institute—college	Academic year program	CU mentoring program
Field trips	Summer Research Institute—high school	CU mentoring program	Pre-matriculation summer session	Academic and career counseling
Resource speakers	Academic year Saturday Academy	Financial aid dissemination	Rural clinical outreach opportunities	Tutoring
Hands-on activities	Tutoring	Counseling	Personal Wellness program	Cultural competency seminars/training
Expanding Your Horizons conferences	Focus on Health Professions monthly activities	Social and academic support group activities	CU mentoring program	Other academic support

Parent groups	Financial aid dissemination	Cultural competency opportunities	Counseling support	Outreach opportunities
EPCOR Discovery Program	CU mentoring program	Volunteerism	Scholarship availability	Scholarship/grant opportunities
Cultural competency development	Community volunteerism	Tutoring	Tutoring	Common ground presentations
	Cultural competency development	Cultural competency development	Cultural competency development	Cultural competency development
				Community-oriented primary care research opportunities COE Summer Research

multiculturalism in the United States, (d) increase their knowledge of cultural perspectives as related to the health professions, and (e) develop the skills necessary to prepare them for culturally competent health professions practice in urban and rural communities in the United States.[6]

Middle school students are often unaware of the differences in beliefs, values, and customs of diverse populations. To develop their awareness, issues related to cultural competence is incorporated into the curriculum of the Health Careers Exploration Club in our HCOP program. Students are led in discussions and activities in the classroom to discover personal predisposition and bias. They participate in discussions about being left out and empathizing with others.

The cultural competency training component for high school students includes didactic sessions on cultural diversity; incorporation of cultural competency issues into the overall curriculum at monthly HCOP meetings, including discussions about the cultural practices in the Omaha community that would be a barrier to seeking good health care in rural and urban communities; and field trips to Black History Celebration events, Hispanic Awareness activities, Native American Pow Wows, and other events, such as culturally significant plays.

During the HCOP collegiate summer session, students are taught to look for biases that impact health care delivery and to explore differences that may affect that care. During field trips to the local Indian-Chicano Health Center and the Charles Drew Health Center, health care professionals discuss the importance of cultural competence in administering care to a multicultural community. Students discuss and write term papers on their experience with cultural immersion.

The cultural competency training component for postbaccalaureate students includes the following:

1. Self-assessment: All postbaccalaureate students undertake a self-assessment designed to explore issues of prejudice and bias.
2. Didactic sessions: Didactic sessions are held once during the diagnostic summer session, once each semester during the academic program, and once during the Pre-Matriculation Program.
3. Postbaccalaureate program reading group: The participants in this group meet monthly over the noon hour to discuss culturally relevant reading material including articles, poems, and books with cultural themes. An attempt is made to incorporate materials that are relevant to health care, such as Louise Erdrich's *The Bingo Palace* and William Gudykunst

and Young Yun Kim's *Communicating with Strangers: An Approach to Intercultural Communication*. The reading group is facilitated by faculty from Creighton's Department of English.

4. Primary care experiences: All postbaccalaureate students participate in two field trips during the diagnostic summer session—one to the Indian-Chicano Health Center and one to the Charles Drew Health Center. Both centers serve a predominantly underrepresented minority population. Students also participate in physician shadowing experiences monthly during the academic year program at the Charles Drew Health Center. Preceptors are encouraged to discuss culturally relevant issues with the postbaccalaureate students.

5. Diversity panel: Once each June (with students from both the diagnostic summer session and the pre-matriculation summer session) and again in December of each year, a panel of health care providers who represent diverse cultures and religions are formed. All postbaccalaureate program students are required to participate in presentations and discussions with the panel to increase their awareness and sensitivity to cultural issues in health care in rural and urban settings.

Proposed Cultural Proficiency Elective for Health Care Professions Schools

Culturally competent care has become a critical component of successful outcomes in the delivery of health services in rural and urban communities. In addition, health care providers are being judged as individuals and given "grades" and report cards by the patients and their families; therefore it is paramount that we are flexible and sensitive in dealing with individuals whose needs are outside of the mainstream.[7–10]

Although cultural diversity issues in health care might seem beneath the pressing concerns of our highly regulated health care system, in fact they end up being bottom-line issues as well. Individuals from other cultures now compose a large segment of the United States, and many of them live in rural or urban poor areas. In fact, the numbers of underrepresented minorities are growing quickly as demographics shift. To provide the best care for our changing subject base, we need to make important changes in our daily interactions with many patients and, on a more fundamental level, in the training of health care professionals to serve the growing need of diverse multicultural, underserved, and rural communities.[11–17]

To ensure appropriate focus on cultural awareness issues, we propose a 2-week elective for students in all the health professions schools before their exposure to clinical practice. Students will not have clinical responsibilities during this time (see Appendix B).

CONCLUSIONS

Interprofessional education is not a new methodology.[18–23] It is an old paradigm newly defined. The existence of cultural bias, underrepresented minorities, and underserved populations is not a new reality; in fact, the existence of bias in the health professions and in health care delivery has been well documented in the literature. HS-MACA's office and its programs are a comprehensive response to the problem of underrepresentation of economically and/or educationally disadvantaged persons in the nation's health care workforce. This chapter provides several examples of how such an infrastructure can be used to facilitate collaboration across the health professions.

REFERENCES

1. Engel C, Gursky E. Management and interprofessional collaboration. In Leathard A, ed. *Interprofessional Collaboration; From Policy to Practice in Health and Social Care.* Hove, UK: Brunner-Routledge; 2003;44–55.
2. www.creighton.edu/administration/mission
3. Cooney R, Kosoko-Lasaki O, Wilson MR, Slattery B. Proximal versus distal influences on underrepresented minority pursuing health professions careers. *JAMA.* 2006;98:1471–1475.
4. Houtz L, Kosoko-Lasaki O. Creighton University Health Professions Partnership Initiative: results of a successful collaboration. *Acad Med.* 2006;81(Suppl):S28–S31.
5. Houtz LE, Kosoko-Lasaki O. Creighton Collaborative Health Professions Partnership: assessing impact beyond the numbers. *J High Educ Outr Engag.* 2006;11:147–162.
6. Cultural Awareness Seminar for Medical Students. Creighton University Medical Center, Omaha, Nebraska; 2006.
7. Betancourt JR, Like RC. A new framework of care [editorial]. *Patient Care.* 2000;9(special issue):10–12.
8. Carrillo JE, Green AR, Betancourt JR. Cross-cultural primary care: a patient-based approach. *Ann Intern Med.* 1999;130:829–834.
9. National standards on culturally and linguistically appropriate services in health care. *Federal Register.* 2000;65.
10. Tervalon M, Murray-Garcia J. Cultural humility versus cultural competence: a critical distinction in defining physician training outcomes in multicultural education. *J Health Care Poor Underserved.* 1998;9:117–125.

11. Stuart MR, Lieberman JA. *The 15-Minute Hour: Applied Psychotherapy for the Primary Care Physician,* 2nd ed. Westport, CT: Praeger; 1993.

12. Ponterotto JG, Pedersen P. *Preventing Prejudice: A Guide for Counselors and Educators.* Newbury Park, CA: Sage Publications; 1993.

13. Root MPP, ed. *The Multiracial Experience: Racial Borders as the New Frontiers.* Thousand Oaks, CA: Sage Publications; 1999.

14. McAdoo HR, ed. *Family Ethnicity: Strength in Diversity,* 2nd ed. Thousand Oaks, CA: Sage Publications; 1999.

15. Levin SJ, Like RC, Gottlieb JE. ETHNIC: a framework for culturally competent clinical practice. *Patient Care.* 2000;9(special issue):188.

16. Lu FG, Lim RF, Mezzich JE. Issues in the assessment and diagnosis of culturally diverse individuals. In: J. Oldham & M. Riba, eds., *Review of psychiatry* (Vol. 14). Washington, DC: American Psychiatric Press.

17. Goldman RE, Monroe AD, Dube CE. Cultural self-awareness: a component of culturally responsive patient care. *Ann Behav Sci Med Educ.* 1996;3:37–46.

18. Andrulis D. The cultural competence self-assessment guide. In McCullough-Zander K, ed. *Caring Across Cultures: The Provider's Guide to Cross-Cultural Health Care.* Minneapolis, MN: The Center for Cross-Cultural Health, Stanton Publication Services Inc; 1997.

19. Berlin EA, Fowkes WC Jr. Teaching framework for cross-cultural health care. Application in family practice. *West J Med.* 1983;139:934–938.

20. Brach C, Fraser I. Can cultural competency reduce racial and ethnic health disparities? A review and conceptual model. *Med Care Res Rev.* 2000;57(Suppl 1):181–217.

21. Cohen E, Goode TD. *Policy Brief 1: Rationale for Cultural Competence in Primary Health Care.* Washington, DC: Georgetown University Child Development Center, National Center for Cultural Competence; Winter 1999.

22. Helman C. *Culture, Health, and Illness,* 4th ed. Oxford: Butterworth-Heinemann; 2000.

23. Huff RM, Kline MV, eds. *Promoting Health in Multicultural Populations: A Handbook for Practitioners.* Thousand Oaks, CA: Sage Publications; 1999.

CHAPTER 20

Interprofessional Curriculum: Preparing Health Professionals for Collaborative Teamwork in Health Care

Irma Ruebling, MA, PT
Judith H. Carlson, RN, MSN
Karen Cuvar, PhD, RN
Jeanne Donnelly, PhD, MBA, RHIA
K. Jody Smith, PhD, RHIA, FAHIMA
Nina Westhus, PhD, MSN, RN
Rita Wunderlich, PhD, RN

INTRODUCTION

As the health care system and the delivery of health care have become more complex, appropriate collaboration and communication among health professionals is considered increasingly more critical to improve the health of society.[1] An Institute of Medicine report recommends that all organizations engaged in the education of health professionals include training as members of an interprofessional team.[2] In another report, *Recreating Health Professional Practice for a New Century*, the Pew Health Professions Commission included the ability to work in interprofessional teams among the competencies needed by health professionals for the 21st century.[3] Specifically, the report states (p. 39)

Comprehensive care of individuals and populations requires a wide range of knowledge and skills and involves a variety of delivery settings. To assure effective and efficient coordination of care, health professionals must work interdependently in carrying out their roles and responsibilities, conveying mutual respect, trust, support and appreciation of each discipline's unique contributions to health care.

The purpose of this chapter is to describe one institution's (The Edward and Margaret Doisy College of Health Sciences at St. Louis University) development of an interprofessional education curriculum. With the merger of two schools in 2005, the School of Allied Health Professions and the School of Nursing, the development of this curriculum was the result of a strategic initiative to bring health professions programs to work together in the formation of a single college unit. Forty members of the Doisy College of Health Sciences of Saint Louis University, in some meaningful manner, participated in the design, implementation, and assessment of the Doisy College of Health Sciences interprofessional curriculum.

The interprofessional education curriculum consists of a series of five interprofessional courses. Students begin the interprofessional curriculum when they enter their health profession program. An interprofessional faculty team leads an interprofessional mix of students in discussion of issues of common concern in the context of practical cases, observation of and practice in interprofessional collaborative teams, and reflective discussions of the value of the shared expertise in coming to best decisions. The curriculum culminates when students engage in an integrative interprofessional practicum experience. This chapter includes a discussion of four important concerns during curricular design: the nature of interprofessional curriculum, the learner, the learning activities, and the institution.

INTERPROFESSIONAL CURRICULUM

As the importance of interprofessional teams gains greater recognition, the value of the individual patient or client as an active participant in the health care process and, therefore, as a member of the team is demanding more attention.[1] Researchers for Health Canada proposed a conceptual framework, Interprofessional Education for Collaborative Patient-Centered Practice. This framework highlights the interdependence between interprofessional education and learner outcomes and interprofessional practice and patient outcomes.[4] D'Amour and Oandasan describe this "emerging concept" as interprofessionality defined as "the development of a cohesive practice between professionals from different disciplines. It is the process by which professionals reflect on and develop ways of practicing that provides an integrated and cohesive answer to the needs of the client/family/population."[4] These authors further state, "We need to look at education and practice across the professions and how education and practice are interdependent upon each other in order to enhance patient-centered care. Interprofessionality is then an education and practice orientation, an approach to care and education where educators and practitioners collaborate synergistically."[4] The challenging question is, How best can interprofessional competence enhance interprofessional practice in health care settings? Equally important, how best can interprofessional competencies be taught effectively in health professions education in the United States?

An authentic interprofessional curriculum focuses on issues and concerns addressed collaboratively with the patient or client and in common with several professions. It specifies the professional scope of practice that is unique as well as that which overlaps among the professions and seeks to develop the skills of interprofessional teamwork.[5] The goal of an interprofessional education program is to transmit knowledge and skills basic for the development of interprofessional competencies required by interprofessional teams in delivering patient- or client-centered care. This collaborative practice does not occur by good will, intent, desire, or chance alone, and as most commonly implemented, neither does it occur by one health professional teaching an interprofessional mix of students nor by an interprofessional team of teachers teaching the students representing only one health profession.[6] Rather, such collaboration occurs when an interprofessional team of educators deliberately plan and implement courses taught to an interprofessional mix of students in which the learning activities engage the students in working together[7] while focusing on the needs of individuals and society to improve health.

Learner

Important perspectives concerning the learners in the interprofessional education experience can be gleaned from the literature. Students become socialized to the concept of interprofessional team activity when it is included as part of their academic and clinical preparation.[8–11] Several authors have noted that health professionals must have an understanding of the unique work and contributions of the various professions.[12–14] Others have noted that health care professionals often do not work cooperatively and that they know little about the roles of other health professionals.[15,16] The ability to communicate with each other is an essential skill that is facilitated when students from different health disciplines are educated in an interprofessional environment.[17] The various perspectives brought by the individual professions enriches the educational experience and enhances the care of the patient through the effective collaborative skills that can be learned.[18] Oandasan and Reeves summarize the competencies for collaborative health care practice to include knowledge about roles, communication and negotiation skills, trust of another's competence, and respect.[19]

Learning Activities

To support developing communication skills and facilitating the sharing of expertise and values among interprofessional student teams, close attention needs to be paid to the learning activities. Several authors have noted the importance of particular learning activities that contribute to the development of interprofessional competence and collaboration. Activities must include those that engage the students actively in learning[19] and reflection.[20] Case studies, problem-solving activities, and group projects are appropriate.[19] Encouraging informal interaction outside the classroom contributes to development of collaboration.[7,21] Such experiences are included in the interprofessional curriculum. For example, students attend interprofessional grand rounds sessions beginning in their first year in their health professions program as an assignment based in the introductory interprofessional course in which they are enrolled. An interprofessional team of health professions faculty and clinicians present and discuss the particular issues, possible interventions, and desired outcomes. The team demonstrates the particular knowledge and the reliance on other members for information leading to a comprehensive and best decision. The students participate by observations focused through questions provided for their reflection. During the introductory course the students also work in interprofessional teams to develop a consumer education brochure on a health topic of interest to the general public. Students gather informally outside the class time to develop the brochure designed for the general public on a health-related topic. They keep an individual log of the stages of team development as they experience each stage and how each member of the team contributes to the completion of the project. The interprofessional education experience culminates with an interprofessional team experience with a patient or community agency working to overcome an identified need to improve the health condition of the individual or community.

Interprofessional learning experiences are developed around topics of mutual interest and concern. These concerns and interests are highlighted focusing on collective action in which all participate. These interprofessional activities are embedded and integrated in the curriculum of each health profession program.[18] As Hilton and colleagues suggest, early shared learning experiences do not need to be based on clinical knowledge but rather should emphasize collaborative health professions relationships.[22]

Institution

Institutional factors guide the development of the interprofessional curriculum plan. Our institution, Saint Louis University, is a private university under Catholic and Jesuit auspices. The center of the Jesuit mission is educating women and men for and with others. This philosophy embraces the ability to adapt to the changing needs of individuals and society. The 34th General Congregation of the Society of Jesus concluded that

> *Jesuit universities will promote interdisciplinary work; this implies a spirit of cooperation and dialogue among specialists within the university itself and with those of other universities. As a means of serving the faith and promoting justice ... they can discover new perspectives and new areas for research, teaching, and university extension services, by means of which they can contribute to the transformation of society towards more profound levels of justice and freedom.*[23]

The interprofessional education program builds on and supports the knowledge, inquiry, communication, leadership, service, community building, and social justice aspects of the Saint Louis University mission.

The Doisy College of Health Sciences of Saint Louis University includes health profession degree programs in athletic training, clinical laboratory science, cytotechnology, health informatics and information management, nuclear medicine technology, nursing, nutrition, occupational therapy, physical therapy, physician assistant, and radiation therapy. Most health or health-related programs of the Doisy College enroll students as freshmen who continue through to completion of their appropriate entry level professional degree, baccalaureate, masters, or doctorate. An alternative curriculum plan was developed to accommodate health professions programs that enroll entry level students who hold a bachelor degree not in the specific professional program. These students include physician assistant and accelerated nursing from within the Doisy College of Health Sciences and medicine and social work external to the Doisy College. Because of compressed time frames of these programs and necessary scheduling not consistent with the other programs, an alternate, more flexible, modular program, in contrast to the course format, was developed. This format allows these health professions students to have the opportunity to develop the interprofessional competencies that have been identified for the graduates.

Interprofessional education is not an entirely new venture at Saint Louis University. The Center for Interprofessional Education and Research was established over 10 years ago.[24] Various interprofessional activities were established and sustained for 7 to 10 years. The educational activities include an interprofessional course, "Issues in Health Delivery," in which students and faculty from four professions participate; an interprofessional team seminar, which includes nine professions; and several community service learning activities.

A significant precipitating factor in the impetus toward an interprofessional education program was the merger of the School of Nursing and the School of Allied Health Professions to form the Doisy College of Health Sciences. The challenge to Doisy College after the merger of the previously independent School of Nursing and School of Allied Health Professions for the university administration was to work together to enhance the quality of the existing programs and to provide a unique educational offering for the students. A faculty team of volunteers was enlisted to begin developing and extending interprofessional educational possibilities. After an extensive series of summer meetings, the curriculum team presented a report that described and recommended the interprofessional education curriculum. The report addressed, in addition to the curriculum plan, the organizational structure and funding. With the approval of the Dean of the Doisy College, faculty forums were held for discussion of the curriculum plan and identification of concerns of the faculty to be addressed. Concerns included accreditation, heavy-course curricula, and faculty work load.

The faculty who developed the interprofessional education curriculum, with addition of four new members, continues to serve as the oversight body for the implementation of the curriculum; the group is titled the interprofessional teaching and learning team. The team is responsible for forming faculty work groups, primarily with faculty volunteers, to develop the courses and other learning experiences of the program. Each course and interprofessional grand rounds has a work group responsible for developing and implementing the course.

The concerns expressed by the faculty were addressed by the team. The accreditation concern was expressed primarily by nursing and was addressed with the appropriate agencies by presenting the curriculum plan and course descriptions. The interprofessional education curriculum was adopted as a graduation requirement for the College of Health Sciences. An internal paper describing possible options for integrating required interprofessional education courses into the professional curricula was distributed. By the end of the year all programs had integrated the courses into their respective curricula. A flexible reimbursement program for faculty participation in the teaching of the interprofessional curriculum was approved and implemented. The faculty participation policy and procedure allowed faculty to negotiate with their program chair a stipend reimbursement as overload or a payment to the program that could be designated for their professional development.

The Dean of the Doisy College was instrumental in the development of the interprofessional education program by encouraging faculty participation and with presentation of the program to higher administration. The President and Provost have supported this initiative with seed monies for initial planning and development and then identifying interprofessional education as a designated line item in the Doisy College budget. The budget helps to support dedicated faculty and staff and provides reimbursement for faculty teaching, supplies, and travel. Overall, about 50% of the Doisy College faculty has participated at some level in the development and implementation of the interprofessional education curriculum.

THE CURRICULUM PLAN

Interprofessional education is consistent with the mission of Saint Louis University and the values of the health professions. To accomplish its mission, interprofessional education should be embedded throughout the academic and clinical programs. The curriculum plan involves five interprofessional courses that the students must complete. The students enroll in the first course when they enter the health profession program. The program culminates with an interprofessional practicum experience. The students are recognized for the completion of this curriculum with a designation of Certificate in Interprofessional Education.

The interprofessional education curriculum evolved through discussions during a 2-month period at 11 meetings of the curriculum team lasting 2 to 3 hours each. The discussions included review of existing courses that may be of interprofessional nature, review of common content among the health professions programs, the University mission, missions of the various health professions, commonalities among existing curricula within Doisy College and missions, review of literature, expected interprofessional competencies, the entry level degree of the students, and barriers and facilitating factors for interprofessional education.

During this period of discussions, faculty was provided status reports and could give feedback to the team. A report was given to the Dean at the end of the summer with recommendation for endorsing the interprofessional education curriculum. As the concept for the interprofessional education curriculum outlined in the report to the Dean was considered, a series of faculty forums was held to describe the curriculum plan and obtain feedback. On the basis of faculty comments and our conclusions, assumptions were formed that became the premises for the interprofessional education curriculum. The premises helped develop the purpose, themes, student competencies, course development and implementation, and policies under which the interprofessional education curriculum operates. The concept of the interprofessional curriculum was endorsed and planning of courses began. As the course planning became more in-depth, course objectives and content were adjusted but always being true to the interprofessional nature of the course. The components of the curriculum plan is described in terms of definitions, purpose, themes, competencies, courses, and learning activities in relation to the grounding assumptions or premises identified by the faculty.

Definitions

The first task of the planning group was to establish common definitions for interprofessional education and other terminology related to the concept. It was evident that a distinction needed to be articulated between the definition of multiprofessional education and interprofessional education. In general, multidisciplinary education is defined as shared experiences without the expectation of interaction and participative decisions on planning, goals, and designing of the activities. The definition of interprofessional education refers to activities that occur in a setting where there is interaction between students and faculty of different professions to enhance understanding of patient or population conditions and involves joint participation and responsibility for problem-solving and the planning and implementing of activities. The outcomes of the educational process are (a) an articulation of knowledge and demonstration of respect for the role and unique contribution of the health professions and (b) effective practice of skills required for collaborative client-centered teamwork. An interprofessional education curriculum requires that learning experiences have specified objectives and content directly concerning roles of health professionals and teamwork. Learning experiences must be planned within courses and in other situations in which students are interactive and work together in planning, making decisions for resolving some issue, or completing a project. In a multiprofessional education experience the students may encounter the objectives and content of a course but there is no expectation that they interact with each other in discussions or completing assignments for the course.

Interprofessional practice is defined as health care activity that requires the collaborative, interdependent use of shared expertise directed toward a unified purpose of delivering optimal patient care. Collaboration in interprofessional practice is defined as a process of joint decision making among interdependent parties that involves joint ownership of decisions and collective responsibility for outcomes.[25] In multiprofessional practice individuals may request information from each other but not usually with the purpose of discussion about decisions which are made most times unilaterally.

Purpose

A basic premise of the curriculum is the conviction that interprofessional education promotes better patient and client care and that interprofessional practice is best practice. In the development of this curriculum the view is held that interprofessional education is the future of effective delivery of increasingly complex health care. The purpose of the interprofessional education curriculum is to prepare graduates of Doisy College of Health Sciences for interprofessional patient- and client-centered practice, effective and efficient delivery of health care services, and advocacy for the improvement of health and health services. From this purpose, seven themes were identified for the interprofessional curriculum.

Themes

Interprofessional curricular themes are interwoven throughout the curriculum in interprofessional courses designed to produce a specific educational outcome. Using a developmental model courses are designed to build on preceding courses, culminating in the ability to operationalize and apply the themes in the care of patients and clients in the clinical or community setting. The themes are advocacy, communication, evidence-based practice, health care ethics/professionalism, informatics, client safety/risk reduction, and social justice (Table 20-1). Each theme is defined and includes a student learning outcome applicable across all professions.

Competencies

The interprofessional education curriculum identifies student learning outcomes related to the development of interprofessional competence and the

Table 20-1. Interprofessional Education Curriculum Themes

Theme	Description	Outcome
Advocacy	Focuses on problem solving, communication to help patients and providers make good decisions together, and ensure access to the desired care or treatment[29]	Help patients make their own decisions through careful, informed deliberation; identify available resources and access appropriate care
Communication	Refers to an interactive, multi-dimensional process of delivering and receiving verbal and nonverbal messages	Accurate information is conveyed, with sensitivity for individual differences consciously using appropriate vocabulary, silence, distance, eye contact, timing and body movements.
Evidence-based practice	Refers to the appropriate use of current best evidence in making treatment decision with and for patients[30]	Know how to find, evaluate and use the best evidence in making decisions about patient care, while integrating patient preferences and values in the decision-making process
Health care ethics/ professionalism	Refers to moral reasoning in the context of caring relationships	Conduct consistent with civility, honesty, integrity, fairness, competence, and respect for others. Demonstrate commitment to professional competence, patient confidentiality, improving quality of care and access to care.

Table 20-1. Interprofessional Education Curriculum Themes *(Continued)*

Theme	Description	Outcome
Informatics	Refers to the integration of health science with computer and information systems to support the decision-making process in the delivery and management of health care	Locate and use information and assist clients in assessing and managing care
Client safety/ risk reduction	Client safety refers to the control of factors that place the patient or client at risk of error, failure to rescue or injury. Risk reduction refers to efforts to minimize factors that increase the probability of illness or injury.	Vigilant and communicative about the processes of care that lead to reduced risk and improved safety
Social justice	Refers to the concern for the rights and welfare of all people and working with others to achieve the common good	Recognition of responsibility to act for the good of others and apply their knowledge and skills in helping the most vulnerable

knowledge and skill needed to practice effectively in teams. Interprofessional competencies include (a) knowledge of the unique professional contributions and common responsibilities of the various health professions, (b) implementation of effective team strategies, (c) operationalization of collaboration in terms of interdependence among health professions, and (d) application of professional knowledge and skills to develop effective plans of care responsive to the diverse needs of patients and populations for the improvement of health. The interprofessional instructional units include specific objectives with content that supports the development of these competencies. Each course or other learning experience also addresses in some manner the outcomes related to the interprofessional curriculum themes.

Principles of Interprofessional Course Development

Three premises were among the driving forces in the selection of course content and the organization of course development. Course content was and is selected that (a) is relevant and of value to all health professions, (b) is essential to the existing curriculum, and (c) contributes to the knowledge and skills for interprofessional collaborative practice. Six criteria were identified that characterize an interprofessional course (Table 20-2). For a course to be designated interprofessional, it must meet all or most of the criteria presented in Table 20-2.

Courses

Sources for content of the interprofessional curriculum included review of content of health professions programs, values of the represented health professions, mission of the university, and national reports on the educational needs of contemporary health practitioners. The curriculum team looked for commonalities among documents and areas that pertained to all or most of the professions represented, determined content knowledge that would contribute to effective interprofessional team participation, and defined knowledge and skills that would contribute to improving health care. The content areas identified were organized into five courses: Introduction to Interprofessional Health Care, Health Care System and Health Promotion, Health Care Ethics, Evidence-Based Health Care, and Integrative Interprofessional Practicum Experience. The issues discussed in these courses are common to all the health professions. The understanding and potential solutions for these issues benefit from the input and expertise of faculty and students representing a mix of professions. Each course is described briefly.

Table 20-2. Criteria for Interprofessional Course

Planning and teaching by an interprofessional mix of faculty

A minimum of one course objective indicating that students, upon completion of the course, demonstrate an increase in level of interprofessional competence

Content relating to interprofessional competence is included and preferably threaded throughout the course

A methods section that includes at least one assignment that requires interprofessional group work

The course evaluation includes assessment of growth in interprofessional competence

Students represent at least two health professions but preferably more

Introduction to Interprofessional Health Care

The philosophical and theoretical foundations of interprofessional health care are explored. Interactive learning experiences provide the opportunity to develop knowledge and understanding of each profession's contribution to health care. Students learn about and experience the steps of team development and they complete a team project related to health care.

Health Care System and Health Promotion

This interprofessional course explores the relationship between the health care system, the health of the country, and current strategies for improving the health condition of the population. Students consider the current status of the health care system and the health of the people of the United States through discussion of political and economic environment of health care and the impact on the condition on health care on the practice of the professions. Students examine the significance of health promotion and interprofessional teamwork as means for improving the health status of themselves and others.

Health Care Ethics

This interprofessional course introduces students to the ethical issues confronting health care practitioners. Through examination of important concepts, principles, and values in health care ethics, students are enabled to perform consistent moral reasoning when faced with ethical dilemmas in health care practice. Interactive learning experiences provide students with opportunities to become familiar with the process of ethical decision making as well as to reflect on their own experiences. A particular emphasis is placed on patient-centered and client-centered care within the framework of an ethics of care.

Evidence-Based Health Care

This course examines the incorporation of evidence into health care. Students work together to develop answerable health care questions, efficiently search the literature, critically appraise the findings, and integrate the evidence with clinical judgments and the patient's values.

Integrative Interprofessional Practicum Experience

This course provides the student with a hands-on learning experience focused on client system–centered care as members of an interprofessional team. The team identifies a pertinent health-related issue with their chosen client population and cooperates, collaborates, and integrates care to improve health outcomes. Each professional uses his or her knowledge and expertise to maximize the productivity of the interprofessional team. Seminars provide opportunities for students to discuss and reflect on how service activities express the professional obligation to work as change agents for a more just society.

Integration of Learning Activities Within the Curriculum

Among the beliefs of the faculty concerning learning activities are that interprofessional education requires (a) interactive learning, (b) reflection as an essential element, and (c) a variety of methods to achieve learner outcomes. Also, students who are at different levels in their health professional programs can participate in a learning activity.

Integrative learning activities are used throughout the interprofessional curriculum. For example, each semester students are required to attend two sessions of interprofessional grand rounds. These sessions are conducted by an interprofessional mix of faculty and clinicians and are based on an actual case. Cases are planned so the students are exposed to a variety of types of individual and population conditions; cases highlight the contributions of different health professions and demonstrate the psychological, sociological, economic, and ethical issues as well as the physical and medical concerns that should be considered in making decisions. The interprofessional team gathers in the auditorium in which the students are seated to discuss the case. Students participate by observation of the interactions among the members of the health care team and by analyzing the issues in the case. Students are given directions for written reflection on their observations and own analysis of the situation. The grand rounds is later discussed in class sessions with a focus appropriate for the objectives of the particular course in which the students are enrolled. As students participate in practicum experiences, they may become more active in presenting cases in the grand rounds.

Other interactive and reflection experiences exist in the courses. In "Introduction to Interprofessional Health Care" the students are assigned to a team and sit together as a team during class. This arrangement allows students to interact during class on questions that are posed. Students also arrange meetings of their team outside of class and discuss the attributes of successful teams and incorporate their experience into their project work.

During the first year that the course was offered each team of students developed a consumer information brochure on a current health issue.

In other classes, teams form and operate in various ways so that students learn that teams may function differently but effectively, given the type of work that is to be done. The assignments and collaborative work covers areas in which all professions have interest with respect to their practice, such as ethics, the health care system, and evidence-based practice. By learning together they share information in ways that the students come to appreciate the roles of others, their expertise, the challenges, and the values of each profession.

The culminating course of the interprofessional education curriculum is "Integrative Interprofessional Practicum Experience." This course is designed to provide interprofessional student teams with a learning experience focused on individual patient-centered care or population-based concern. Students are placed in an interprofessional team with a faculty advisor. The team identifies a pertinent health-related issue with their chosen patient, client, or population and collaborates to improve health outcomes. Students consider evidence-based practice, quality improvement approaches, client safety, informatics, and cost management in the decisions and work of their team. Each professional uses his or her knowledge and expertise to maximize the productivity of the interprofessional team. The students discuss and reflect on how service activities express the professional obligation to work as change agents for a more just society.

EVALUATION

The purposes of the evaluation of the interprofessional education program are presented in Table 20-3. The evaluation of these purposes is both formative and summative. The process of evaluation begins with examining and evaluating course development and implementation and ensuring congruence between the program's objectives and the individual courses that make up the interprofessional curriculum. Formative process evaluation activities may include assessment of instructors' performances, students' performances, and peer review to evaluate the congruence of the courses' objectives and teaching methodologies to the interprofessional curriculum competencies. Proposed methods of evaluating the interprofessional education curriculum include faculty assessment of student's interprofessional knowledge at periodic points, qualitative data from student reflections, course evaluations by students, focus groups (students), focus groups (faculty), and peer review of faculty instruction.

Table 20-3. Purpose of Evaluation of the Interprofessional Education Program

To determine the degree of attainment of program objectives

To document strengths and limitations of program for making decisions, changes, and planning

To monitor standards of performance (both student and faculty) and establish quality control mechanisms

To meet the demand for fiscal accountability

To enhance the faculty's skill in providing interprofessional education

To promote positive public relations and community awareness

To contribute to the scientific and educational knowledge about interprofessional education

Adapted from Windsor R, Baranowski T, Clark N, Cutter G. *Evaluation of Health Promotion Health Education and Disease Prevention Programs.* Mountain View, CA: Mayfield Publishing Company; 1994.

The object of summative evaluation is simply to determine if a predetermined set of goals or competencies were accomplished. Summative evaluation attempts to determine the congruence between objectives and performance and isolate the cause(s) of the outcomes whether positive or negative.[26] Proposed methods of summative evaluation include assessment of student's interprofessional knowledge at end of the program, student assessment of the program on completion of the program, student reflection on integrative interprofessional practicum experience, end-of-program survey, 6-month postgraduation survey, clinical site surveys, and employers' surveys.

CONCLUSIONS

Interprofessional patient- and client-centered practice is being identified as a change in the delivery of health care that will improve the effectiveness and efficiency of the health of society.[27] Interprofessional education early in the students' program can work to foster positive attitudes toward other professionals[28] and instill communication skills for collaborative teamwork. Through the context of learning with other health professionals, students become aware of the similarities and distinctions each brings to the encounters with individual patients and clients and community-wide dilemmas. Students have the opportunity to understand the shared values among the health professions and that the "greater good" for improving health care is achieved when they work together.

REFERENCES

1. Institute of Medicine. *Crossing the Quality Chasm.* Washington, DC: National Academy of Sciences; 2001.
2. Institute of Medicine. *Health Professions Education: A Bridge to Quality.* Washington, DC: The National Academy of Sciences; 2003.
3. Pew Health Professions Commission. *Recreating Health Professional Practice for a New Century.* San Francisco: The Center for the Health Professions; 1998.
4. D'Amour D, Oandasan I. Interprofessionality as the field of interprofessional practice and interprofessional education: an emerging concept. *J Interprof Care.* 2005;(Suppl 1):8–20.
5. Schmitt M. USA: focus on interprofessional practice, education, and research. *J Interprof Care.* 1994;8:9–18.
6. Lynch B. Cooperative learning in interdisciplinary education for the allied health professions. *J Allied Health.* 1984;(May):83–93.
7. Freeth D, Nicol M. Learning clinical skills: an interprofessional approach. *Nurse Educ Today.* 1998;18:455–461.
8. Clark P. Participatory health seminars for nursing home residents: a model for multidisciplinary education. *Gerontol Geriatr Educ.* 1984;4:75–84.
9. Erkel E, Nivens A, Kennedy D. Intensive immersion of nursing students in rural interdisciplinary care. *J Nurs Educ.* 1995;34:359–365.
10. Clark P, Spence D, Sheehan J. A service/learning model for interdisciplinary teamwork in health and aging. *Gerontol Geriatr Educ.* 1986;6:3–16.
11. Gelmon S. Can educational accreditation drive interdisciplinary learning in the health professions? *J Qual Improv.* 1996;22:213–222.
12. Mellor M, Davis K, Capello C. Stages of development in the life of an academic interdisciplinary team in geriatrics. *Gerontol Geriatr Educ.* 1997;18:3–36.
13. Brickell J, Huff F, Fraley T. Educating for collaborative practice. *Clin Lab Sci.* 1997;10:311–314.
14. Hayward K, Powell L, McRoberts J. Changes in student perceptions of interdisciplinary practice in the rural setting. *J Allied Health.* 1996;25:315–327.
15. Laatsch L, Milson LM, Zimmer SE. Use of interdisciplinary education to foster familiarization among health professionals. *J Allied Health.* 1986;(Feb.):33–42.
16. Verstraete C, Scudder G, Karni K, Meier M. Developing interdisciplinary courses for allied health students: a retrospective view. *J Allied Health.* 1978;(Spring):99–108.
17. Lary M, Lavigne S, Muma R, Jones S, Hoeft H. Breaking down barriers: multidisciplinary education model. *J Allied Health.* 1997;(Spring):63–69.

18. Hammick M. Interprofessional education: concept, theory and application. *J Interprof Care.* 1998;12:323–332.

19. Oandasan I, Reeves S. Key elements for interprofessional education. Part 1: The learner, the educator and the learning context. *J Interprof Care.* 2005;(Suppl 1):21–38.

20. Reeves S, Freeth D, McCrorie P, Perry D. "It teaches you what to expect in future . . .": interprofessional learning on a training ward for medical, nursing, occupational therapy, and physiotherapy students. *Med Educ.* 2002;36:314–316.

21. Howkins E, Allison A. Shared learning for primary health care teams: a success story. *Nurse Educ Today.* 1997;17:225–231.

22. Hilton RW, Morris DJ, Wright AM. Learning to work in the health care team. *J Interprof Care.* 1995;9:267–274.

23. General Congregation of the Society of Jesus. *Decree 17, item 412.*

24. Saint Louis University. Center for Interprofessional Education and Research. Available at: http://www.slu.edu/centers/interpro/. Accessed September 28, 2007.

25. Liedtka JM, Whitten E. Enhancing care delivery through cross-disciplinary collaboration: a case study. *J Healthcare Manage.* 1998;43:185–203.

26. Windsor R, Baranowski T, Clark N, Cutter G. *Evaluation of Health Promotion Health Education and Disease Prevention Programs.* Mountain View, CA: Mayfield Publishing Company; 1994.

27. Ruebling I, Lavin M, Banks R, et al. Facilitating factors for, barriers to, and outcomes of interdisciplinary education projects in the health sciences. *J Allied Health.* 2000;29:165–170.

28. Carpenter J. Doctors and nurses: stereotypes and stereotype change in interprofessional education. *J Interprof Care.* 1995;9:151–161.

29. Hamel P. Interdisciplinary perspectives, service learning, and advocacy: a nontraditional approach to geriatric rehabilitation. *Top Geriatr Rehabil.* 2001;17:53–70.

30. Centre for Evidence-Based Medicine. Available at: http://www.cebm.utoronto.Ca/glossary. Accessed February 13, 2007.

Interprofessional Training in Telehealth Technologies for Service Delivery and Development of Rural Communities of Practice

Darlene M. Sekerak, PhD, PT
Linn Wakeford, MS, OT
Keith M. Cochran, MS
Joshua J. Alexander, MD

INTRODUCTION

Telecommunication technologies have the potential to connect health professionals and to assist in building communities of practice supporting both professionals and families in rural communities. An important component for success of any telehealth endeavor is adequate training of clinical personnel in the technology and its application. The current project used web-based materials, asynchronous communication networks, virtual clinics, videoconferencing, and supervised opportunities for practice of new technology skills in a rural clinic environment. The project reinforced that an important component for success of any telehealth endeavor is adequate training of clinical personnel in the technology and its application, adequate ongoing technical support, budgetary support, and elimination of disincentives to maintain the program. Centralized coordination to initiate and facilitate communication increases the likelihood that the technology will be used and the "communities of practice" will continue developing and maturing through electronic communication.

BACKGROUND

A major barrier to adequate access to services for children with special health care needs in rural communities is the shortage or maldistribution of qualified health care personnel. Many rural communities in North Carolina have no therapists; have no therapists with expertise related to children with disabilities, their families, and other caregivers; or have a limited number of therapists with the necessary expertise.[1] To further exacerbate the problem, therapists in rural North Carolina are professionally isolated and have limited access to other specialists and subspecialists in their own or related disciplines.

Wenger and colleagues described the concept of a "community of practice."[2] According to Wenger et al. (p. 4),

> [C]ommunities of practice are groups of people who share a concern, a set of problems, or a passion about a topic, and who deepen their knowledge and expertise in this area by interaction on an ongoing basis.

Members of a community of practice

- Find value in their interaction
- Share information, insight, and advice
- Help each other solve problems
- Discuss their situations, aspirations, and needs
- Ponder common issues, explore ideas, and act as sounding boards
- Create tools, standards, and designs
- Develop a body of common knowledge, practices, and approaches
- Gain personal satisfaction in knowing colleagues who understand each other's perspectives and in belonging to an interesting group of people

Members of a community of practice become informally bound by the value they find in learning together. Communities are unique among organizational structures in their ability to deal with a broad variety of knowledge-related issues. They can connect local pockets of expertise and isolated professionals. Communities of practice can (a) diagnose and address recurring problems whose root causes cross facility and geographical boundaries, (b) analyze the knowledge-related sources of uneven performance across practitioners and work to bring everyone up to the highest standards, and (c) link and coordinate unconnected activities and initiatives.[2]

Fifty-two percent of North Carolina's population live in rural communities along the coastal plains, southern piedmont, and Appalachian mountain areas.[3] Thirty percent of our 100 counties are estimated to have populations of 25,000, or less and many of these individuals live and work more than 1 hour from the nearest urban or high amenity center.[4] Therapists in rural areas of North Carolina are geographically isolated from peers, professional organizations, educational institutions, and large medical centers. Their opportunities for ongoing interaction are fewer than those of their urban peers, and they miss the support of a professional community. The need for professional interaction and networking cannot be underestimated. It is interesting that recent findings related to professional competence suggest health professionals who are geographically isolated or work on their own may be at higher risk for being disciplined by their licensure board or for having competency concerns.[5] This research reinforces the value of professional interaction and peer support for health providers in rural settings.

Theoretically, well-developed communities of practice can improve access to care and specialty expertise, which should ultimately lead to improved health status of the children served by professionals within these communities. If improved professional interaction and networking leads to improved competence and if networking increases a professional's knowledge about available services and resources, then the patients served by those professionals will be the beneficiaries. The potential for improved connectivity and a sense of belonging may also make rural settings more attractive to practitioners.

Telecommunication technologies have the potential to provide this connectedness among therapists and to build communities of practice supporting both professionals and families in rural communities. E-mail communication has provided another avenue for interaction among professionals. Web-based resources provide increased access to information, and videoconferencing provides a medium for real-time consultation for patients, families, and professionals who are geographically distant.

Recent data from the e-NC Authority, a grassroots initiative charged by the North Carolina General Assembly to link all North Carolinians—especially those in rural areas—to the Internet, documents that 90% of the population in North Carolina, including the many rural areas of the state, have access to high speed connectivity.[6] A survey of North Carolina businesses found that 83% of computer users in the most rural counties, those without a population center of 10,000 people, are connected to the Internet.[3] Technology for service providers in rural communities is becoming reasonably affordable and accessible. The potential service delivery enhancements offered by technology will remain untapped, however, without properly trained professionals to effectively apply the technology.

The purpose of the current project was to design specialized training for occupational therapists, physical therapists, and speech and language pathologists in the use of new Internet technologies, to assess the application of those technologies in practice, and to support the development of interprofessional communities of practice among rural practitioners.

DESCRIPTION OF THE PROJECT

The project described here, TelAbility Training Allied Health, used web-based materials, asynchronous communication networks, virtual clinics, videoconferencing, and supervised opportunities for occupational therapy, physical therapy, and speech and language pathology students to practice these new skills in a rural clinic environment. The project was a companion program designed to support TelAbility, an innovative interdisciplinary program funded in part by The Duke Endowment and by the North Carolina Departments of Health and Health and Human Services and housed in the Department of Physical Medicine and Rehabilitation at the University of North Carolina at Chapel Hill under the direction of one of the chapter authors, J. Alexander. TelAbility uses real-time videoconferencing and web-based instructional technologies, to provide comprehensive, coordinated, family-centered, clinical consultations to children with special health care needs and education and training opportunities for their care providers across North Carolina.[7] As part of the TelAbility program, the physician holds teleclinics for follow-up visits for his patients living in rural areas of the state. The TelAbility project has served as an umbrella program for several telehealth initiatives, including the interprofessional training program described here.

The specific aims of the training program were to

1. Increase the number of occupational therapist, physical therapist, and speech and language pathologist graduates competent to provide services for children with special needs in underserved rural communities of North Carolina using telehealth technologies
2. Facilitate the placement of graduates in underserved communities in North Carolina
3. Provide training for occupational therapists, physical therapists, and speech and language pathologists and others already practicing in North Carolina in the use of telehealth technologies

4. Increase access to interprofessional educational opportunities, consultation, and information resources
5. Evaluate the ability of current technology to provide a cost-effective mechanism for delivery of quality interprofessional rehabilitation services
6. Contribute to the development of technical standards for delivering occupational therapy, physical therapy, and speech and language pathology consultation via telecommunication technology

Over 3 years, 25 student participants were recruited from the second year classes of each of the three participating professions at the University of North Carolina at Chapel Hill. The third year of the program also included an early education student from Meredith College in Raleigh, North Carolina. Eligibility requirements were:

- Submission of an application for the program
- Participation in one 30-minute interview with at least two project faculty, including the project faculty member from the student's profession
- Good academic standing as determined by the student's home division and all passing grades on the transcript
- Stated interest in employment in rural communities working with children with special needs and their families
- Selection by the project faculty based on application and interview

To receive the certificate of completion students were required to

1. Participate in the training seminars
2. Complete the pre- and posttests
3. Score at least 80% on the technical section of the seminar posttest
4. Complete a pediatric clinical or field placement requirement of 6 to 12 weeks depending on the profession of study
5. Participate in a minimum of two clinical consultations (one source, one remote)
6. Contribute one content article for the TelAbility web page[7]
7. Evaluate two websites related to children and families

The educational seminars and learning experiences were designed to train these students in the technical skills necessary for application but also, more importantly, in the judicious use of the technology for communication and clinical consultation (Table 21-1).

Table 21-1. Interprofessional Telehealth Training Plan

Learning Outcome	Rationale	Learning Activities	Criteria
1. Find, review, and evaluate web-based health information, including web pages, chat rooms, asynchronous threaded discussion groups, blogs, and expertise directories.	Practitioners need skill in assessing the quality and usefulness of information provided by web services for their own use and for guiding families and children to useful resources.	a. Students were required to submit evaluations of two websites or services based on stated criteria, Health on the Net Principles[8] and Bobby WorldWide[9] accessibility ratings.	Services and information assessed for timeliness, accuracy, sensitivity, accessibility and ease of navigation, level of difficulty, applicability, audience, advertising, and conflicts of interest
2. Prepare and format educational materials for web posting.	Early intervention providers may discover new opportunities to use the Internet to share or disseminate information to colleagues and families.	b. Edit a draft of a case description prepared for dissemination on the web as a teaching/information piece. c. Prepare a handout about a topic of interest to families or professionals appropriate for posting on the TelAbility website.	Apply similar criteria to activity no. 1 with special attention to formatting concerns to improved access, readability, and speed navigation.

3. Learn new methods for interprofessional networking and communication.	Same as no. 2	d. Participate in an on-line chat session with students, project faculty, and families.	Demonstrate criteria listed for no. 1 as applicable. Incorporate enhancements like slides, video, Internet sites to support discussion.
4. Develop basic skills in video clinic consultation	The effectiveness of a clinical consultation can be enhanced by an understanding of the technology, impact of lighting, sound, room arrangement, communication skills, and camera presence.	e. Complete a pediatric clinical or field placement serving a rural community. f. Participate in a minimum of two clinical consultations (one source, one remote).	Demonstrate on-camera skills, basic technical skills in use of videoconference equipment, and best practice in coordinating and implementing clinical consultations by videoconferencing.
5. Understand and follow regulatory requirements related to state licensure, federal health information security laws, and insurance reimbursement.	Issues related to jurisdiction, informed consent, confidentiality, and supervision are all relevant to telehealth. Reimbursement varies by payer and jurisdiction.	g. Reading and group discussion. Application of knowledge learned in clinical placements/fieldwork assignments.	Demonstrate understanding of, and comply with, all regulatory requirements during clinical practicum assignments.

(Continues)

Table 21-1. Interprofessional Telehealth Training Plan *(Continued)*

Learning Outcome	Rationale	Learning Activities	Criteria
6. Assess the professional ethical obligations and quality of care concerns related to web-based information sharing and clinical consultation.	Fundamental ethical principles of beneficence, nonmalfeasance, and justice. Codes, standards, and policy statements for each profession apply in telehealth environments and may present unique challenges.	h. Reading and group discussion. Application of knowledge learned in clinical placements/fieldwork assignments.	Demonstrate understanding of, and comply with, all ethical and professional standards during clinical practicum/fieldwork assignments.
7. Expand their understanding of the unique issues associated with rural culture and the special challenges of service delivery for children with special needs and their families.	Early intervention providers need to understand the lifestyle and values of rural populations and the impact of these variables on health care behaviors including barriers to health care and the unique support systems of rural communities and culturally diverse groups.	i. Reading and group discussion. Application of knowledge learned in clinical placements/fieldwork assignments.	Demonstrate commitment to and model advocacy for culturally sensitive practice during clinical practicum/fieldwork assignments.

Initially, these instructional modules were delivered using traditional on-site methodologies over a 3-day weekend. By the third year of the project, all learning modules were accessed by students on-line. The learning modules included content related to the unique aspects of rural health care delivery, cultural competence, families and children with special needs, ethics, licensure, reimbursement, and technology. Students participated in learning exercises related to the Health on the Net Code of Conduct,[8] accessibility issues for Internet websites,[9] Internet communication etiquette and chat room savvy, on-camera skills, observational play-based and transdisciplinary assessments,[10] and verbal instruction in test item administration by a remote caregiver. The three interprofessional cohorts of students and faculty were culturally, ethnically, and racially diverse, adding to the richness of the experience and the learning discussions. Parents of children with special needs were also included as discussion facilitators (Table 21-2).

Each cohort of students completed a written (first and second cohort) or on-line (third cohort) pretest survey of attitudes and beliefs about clinical teleconference services and a self-assessment survey regarding the skills program faculty considered important for successful delivery of clinical telehealth services. Pretesting also included a multiple choice test of knowledge about videoconference technology application. Students repeated the survey and multiple choice test after completion of all program modules. Tables 21-3 and 21-4 provide examples of the types of questions included in the surveys and the multiple choice tests.

Students were required to complete learning assignments that provided practice opportunities and feedback. These assignments related to the skills associated with identifying and evaluating the quality of health information

Table 21-2. Racial Diversity of Faculty and Student Participants

	Faculty	Students
White	4	20
Latino	0	0
African-American	1	2
Asian	0	3
Total	5	25

Table 21-3. Sample Questions From the Pre- and Postprogram Student Surveys

	Strongly Agree	Agree	Neutral	Disagree	Strongly Disagree
Sample questions related to beliefs and attitudes about clinical videoconferencing.					
1. It is difficult to establish a meaningful relationship with a family if services are provided via videoconferencing.	☐	☐	☐	☐	☐
2. I must be in the room with the child and able to touch the child in order to accurately assess a child's needs.	☐	☐	☐	☐	☐
3. Services provided via videoconferencing technology are not as good as services provided on-site.	☐	☐	☐	☐	☐
4. If my child needed services I would probably drive several hours to the medical center than use services provided via videoconferencing.	☐	☐	☐	☐	☐
5. Videoconferencing is inefficient because of frequent technical difficulties.	☐	☐	☐	☐	☐

Sample questions for student self-assessment of technical skills.

1. I feel confident in my ability to interview parents during a telehealth session in order to gather information pertinent to assessment or intervention for their child. ☐ ☐ ☐ ☐

2. I feel confident in my abilities to operate camera, audio, and room logistics to assist in successfully conducting a telehealth consultation session. ☐ ☐ ☐ ☐

3. I know how to modulate my voice tone, volume, rate, and timing of speech in order to be understood by those on the remote end during a telehealth consult. ☐ ☐ ☐ ☐

4. I know how to problem-solve minor technical difficulties during a telehealth consultation, such as loss of audio or video capabilities. ☐ ☐ ☐ ☐

Table 21-4. Examples of Multiple Choice Knowledge Questions Included on the Pre- and Posttests

Select the best option for completing each statement.

1. All the following may be strategies for effective nonverbal communication during videoconferencing except
   [ ] increase your energy level of animation to 125%
   [ ] decrease your level of animation to 75%
   [ ] act naturally
   [ ] decrease the speed of your movements by 25%

2. To simulate eye contact during video communication you should
   [ ] look directly at the center of the monitor when speaking
   [ ] look at the camera when speaking and listening to the remote speaker
   [ ] look at the center of the monitor when the remote person is speaking
   [ ] periodically glance at the top center of the monitor

3. All the following affect the quality of the audio and video transmission except
   [ ] bandwidth available
   [ ] number of router hops
   [ ] quality of the hardware
   [ ] Z73 rate
   [ ] features of the software

4. The lowest acceptable frame rate for clinical videoconferencing is
   [ ] 8 fps
   [ ] 15 fps
   [ ] 22 fps
   [ ] 30 fps

5. The standard for videoconferencing over IP is
   [ ] H.261
   [ ] H.320
   [ ] H.323
   [ ] T120

6. Informed consent for videoconferencing should include (check all that apply)
   [ ] statement of agreement by everyone present
   [ ] statement that the session is being audio or video recorded
   [ ] statement about the purposes for which the recording might be used
   [ ] identification of the agency/person responsible for maintaining the consent agreement

posted on the Internet and writing materials for the Internet that are both professional and family friendly and are appropriate for a variety of Internet mediums. Students also had the opportunity to participate in chat rooms, real-time and asynchronous video presentations, discussion boards, listservs, and clinical videoconferences. Students developed web materials for use by professionals and families that clarified and condensed current information and evidence available about the topic into short, convenient, and useful handouts that could easily be printed or downloaded. Students also participated in scheduled on-line chat room discussions with other practitioners and families on topics of interest, including promoting healthy levels of physical activity for children with special needs, advanced practice and the master clinician, and use of the gross motor function classification system for children with cerebral palsy.[11]

The initial technical laboratory instruction was delivered in person in the videoconference laboratory. Students learned about the effect of lighting, sound delays, camera position, and the technical aspects of the equipment and software. Students also practiced scripted interviews and opening and closing formats and all aspects of managing a videoconferencing session to optimize the experience of the participants.

After completion of the learning modules, students were assigned full-time to one of three collaborating rural child development service agencies (CDSAs) or other pediatric sites for a clinical affiliation or fieldwork placement as part of the normal curriculum in their respective educational program. The supervising therapists at the CDSAs had been trained in use of the technology as part of the project. During the time assigned at the CDSA, each student completed at least two clinical consultations using videoconferencing—one as a consult source and one as a consult recipient. As examples, one student participated in a consultation for a child being served in a child care center in Chapel Hill with a specialized feeding team at one of the CDSAs and assisted in the development of a feeding program for that child. Another student assisted in a videoconference consult regarding motorized seating recommendations for a preschool child with cerebral palsy.

OUTCOMES

Twenty-five students (9 occupational therapy, 12 physical therapy, 3 speech and language pathology, and 1 early education) participated in the training program. Posttest scores on the multiple choice knowledge test related to technology skills increased 56% over pretest scores. Based on a five-point Likert scale survey, agreement with positive statements about the use of technology and self-assessment of the students' own skill level also increased an average of two rating levels over pretest ratings with all students showing positive changes in attitudes at completion of the program. Disagreement with negative statements about the use of technology increased by one rating level over pretest ratings.

The first year after graduation, all program participants were providing services to families in underserved areas of the state in public schools, early intervention, and home health programs. Few reported having easy access to videoconferencing technology or administrative support to use the systems that were available in their communities. They were using the Internet for networking and as a source of information for self, peer, and family education. The CDSAs currently use videoconferencing for staff development and clinical consultation on a limited but regular basis or for consultation with the physician for follow-up with children who are his patients. Unfortunately, the North Carolina Medicaid program does not reimburse clinical services or consultation by therapists so participation by these practitioners in providing or requesting videoconference services is still limited to facility or grant-funded services or unfunded visits.

The North Carolina Department of Health and Human Services negotiated separate contacts for project staff to expand training to the other 15 CDSAs in the state system and for follow-up and advanced training for previously trained staff. Videoconferencing technology was installed in all the remaining CDSAs as part of the TelAbility project funded by a grant from the Duke Endowment.

The use of technology for clinical consultation and collaboration has been less than project staff originally hoped. Graduates of the program cite limited time, lack of reimbursement for telehealth services by therapists, connectivity issues, and limited technical support as barriers to full implementation in their postgraduation practice settings. As a spin-off to the above projects, the John Rex Foundation has funded a focused project (Wake Area Telehealth Collaborative Helping children with special needs, or WATCH) designed to build a technology-based community of practice among service provider programs serving children in Wake County, North Carolina.[12] The lessons learned in previous projects related to the need for coordination and multiple structured and unstructured opportunities to facilitate professional networking and collaboration are being applied successfully in the WATCH project.

DISCUSSION

The project reinforced that an important component for success of any tele-health endeavor is adequate training of clinical personnel in the technology and its application, adequate ongoing technical support, budgetary supports, and elimination of disincentives to maintain the program. We found that centralized coordination to initiate and facilitate communication increases the likelihood that the technology will be used and the "communities of practice" will continue developing and maturing. Wenger and colleagues suggest that alive communities have a coordinator or leader who organizes events and connects community members.[2] Also, a core group of active community leaders is essential to provide the heart for the group. To sustain a virtual community of practice connected via technology, a coordinator is necessary to plan and organize activities, respond to technical issues, and encourage and nurture participation at all levels. It is our experience that, in the absence of a coordinator, a virtual community is unlikely to mature. Likewise, a core group of committed and passionate leaders is essential to sustain and grow a community. This level of leadership requires financial support, especially for the coordinator's time. Easy and timely access to technical assistance is also key. Given identified leaders and the necessary financial supports, however, Internet technology can provide the tools to link isolated providers into vibrant and dynamic virtual communities of practice.

An activity that many health professionals find rewarding is brainstorming ideas focused on an individual patient's needs. This can happen spontaneously in a clinic setting supporting multiple providers or as a scheduled case conference. Videoconferencing can allow for these brainstorming sessions and patient problem-solving sessions by linking clinicians in distant sites to a patient in a home or clinic setting. Videoconferencing technology can also link specialists and subspecialists in urban medical centers to rural clinics. For most therapists in most states, however, these telehealth services are not reimbursed by private insurance or by government programs like Medicaid. The convenience and cost saving associated with reduced travel and wait times are appreciated by the families involved, but the cost is equal to or greater for the professional delivering the care in this manner. We need to develop funding models that demonstrate the long-term cost savings associated with the improved access to care that telehealth services can provide. The security measures associated with the Health Information Portability and Accountability Act[13] have also created problems for telehealth programs because of the firewalls installed by hospitals and other health care centers to protect the privacy of protected health information. Penetrating or circumventing these firewalls for videoconferencing to external sites is problematic. These barriers add to the challenges of virtual health professional communities of practice.

As with other innovations, teleheath technology also presents the opportunity for misuse or improper application. Early education and training offers one strategy to encourage discriminate application of promising new professional networking service delivery options by competent practitioners who understand the capability and limitations of the technology and the ethical, legal, and practice issues associated with its use.

CONCLUSIONS

TelAbility Training Allied Health offers a model for instruction to prepare graduates for incorporation of telehealth technologies in practice and for the use of technology to develop and maintain professional communities of practice to support the delivery of quality health care services in rural environments. Including technology skill training in professional education programs is an innovative approach to preparing professionals for successful practice and interprofessional networking in rural and underserved communities.

REFERENCES

1. Thaker S, Fraher E, King J. *Allied Health Job Vacancy Tracking Report. An Examination of Job Vacancies in Selected Allied Health Professions in North Carolina.* Chapel Hill, NC: North Carolina Health Professions Data Systems; 2006. Available at: https://www.shepscenter.unc.edu/hp/alliedhealth/2006ahvacancy.pdf
2. Wenger E, McDermott R, Snyder W. *Cultivating Communities of Practice: A Guide to Managing Knowledge.* Boston: Harvard Business School Press; 2002.
3. Population in North Carolina, North Carolina Rural Economic Development Center. Available at: http://www.ncruralcenter.org/databank/trendprint_population.asp. Accessed September 5, 2007.
4. *State and County QuickFacts.* U.S. Census Bureau. Available at: http://quickfacts.census.gov/qfd/states/37000lk.html. Accessed September 5, 2007.
5. Austin Z, Marini A, Croteau D, Violato C. Assessment of pharmacists' patient care competencies: validity evidence from Ontario (Canada)'s Quality Assurance and Peer Review Process. *Pharm Educ.* 2004;4:23–32.
6. North Carolina's e-NC Authority. Available at: http://www.e-nc.org/e. Accessed January 31, 2007.
7. TelAbility. Available at: www.telability.org. Accessed January 31, 2007.

8. Health on the Net Foundation. Available at: http://www.hon.ch/. Accessed January 31, 2007.

9. Bobby WorldWide Web Accessibility Tool. Mardiros Internet Marketing. Available at: http://www.mardiros.net/bobby-accessibility-tool.html. Accessed September 7, 2007.

10. Early Childhood LINK. Available at: http://www.cdl.unc.edu/link/What%20is%20TD%20Definition.htm. Accessed September 10, 2007.

11. Bodkin AW, Robinson C, Perales F. Reliability and validity of the gross motor function classification system for cerebral palsy. *Pediatr Phys Ther.* 2003;15:247–252.

12. Wake Area Telehealth Collaborative Helping children with special needs (WATCH). Available at: http://www.telability.org/watch/. Accessed January 31, 2007.

13. Public Law 104-191. Health Insurance Portability and Accountability Act of 1996. Available at: http://aspe.hhs.gov/admnsimp/pl104191.htm. Accessed January 31, 2007.

SECTION 5

Best Practice

The View From 30,000 Feet: Rural Interprofessional Education at the Academic Health Center Level

Barbara F. Brandt, PhD
Gwen Wagstrom Halaas, MD, MBA

INTRODUCTION

Recent policy reports have recommended transforming academic health centers to respond to critical issues in health care and, specifically, in rural health. An Institute of Medicine report on the future of rural health care recommends the need to expand experientially based workforce training programs in rural areas to ensure that all health care professionals master core competencies, including working in interdisciplinary teams.[1] The care delivery system has recognized the need for health professionals who understand systems and their roles in them, make decisions based on evidence and best practices, use electronic information systems, value and promote patient-centered care, and effectively work with other providers as needed. To graduate health professionals with these competencies, the Institute of Medicine report on academic health centers recommends that academic health centers should reorganize to work across professions and across settings of care to develop organizational structures that facilitate team approaches to care, incorporating those changes into clinical and experiential education.[2] To enhance learning about new approaches to care, curricular content and methods of education should cross professional schools.

In 2000 the University of Minnesota Academic Health Center created a strategic plan that proactively addresses the issues of educating the next generation of health professionals who can work in teams to meet the health care needs of Minnesota while addressing the state's growing health challenges. The University of Minnesota is the sole comprehensive Research I higher education institution in Minnesota that prepares physicians, pharmacists, advance nurse practitioners, dentists, public health professionals, and veterinarians for the state. Subsequent analysis of greater Minnesota health needs revealed gaps in the University's track record of supplying the health professions workforce across the state. As a result, strategic efforts in dentistry, pharmacy, and nursing were initiated to increase class sizes and address the workforce maldistribution in greater Minnesota.

One key outcome of the Academic Health Center's strategic plan is the Minnesota Area Health Education Center. Established with federal and state funding in 2002, Minnesota Area Health Education Center was positioned in the Academic Health Center's central administration and charged to work across the six health professions schools, due in part to the importance of health professions workforce development to the health of Minnesota citizens and economy of the state.

As Minnesota is the 46th state to host an Area Health Education Center, Minnesota Area Health Education Center leaders have had the advantage of building on lessons learned by others since the Area Health Education Center movement began in 1970. Minnesota Area Health Education Center has focused on addressing the state's specific workforce needs while integrating emerging recommendations for rural health care. In this chapter we describe how the University of Minnesota Academic Health Center has strategically positioned Minnesota area health education center to respond to critical issues in rural health and rural health care, making it a model for the next generation of community–campus partnerships.

RURAL MINNESOTA: CHANGING DEMOGRAPHICS AND HEALTH DISPARITIES

Since 1990 America's Health Rankings™[3] has rated Minnesota as among the top two states listed as the "healthiest" in the nation. However, this designation conceals significant disparities between rural and urban population health statistics, variations between the distribution of rural and urban health professions workforce, and ethnic and racial differences in health.

Urban Versus Rural Health Disparities

Rural areas of Minnesota, often referred to as "greater Minnesota," experience among the most critical health care access needs and health disparities in the state. Compared with urban areas, rural residents have higher poverty rates, tend to be in poorer health, have access to fewer health professionals and other health resources, face more difficulty traveling to health services, are less likely to obtain certain preventive services, and are further behind in meeting Healthy People 2010 objectives.[4] A 2005 Minnesota Department of Health study documented significant disparities in health and well-being between citizens who live in the 7-county metropolitan area and those in the 82 counties of rural Minnesota.[5]

Health Professions Workforce Shortages

Health professions workforce shortages may significantly contribute to Minnesota's health disparities. In several categories of health professionals, Minnesota has experienced some of the least favorable ratings in the United States. There is a particular crisis in the allied health professions; for example, it is estimated that 150 to 200 additional clinical laboratory scientist graduates are needed annually in Minnesota to support the health care system and biomedical industry.[6] Rural areas of the state are particularly affected by health professions workforce shortages and maldistribution. Many Minnesota counties lack sufficient health care providers to meet the needs of their residents—nearly 90% of all or portions of Minnesota counties, many of them rural, are designated health professional shortage areas or medically underserved areas.

In nearly every health professions category, the ratio of provider to population is significantly lower in rural Minnesota than in urban areas (Table 22-1).[6] Additionally, the rural health professions workforce is significantly older and includes a larger percentage nearing retirement than its metropolitan counterpart.[7] This maldistribution is likely to continue. Graduate exit survey data collected by the Minnesota Department of Health demonstrates that very few respondents had committed to practices in rural areas (Table 22-2).[8]

Changing Demographics

Minnesota's rapidly changing demographics also contribute to health care disparities. Minnesota's population is becoming increasingly racially and

Table 22-1. Minnesota Distribution of Health Professionals: Urban and Rural

	Urban	Rural
Population	59%	13%
Physicians	80%	5%
Primary care	73%	8%
Specialists	87%	2%
Physician assistants	69%	11%
Registered nurses	74%	8%
Licensed practical nurses	48%	18%
Physical therapists	71%	9%
Dentists	69%	8%
Dental hygienists	70%	7%

Minnesota Distribution of Health Professionals: Metropolitan, Micropolitan, and Rural

	Metropolitan Counties	Micropolitan Counties	Rural Counties
Population	72%	15%	13%
All physicians	84%	11%	5%
Primary care	79%	13%	8%
Specialists	89%	9%	2%
Registered nurses	80%	12%	8%
Licensed practical nurses	59%	23%	18%
Dentists	78%	14%	8%
Dental hygienists	71%	14%	15%
Physician assistants	79%	12%	9%
Physical therapists	68%	13%	19%

Sources: Minnesota Department of Health, Office of Rural Health and Primary Care. *Demographics of Physicians, Nurses and Dentists: Urban-Rural Comparisons of Minnesota's Health Care Workforce.* Available at: http://www.health.state.mn.us/divs/orhpc/pubs/workforce/demo.pdf. Accessed November 2005. Minnesota Department of Health. *Healthcare Workforce Data and Reports.* Available at: http://www.health.state.mn.us/divs/orhpc/workforce/data.html.

Table 22-2. Minnesota Health Professions Trainee Exit Survey: 2001–2003

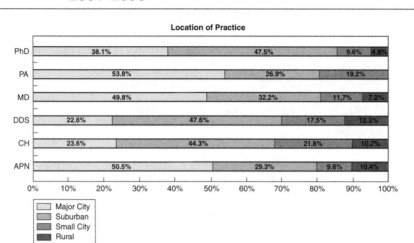

Source: Health Economics Program, Health Policy, Information and Compliance Monitoring Division, Minnesota Department of Health. *Minnesota: Results of the 2001–2003 Minnesota Health Professions Trainee Exit Surveys, March 2005.* Available at: http://www.health.state. mn.us/divs/hpsc/hep/merc/workforce/extsrv03.pdf

ethnically diverse. Between 2005 and 2015, the non-White population is projected to grow 35%, compared with 7% for the White population. The Hispanic population is expected to increase 47%.[9] A contributing factor to this population growth and diversification is international immigration and refugees. In one single year, 2002, 14,000 new immigrants from 160 different countries moved to Minnesota.[10] A majority of these immigrants originate from Latin America (24%) and Asia (40.4%). Neighborhoods and enclaves of Latino, Hmong (originating from Laos), Somali, Vietnamese, Russian, Laotian, Cambodian, and Ethiopian populations are found throughout the state. Large segments of these populations reside not only in Minneapolis, St. Paul and surrounding suburbs but in rural areas where public and social services tend to be ill prepared to meet their specific needs.

Although the proportion of Minnesotans who are 65 or older is only slightly lower than the national average, the projected growth for this age group is on the rise.[11] Minnesota's 65-plus age group is projected to grow by almost 700,000 between 2000 and 2030, a growth rate of 117%. The greatest concentration of Minnesota's older citizens is in rural areas. This is attributed to both a decrease in the number of adults with children and an attraction for retirees to move to recreational areas of the state. The 10 counties that make up the lakes region in north central Minnesota attract retirees ages 65 to 74 in large numbers. The aging population is straining the already burdened health care system, especially long-term and chronic care.[12]

THE UNIVERSITY OF MINNESOTA ACADEMIC HEALTH CENTER

The University of Minnesota Academic Health Center is one of a small number of land-grant universities with six health professions schools in one institution: School of Dentistry, Medical School, School of Nursing, College of Pharmacy, School of Public Health, and College of Veterinary Medicine. In addition, the Academic Health Center is developing a Center for Allied Health Programs with a long-range goal of working with higher education and health system partners to develop a statewide School of Allied Health Professions to address serious and volatile workforce needs. The Academic Health Center plays a unique role in the state of Minnesota. The Academic Health Center educates two-thirds of Minnesota's health professionals (dentists, physicians, advanced nurse practitioners, pharmacists, public health professionals, and veterinarians). In the 2006–2007 academic year, the Academic Health Center had more than 6,000 health professional students in 64 undergraduate, graduate, first professional, and advanced professional degree programs. Several Academic Health Center schools have a statewide and regional scope. The College of Pharmacy is the only pharmacy school in the state. The School of Dentistry, School of Public Health, and College of Veterinary Medicine are regional schools or the only health professions school serving several surrounding states. Currently, the School of Nursing offers the only doctoral degree in nursing in the state.

In 2000 the University of Minnesota Academic Health Center senior leadership engaged faculty, staff, students, and the broader University and Minnesota community to develop a strategic plan. This plan proactively addresses the issues of educating the next generation of health professionals who can meet the health care needs of Minnesota while addressing the state's growing health challenges. Strategies include increasing class sizes in some health professions schools, such as nursing, pharmacy and dentistry, as well as regionalizing programs to other areas of the state where workforce needs are the most severe. The plan emphasizes the importance of developing new models of health care and incorporating innovative educational models across the health professions.

In 2006 the University's strategic repositioning effort commissioned an Academic Health Center Health Professions Workforce Task Force. The Task Force's charges included defining the role and best use of interprofessional education in training the next generation of health professionals and with delineating new interprofessional education and care delivery models. The Task Force made a series of recommendations, including one that the Academic Health Center should transform its culture to embrace interprofessional education, develop sustainable systems to ensure exemplary interprofessional educational programs, adopt the United Kingdom Centre for the Advancement of Interprofessional Education definitions of interprofessional education to guide further development of education and practice, and designate a central coordinating entity and manager of interprofessional education activities in the Academic Health Center.

Minnesota Area Health Education Center

One key outcome of these planning processes is the Minnesota Area Health Education Center. Minnesota Area Health Education Center is a statewide network of community and academic partners committed to meeting the health professional workforce and community health needs of greater Minnesota. Established in September 2002 with federal and state funding, Minnesota Area Health Education Center promotes rural health educational experiences for students across a continuum, addressing the needs of K–12 students, undergraduates, health professions students, health professionals, and community members. Minnesota Area Health Education Center has established four regional area health education centers in the northeast, northwest, central, and southern Minnesota. These regional area health education centers operate as independent nonprofit organizations with community boards and work with the University of Minnesota to form community–campus partnerships.

In 2002 Minnesota Area Health Education Center staff developed the "Greater Minnesota Strategy" not only to address the workforce challenges but to proactively incorporate activities that would address national recommendations for transforming health professions education and rural health.

The Greater Minnesota Strategy's vision for rural health education programs in Minnesota is to

- Promote health outcomes by developing future health professionals who value community engagement
- Ensure a vital health professions workforce through community–campus partnerships with the University of Minnesota
- Contribute to a vibrant rural economy by eliminating health professions shortage areas

To achieve these outcomes, Minnesota Area Health Education Center works to bring together a variety of partners to maximize resources both internal and external to the University of Minnesota. Internally, Minnesota Area Health Education Center staff link existing programs in the Academic Health Center and University such as the University of Minnesota Extension, 4-H, various colleges and schools educational programs, and centers to rural health and the education of health professionals. For example, Minnesota Area Health Education Center shares a liaison position with the University of Minnesota Extension to coordinate programs in specific rural communities. Externally, staff work to build the next generation of community–campus partnerships focused around health professions education and training using the philosophy of "shared resources, shared risks, and shared rewards." This guiding principle acknowledges the reality of diminishing resources for health professions education and rural health.

Building On Success: The Rural Physician Associate Program

Minnesota Area Health Education Center builds on the success of the Rural Physician Associate Program, a University of Minnesota Medical School program that has trained medical students in rural communities since 1971. With an eye toward maximizing internal resources, Minnesota Area Health Education Center recognized the history and success of the Rural Physician Associate Program as well as the recent strengthening of the program's community health experience beyond a traditional clinical practice focus. The development of structured student community health assessment projects designed to create a learning experience that would return value to the community provided an opportunity for area health education centers in interprofessional education.

Rural Physician Associate Program was established through support from the Minnesota state legislature to address a shortage of primary care physicians in rural Minnesota. This is a 36-week elective program to which students apply and are accepted. Thirty to 40 students are placed each year in Minnesota communities that range in population size from 1,000 to 30,000. Since 1971, 110 Minnesota communities have served as Rural Physician Associate Program sites. Some 1,127 students have completed the program, with at least 892 former students currently in medical practice. Minnesota Area Health Education Center supports Rural Physician Associate Program students through additional financial stipends to help with the cost of housing in relocating, through information about the community and the local health care system, and by providing or enhancing community health educational experiences. Minnesota Area Health Education Center also helps medical students in earlier years connect with clinical experiences in greater Minnesota, which may help the Rural Physician Associate Program pipeline of the future and also helps develop interprofessional education experiences that will enrich the Rural Physician Associate Program student experience. Sixty percent of 892 former Rural Physician Associate Program students currently practice in a rural setting nationally or internationally. Of those Rural Physician Associate Program physicians in rural practice in Minnesota, 89% are in primary care and 82% are in family medicine.

In an effort toward designing a system to address workforce needs while focusing on community health, the Director of Rural Physician Associate Program now also serves as associate director of Minnesota Area Health Education Center. Charged with improving interprofessional practice and community health outcomes, the associate director has supervised grant opportunities from Minnesota's Medical Education and Research Costs pool to communities, many which have been Rural Physician Associate Program teaching sites. For 3 years, Rural Physician Associate Program students have conducted community health assessment projects designed to bring value to the Rural Physician Associate Program community. The health issues chosen for these projects were based on Healthy People 2010 leading indicators or on priority health issues apparent in the community. The wide range of topics includes the following:

- Improving diabetes care
- Access to dental care
- Adolescent wellness, education on sexual behavior, and teen pregnancy prevention

- Advance directives
- Geriatric risk assessment, depression, and falls prevention
- Early childhood education for fathers
- Exercise in rural Minnesota
- Improved health access and health care for the Latino population
- Obesity education and care improvement for children, families, and patients after bariatric surgery
- Smoking cessation in pregnant women, high school students, and communities
- Recreational and agricultural accidents and injuries

Minnesota Area Health Education Center Faculty Leadership Council

To further assist communities as they develop effective interprofessional practice teams, Minnesota Area Health Education Center recently developed the Faculty Leadership Council, which is composed of faculty from the schools of medicine, nursing, dentistry, pharmacy, and public health, appointed by their respective deans. The Council functions as a liaison between the health professions schools and Minnesota Area Health Education Center and provides strategic oversight and coordination of rural health educational opportunities through the Minnesota Area Health Education Center network. It is charged as follows:

- To cultivate and engage academic programs for rural and underserved health professions education opportunities by connecting existing educational opportunities to community-based interprofessional practice experience
- To lead collaborative development of interprofessional education opportunities for health professions students in rural and underserved areas

The Council meets regularly with the associate dean(s) of the school about rural and interprofessional education to help develop strategies and to develop a coordinated system that will receive and address community requests for health professions students. Among other functions, the Council engages and advises the professional schools in developing rural educational opportunities through Minnesota Area Health Education Center.

Minnesota Area Health Education Center and the Faculty Leadership Council are partnering with rural Minnesota communities to develop interprofessional learning experiences for health professions students. In 2004 Minnesota Area Health Education Center requested proposals from Minnesota communities for grant funds from the Minnesota Education and Research Costs to strengthen interprofessional practice teams that could become experiential interprofessional education sites for health professions students. Moose Lake and Montevideo were the initial two sites selected. Two additional sites, Hibbing and Fergus Falls, were selected in 2005. The following is a summary of the current sites and their projects.

Fergus Falls—Central Minnesota Area Health Education Center

The primary goal of this group is to provide public and health professional awareness of the impact of falls, particularly in the elderly, and assess those at risk. The core program elements entail a focus on the underserved or frail elderly and/or those with multiple medical problems and significant polypharmacy. The work of the interprofessional team is to identify those at risk for falls, assess the risk in nonfallers and in those who have already fallen, advise on how to lessen the risk of falls and make necessary health care modifications, lead an effort for home and environmental hazard improvement, and measure outcomes data of the success of the project.

Hibbing—Northeast Minnesota Area Health Education Center

Fairview Mesaba Clinics/Range Regional Health Services identified diabetes as their community-based initiative for an interprofessional project. The goal is to provide a team approach to deliver preventative diabetes education and diabetes management. The desired outcome is to enhance quality of life of the served population by teaching them to stay healthy and learn to live well with diabetes.

Moose Lake—Northeast Minnesota Area Health Education Center

The focus of the interprofessional project has been defined as hospital, home care, assisted living, and community working together to reduce hospitalizations and rehospitalizations among the elderly population in Moose Lake. The primary goal of the Moose Lake Community Geriatric Project is to decrease hospitalization/rehospitalization of the elderly, decrease emergency room and urgent care visits, and strengthen the ancillary services that the hospital provides.

Montevideo—Southern Minnesota Area Health Education Center

The goals for this program include decreased preterm labor and complications, improved birth outcomes, and health promotion education for vulnerable rural citizens based on individualized assessments. Reaching the Latino population in the communities and offering educational opportunities for these families is a key priority. The Montevideo project will enhance currently available services provided by the hospital and the local county public health services. The interprofessional team has changed from the first year; however, they are currently reporting positive results on team function. In 2006 the following six additional sites were selected: Mountain Iron, New Ulm, St. Cloud, Park Rapids, Willmar, and Brainerd. Projects at these sites will support the development of an interprofessional practice and health professions students training in addressing obesity, Alzheimer's dementia, and cultural competence.

Challenges and Opportunities of the Interprofessional Education Projects

The challenges these communities face in achieving expert interprofessional collaboratives are not unexpected from newly developing projects. Although each of the communities has experienced small successes, progress remains slow. Because of the uniqueness of each community's needs, it is difficult to pinpoint major barriers. Common themes identified by the interprofessional education sites include administrative constraints, project and membership definition, and successful incorporation of interprofessional learners into the project. Rural communities often present opportunities for change and improvement in health care that are a result of the need to meet local needs with fewer bureaucratic hurdles to cross. With guidance from Minnesota Area Health Education Center and the Faculty Leadership Council, these concerns and opportunities are being addressed. In July 2007 a statewide community project conference was held to share experiences and plan for interprofessional education site coordination.

The interprofessional teams in these communities are local health care providers and staff who face the daily demands and responsibilities for health care needs in small communities. There is little opportunity for protected time. The counterbalance is that in a small community teamwork is natural, essential, and understood as the way to get work done. Communication between health care providers is easier because they interact with each other in the course of daily life and work. The impact of team practice is more visible and meaningful because providers know the patients, their families, and their context well.

Formal systems are seldom in place to support interprofessioonal teams. Informal systems are ubiquitous and can help or hinder interprofessional teamwork. Increasingly, rural communities are recognizing systems needs and developing the skills and the practice of systems-based care. The Faculty Leadership Council members are leveraging this recognition to develop community teams and teaching sites.

University of Minnesota formal education is not well understood and is somewhat intimidating to rural community providers. Informal education is ongoing in communities where patients are more informed and health care teams feel the responsibility for the health of their community. We found that pride in participation in the formal education of University of Minnesota health professions students is tremendous from providers and patients alike.

Community attitude toward the University is often a barrier. When the University is seen as a large, urban, unapproachable institution that is not connected to the needs of communities, we have experienced an intentional avoidance of our work. By contrast, the personal attention developed over a number of years connects the University to communities. The most common facilitator of the work is an enthusiastic alumnus who has a desire to make the connection and to participate in ongoing education. Strong relationships such as those developed over years with the Rural Physician Associate Program are a tremendous asset toward reconnecting with campus and creating interprofessional experiential education.

A sense of teamwork is generally stronger in small communities where working together is essential. Flexibility in roles is also an advantage as the work of rural health care providers often involves a broader scope, and there is always need for cross-coverage. We believe these rural teams are powerful role models for students learning interprofessional skills.

Education is often seen as classroom-based or didactic rather than experiential or interactive group learning. The Rural Physician Associate Program is a familiar model in Minnesota for apprentice-style experiential learning that is an opportunity to translate or to develop aspects of the Rural Physician Associate Program experience for interprofessional students.

Technology offers challenges and opportunities. Although some communities may still be limited in terms of Internet bandwidth or cable access, other communities are early adopters by necessity. This might involve telemedicine or tele-education, electronic health records, early adoption of technology-assisted health care, and other technology innovations.

Although accessing care is often an issue in rural communities, expectations of the care provided may not be as rigid. Although there are still preferences and personality issues, there is an acceptance of what is available and a reluctance to travel too far for what is not available. Word of mouth is particularly important, and if there is an appreciation of team-based services, this will quickly become the norm.

Provider expectations are personality dependent and variable, but there is also often a recognition of the value of teamwork to make life easier and more enjoyable in the constantly demanding world of health care services.

Without health care providers or services, it is difficult for rural community members to remain healthy physically or for communities to survive economically. Rural health practitioners have an increased professional satisfaction with an opportunity to teach and/or mentor students, which leads to greater retention. Practitioners, health care staff, patients, and community members see the real or potential impact of making an investment in the education of health professions students when they see them return to the community.

LESSONS LEARNED: STRATEGIES FOR BUILDING THE NEXT GENERATION OF COMMUNITY–CAMPUS PARTNERSHIPS

Work From the Center, Not the Fringe

The University of Minnesota previously had not made a commitment to a rural health education vision from a senior leadership perspective. Workforce maldistribution and low percentages of health professional graduates selecting rural practice demonstrated this lack of strategic attention. Since 2000 a major University effort has been expended on addressing the workforce needs of greater Minnesota. This effort is beginning to demonstrate results. Before 2002, only 16% of the College of Pharmacy graduates selected rural practice. Today, a relatively large percentage of the first Duluth expansion pharmacy graduating class is selecting to practice in greater Minnesota. We believe policy decisions about rural health professions education that occur at the senior leadership level, engage deans and faculty, advocate at the state legislature successfully, and involve city and state government officials are necessary and essential for successful long-term outcomes.

Create Synergy by Building on Success

We have found that by partnering a successful program, Rural Physician Associate Program, with a new one has created a synergy for both programs. As a result, Rural Physician Associate Program has created new models of community health assessment projects that have become a launch for interprofessional education. Academic Health Center faculty colleagues have provided vitality for collaboration and development of a comprehensive interprofessional community teaching site for the future. Previous attempts at establishing rural health professions education programs met with limited success because of a lack of organizational support and full engagement of successful programs such as Rural Physician Associate Program.

Encouraging Innovation Through Shared Resources

No one organization, including public universities, has adequate resources to support health professional student's experiential education in rural communities. Yet, the future workforce depends on exposing students to rural and community practice. We now work to leverage resources to design community teaching sites where students can learn their clinical and community skills while contributing to community health outcomes. Our best examples involve starting with co-created financial plans and garnering resources together. Providing grant funding with expected in kind contributions, seeking out communities that had successful interprofessional practice models or experience with participating in the Rural Physician Associate Program, and working together in campus–community partnerships in which there are shared ideas and resources created a breeding ground for innovative interprofessional education. We are cultivating relationships with our community partners by creating innovative and meaningful interprofessional experiential education. The ultimate goal is to attract students, faculty, and community health practitioners who are committed to successful models of future practice.

Build Meaningful Partnerships

We have learned that money alone does not result in success. Previous experience with grant funds to develop a meaningful interprofessional experience did not result in a significant impact on students or communities. The numbers of students involved were small, and the experience was traditional classroom education. Having the area health education center regions established with experienced staff to support and be the interface in a campus–community partnership is fertile ground. The successful model of Rural Physician Associate Program has demonstrated valuable community–university partnership and successful educational and rural physician workforce outcomes. The area health education center interprofessional practice and education projects are developing community-specific experiential education opportunities with the partnership of university faculty and the support of the regional area health education centers.

Personality-Specific Work

Community–campus partnerships are often driven by specific individuals who have a passion for the work and, specifically in our case, rural health in Minnesota. Historically, rural health education in Minnesota has been driven by a few visionaries who have been instrumental in the success of the Rural Physician Associate Program over time. We recognize that continued development of rural interprofessional education and practice associated with the work of the Minnesota Area Health Education Center will require expanding the circle of committed faculty, students, health professionals, university administrators, and communities.

CONCLUSIONS

The leadership view from 30,000 feet allows a full perspective looking back over history, critically at the present, and toward the future. Although the interest in interprofessional education has existed for decades, the time is right to use the knowledge and resources we have to address the impending workforce shortage and the health care challenges of aging and increasingly diverse communities. This view is aimed at achieving success for the University and meeting the needs of the citizens of Minnesota. It includes a vision of transforming health professions education toward interprofessional teamwork that will be patient-centered and effective, using the evidence to improve the health of individuals and communities with team-based skills enhanced by the use of information and other technology. This transformation will be facilitated by a new Center for Interprofessional Education. The work of this Center will include the right educational methodology and faculty for teaching common ground topics of leadership and teamwork, quality improvement and patient safety, health informatics, health policy and care systems. Students will be taught in interprofessional teams throughout their educational experience on campus and in communities. Faculty and community health care practitioners will learn alongside students and patients. The goal is to develop new models of care delivery to address the growing problems of chronic disease and critical care and to improve our outcomes in health promotion and disease prevention. This will be a challenge, but the commitment to this goal is strong from the deans of the schools, faculty, students, and Minnesota communities—ready for teamwork toward a healthier Minnesota.

REFERENCES

1. Institute of Medicine, Committee on the Future of Rural Health Care. *Quality Through Collaboration: The Future of Rural Health Care.* Washington, DC: The National Academies Press; 2005.
2. Institute of Medicine. *Academic Health Centers: Leading Change in the 21st Century.* Washington, DC: The National Academies Press; 2003.
3. United Health Foundation. America's Health Rankings. Available at: www.united-healthfoundation.org/shr2005/Findings.html. Accessed March 31, 2007.
4. Casey M, Call K, Klinger J. Are rural residents less likely to obtain recommended preventive healthcare services? *Am J Prevent Med.* 2001;21:182–188.
5. Minnesota Department of Health. Office of Rural Health and Primary Care and Center for Health Statistics. *Health and Well-Being of Rural Minnesotans: A Minnesota Rural Health Status Report.* Available at: http://www.health.state.mn.us/divs/chs/reports/hwb.pdf. Accessed March 31, 2007.
6. Minnesota Department of Health. Office of Rural Health & Primary Care Health Workforce Analysis Program. *Demographics of Physicians, Nurses and Dentists: Urban-Rural Comparisons of Minnesota's Health Care Workforce.* Available at: http://www.health.state.mn.us/divs/orhpc/pubs/workforce/demo.pdf. Accessed March 31, 2007.
7. Brandt B, Ling L. *Final Report of the Academic Health Center Task Force, Transforming the University.* Minneapolis, MN: University of Minnesota; 2006.
8. Minnesota Department of Health. *Health Professions Education in Minnesota: Results of the 2001–2003 Minnesota Health Professions Trainee Exit Surveys.* Available at: http://www.health.state.mn.us/divs/hpsc/hep/merc/workforce/extsrv03.pdf. Accessed March 31, 2007.
9. Gillaspy T. Minnesota State Demographic Center. *Minnesota Population Projections by Race and Hispanic Origin 2000–2030.* Available at: http://www.demography.state.mn.us/DownloadFiles/PopulationProjectionsRaceHispanicOrigin.pdf. Accessed March 31, 2007.

10. Ronningen BJ. Minnesota State Demographic Center. *Estimates of Selected Immigrant Populations in Minnesota: 2004*. Available at: http://www.demography.state.mn.us/PopNotes/EvaluatingEstimates.pdf. Accessed March 31, 2007.

11. McMurry M. Minnesota State Demographic Center. *Elderly Minnesotans: A 2000 Census Portrait*. Available at: http://www.demography.state.mn.us/PopNotes/ElderlyMinnesotans2004.pdf. Accessed March 31, 2007.

12. Faculty Workgroup on Peopling Long Term Care. *Peopling Long-term Care: Assuring an Adequate Workforce for Minnesota*. Minneapolis, MN: University of Minnesota; 2001.

Training for Interprofessional Services to Appalachian Adolescents with Mental Health Needs: Lessons Learned from PRISYM

Doris Pierce, PhD, OT, FAOTA
Amy Marshall, MS, OT
Stephanie W. Adams, MSW
Carol W. Cecil, MA, EdD
Brent Garrett, PhD, MPA
Marlene Belew Huff, PhD, LCSW
Carmilla Ratliff

INTRODUCTION

Originally scheduled to run from 2004 to 2007, congressional budget cuts under Title VII of all Quentin N. Burdick Interdisciplinary Rural Health Training Programs reduced the Providing Rural Interdisciplinary Services for Youth with Mental Health Needs (PRISYM) Project by 1 year. Thus it ran from 2004 to 2006. Although this was disappointing to the highly invested interprofessional PRISYM team, the project still generated many lessons, accomplished its objectives, and has served to launch other initiatives that continue emphasis on the development of services to Appalachian at-risk youth. PRISYM's program objectives were, in general, the development of exemplary interprofessional rural training experiences, provision of services to Appalachian youth with mental health needs, research contributions in this area, and making rural practice a more attractive career choice. We focus this chapter, however, on PRISYM's training objectives and the lessons they generated for PRISYM's leadership team, trainees, training sites, and state agencies. PRISYM training objectives were as follows:

1. Trainees will be competent in interdisciplinary collaboration.
2. Trainees will be prepared to provide culturally sensitive services to rural Appalachian clients.
3. Trainees will examine the advantages and disadvantages of rural practice as a personal career choice.
4. Trainees will collaborate within an action research approach to training and service program development.

The three professions trained through PRISYM were occupational therapy, social work, and psychology. The social work trainees were undergraduates, whereas the occupational therapy and psychology trainees were graduate students. The PRISYM plan of study (Table 23-1) fit into all students' final year requirements in their professional training and was shaped by the themes of the training objectives previously stated.

Trainees completed all aspects of the plan of study together in annual cohorts. Sharing all training experiences as a bonded cohort built a history of

Table 23-1. PRISYM Plan of Study

PRISYM Semester	PRISYM Courses (Credits)	Other Credits (not PRISYM)
Fall	OTS 520/720 Providing Health Services in Appalachia (3) OTS 875 PRISYM Seminar I (1)	OT: 9 Psychology: 10 SW: 9

Spring	Interdisciplinary Rural Immersion Practice Experience:
	   OTS 847 Professional Fieldwork (2)
	   PSY 899 Internship (6)
	   SWK 490 Final Social Work Field Practicum (12)
	   OTS 875 PRISYM Seminar II (1)
		OT: 7
		 Psychology: 3
		 SW: 0

OTS, Occupational Therapy.
PSY, Psychology.
SWK, Social Work.

understanding of each other as persons, as disciplinary practitioners, and as interprofessional team members with specific strengths and needs. There were 15 trainees in cohort 1 during the 2004–2005 academic year, which was kept purposefully small for program development. In 2005–2006 there were 25 trainees in cohort 2. We provide descriptive data here for this second, larger cohort. Although PRISYM was defunded for 2006–2007, by incorporating aspects of the PRISYM plan of study and developed field sites into the existing educational programs of the occupational therapy and social work programs, a small cohort of trainees is currently being supported.

Carmilla's Story: My Challenges and Successes With My Mental Illness

We start this chapter with the story by a member of the PRISYM leadership team about her own experiences with mental health services as she grew up in a small town in Kentucky. It illustrates in a very real way how complex services to Appalachian youth with mental health needs can be and the primary challenges to the PRISYM training program: creating an effective interprofessional service team, working appropriately within mountain culture, the shortage of skilled rural service providers, and issues of justice and power at many levels. Carmilla's story is not unusual for at-risk youth in Kentucky, except that she has managed to make a great success of her life, which is certainly not the typical case.

I have an older sister who stayed gone a lot. . . . My mom went to bars with her friends, leaving me home with my dad. My dad was emotionally abusive to me for years and no one knew. . . .When I was twelve I started having headaches and back pain. I went to the doctor and he started doing different tests and didn't find anything so he sent me to different doctors. They didn't find anything. My parents accused me of faking it. My doctor told me and my mom that I need to see a psychiatrist. I refused to go, I cussed and yelled that's for crazy people, I'm not crazy there's nothing wrong with me! My family has something wrong with them! I agreed to go so I could prove that there's something wrong with my parents not me. The psychiatrist was the first person I told what my parents were doing. I've never had headaches or back pain since.

I always felt like no one believed me when I told them what my parents were doing to me. I always got nervous meeting new therapists, because I felt like I had to start all over. I always struggled with taking medicine because it meant something was wrong with me. I'm not normal. It was explained to me by saying a diabetic takes medicine to produce the insulin they need, and you need medicine because your brain isn't producing the chemicals needed. This was not the same thing to me! I never heard anyone making fun of a diabetic, calling them names or acting like something was wrong with them. I was hospitalized off and on from twelve years old.

My first year of high school, I was put in the hospital for a month. Every time I returned to school from being at the hospital, students were rude to me. I didn't make friends. The school charged me with truancy. They said they would drop the charges if I went to alternative school. I didn't feel I had any choice but to go. I went there for the rest of school. We did worksheets and copied stuff out of old books. I made copies, filed papers, and answered the phone. The highest grade I could make was a C. Most of the kids had behavior problems. There were no doors on the rooms. There were five teachers for about fifty students. I thought they were teachers, it turns out that at least two were instructors. It leaves me wondering if any of them had any teaching degrees.

My family doesn't understand about mental illness. My dad is prescribed medicine by the same doctor I see, but refuses to take the medicine because he says there's nothing wrong with him. I tried to talk to him about my social anxiety, and he said that he's not like that. How did I get that? My mom also thinks that she's not like me and it's not her fault. My sister recently said to me that she thinks it was wrong for therapists and doctors I have seen to not tell me that I would not always need medicine. . . . Without my parents' support, I had to learn to advocate for myself and find support in others. I received services through Kentucky Impact, which helps young people with serious emotional disturbances. You have a service coordinator who works with a team of people including family members and the consumer to get the help you need. The services I received helped me. I attended youth groups, and had a big buddy type person that did things with me. The services I received helped me. After I was out of the Impact program I joined a youth council to help reduce the stigma of mental illness. I learned even more about advocating for myself and others.

LESSON ONE: DEFINING A STRONG SERVICE TEAM FOR APPALACHIAN AT-RISK YOUTH

What Do We Mean by a Team?

When PRISYM was conceptualized, the grant-writing group was thinking very much as health care providers. To us, a strong interdisciplinary team included health professionals from as many different professional perspectives as possible. Occupational therapy, psychology, and social work joined forces within PRISYM because the three professions had shared interests in at-risk Appalachian youth, community-based services, and client-centered perspectives.

The PRISYM leadership team, or management group, initially included the project director, training coordinators for each profession, a representative from the Kentucky Department of Mental Health and Mental Retardation Services, two service coordinators from the two state mental health regions who had subcontracts to provide the training sites for the students, a cultural competency coordinator who was also the director of Eastern Kentucky University's Center for Appalachian Studies, and the director and a consumer from an advocacy group for this population, the Kentucky Partnership for Families and Children. The team alternated between meeting face-to-face, often over potlucks, and via the Kentucky Tele-Link Network (KTLN).

As the leadership team began working in the participatory action research cycles that were planned for development of PRISYM, one of the first topics for critical discussions was what we meant by an interdisciplinary team and preparation of trainees for interdisciplinary collaboration. This questioning of our health care–shaped definition of an interdisciplinary team was very beneficial and resulted in rippling improvements to the entire project. Through discussion, literature review, and examination of the types of teams at the wide variety of service sites in the rural mountain regions targeted and being considered for training use, we came to redefine the optimal service team for adolescents with mental health needs. Neither "interdisciplinary" nor "interprofessional" were appropriate terms, for several reasons. They were too identified with health care, thus excluding from our conceptualization of the team the many educators, family members, juvenile justice professionals, and other community members who played important roles on the support teams of adolescents with mental health needs. They did emphasize sufficiently the importance of the team being family and child driven. This was not only a critical issue of justice and power in managing services to at-risk youth but also influenced the effectiveness of the team in prioritizing the goals of service and selecting the most useful strategies. Finally, one of the most difficult aspects of providing services to at-risk rural youth was the degree to which they were involved with multiple agency types that were all underresourced. That is, these young people were dealing with, at minimum, both alternative educational programs and medical services. Often, they also had involvement with the social services and juvenile justice systems as well. Strong teamwork required professionals who could work effectively in an interagency fashion, despite striking differences in the cultures and missions of their agencies.

PRISYM settled on defining a strong service team for adolescents with mental health needs as unique to the needs and circumstances of each individual served, youth guided and family driven, and effectively coordinated across multiple agencies. State policy and system reform in the children's mental health system were important components of this picture. A statewide program, Kentucky IMPACT, grew out of the need for more community-based intervention for children and adolescents with severe emotional disabilities. Kentucky IMPACT, established in 1990, is a statewide program which coordinates services for children with severe emotional disabilities and their families. In addition to establishing a coordinated, interagency approach to service delivery, this model provides funding for services not traditionally available, such as mentoring and intensive in-home therapy. The Kentucky Bridges Project, built on the infrastructure of IMPACT, extends school-based mental health services beyond school-based therapy to a continuum of positive behavioral interventions and supports and a wraparound approach across multiple environments. Kentucky is fortunate in having such an interagency and family-driven system of care across most agencies serving this population. Efforts to implement structures that support this model from the state to the local level are growing and have different degrees of effectiveness depending on locality.

The PRISYM leadership team was also changed by this examination of the meaning of a service team. We found it beneficial to add parent advocates from both service regions, the field placement coordinators from each academic department, the instructor for the Health Care Services in Appalachia course, and state agency representatives beyond mental health.

Training for Strong Service Team Participation

PRISYM intentionally prepared trainees to understand, observe, analyze, experience, and continually improve team collaboration and to develop interdisciplinary insight. This was accomplished through study of the literature on interdisciplinary collaboration, shared learning in the interdisciplinary training cohort over a full academic year, interdisciplinary student teams within shared rural practice and living experiences, observation of and participation in the PRISYM leadership team, interdisciplinary teaching of the seminars by the training coordinators, participation on diverse teams providing services to adolescents with mental health needs, and sharing written reflections on team processes and experiences with their training cohort.

To assess student growth in team collaboration skills, we used a pre- and posttest student survey (Table 23-2). The pre- and posttesting of training objectives was field tested with cohort 1 and revised. The pretest was administered to cohort 2 in August 2005 and the posttest was administered in April 2006. Each of the five items had a statistically significant increase between pre- and posttest. The greatest degree of change was with the item, "I feel prepared to work as part of an interdisciplinary team," which was a key PRISYM outcome.

Site supervisors were also asked to rate to what degree students were able to work as part of a strong service team at the end of their internship. Sixty-five percent of the supervisors strongly agreed with the statement, "students were well prepared to work as part of an interdisciplinary team."

Student feedback focused on the importance of collaboration across disciplines. Students want more time to communicate with and become more familiar with students from other disciplines, both in classroom settings and at internship sites. One student suggested that it would be helpful to rotate among sites to get more experience at different types of sites. Another student proposed that more collaborative case studies be used in class as part of interdisciplinary small group work. Students suggested that these changes would lead to a greater understanding of the "techniques" of different disciplines and they would gain more information and opportunities for interagency networking and the gathering of community resources.

The need to increase the sharing of service team experiences and variety for the trainees resulted in the evolution from a small effort in the first year to formal adoption in the second year of cluster meetings. The clusters served as an additional place that students in service sites within an area of one region could meet every 2 weeks and discuss their team experiences and cases.

Table 23-2. Student Data Related to Interdisciplinary Collaboration

Items	Pretest		Posttest		Paired Samples t-Test		
	Mean	SD	Mean	SD	Mean	t Score	Significance
1. Trainees will be competent in interdisciplinary collaboration.							
1a. I understand the difference between the roles of members in a multidisciplinary, interdisciplinary, and transdisciplinary team.	3.56	0.82	4.22	0.80	+0.65	2.812	0.010
1b. I have a clear understanding of the roles of the health professions that are represented in PRISYM.	3.84	0.55	4.43	0.59	+0.57	3.725	0.001
1c. I feel prepared to work as part of an interdisciplinary team upon graduation.	3.84	0.62	4.65	0.49	+0.74	4.715	0.000
1d. I think it is beneficial to work as part of an interdisciplinary team.	4.28	0.68	4.7	0.56	+0.48	2.712	0.013
1e. I believe that team interaction is as important as the skills of an individual health provider in influencing the outcomes of clients.	4.44	0.51	4.74	0.45	+0.35	2.336	0.029

SD, standard deviation.

LESSON TWO: APPRECIATING AND PROVIDING SERVICES WITHIN APPALACHIAN CULTURE

A Culture Both Exploited and Valued

Provision of effective services in rural eastern Kentucky requires an appreciation of Appalachian culture. A unique set of abilities to understand, communicate with, and provide services to individuals and families of Appalachian descent is required. From practitioners, Appalachians regularly encounter a degree of ridicule and blame for their poverty and illiteracy that most practitioners would consider to be completely inappropriate when providing services to disadvantaged populations of more obvious ethnic difference. This results in misinterpretations of client actions and values, ongoing prejudice, and significant failures of intervention.

The impact of stigma and governmental neglect of the needs of rural Appalachia is an historical pattern that has broad effects. During the early 20th century, Appalachia was described as "a strange land of peculiar people." Appalachia has been stereotyped as unequal and separate from the rest of the country ever since.[1] However, this stigmatizing "idea of Appalachia" ignores historical realities.[2] The region has been dominated by the coal industry since the early 20th century and was the site of some of the earliest and most hard-fought labor union battles in the United States. Because of increasing mechanization of the coal extraction process, however, few mining jobs are now available for its residents. Those who do have mining jobs are increasingly unsafe in the current period of weakened safety regulation of the industry. Decades of corporate abuse related to the mining industry have undermined civic structures. Families and communities have been weakened by generations of outmigration in search of work. Further, the region's environment has been destroyed by exploitation of natural resources by absentee international landowners. For example, over 600 miles of the Kentucky River are unsafe for human use.[3] Given this history, it is not surprising that Appalachian people are mistrustful of outsiders who come for a time to their communities to serve, educate, photograph, improve, or convert them.

Lost in this picture of disadvantage and poverty is the richness of Appalachian culture. Appalachian crafts, music, dance, food, auto and horse racing, and art are all central to the American identity. Though many Americans define themselves as "not that" in terms of the "hillbilly" stereotype so widely disseminated by the media, the image of the proud mountaineer is also central to our positive consciousness of what it means to be an

Table 23-3. Student Data Related to Cultural Competence

Items	Pretest		Posttest		Paired Samples t-Test		
	Mean	SD	Mean	SD	Mean	t Score	Significance
2. Trainees will be prepared to provide culturally sensitive services to rural Appalachian clients.							
2a. I have insights into how my own cultural background shapes my interactions with others on a daily basis.	4.24	0.44	4.87	0.34	+0.61	5.850	0.000
2b. I understand and easily accept differences in other cultural groups although I may not personally agree with their beliefs.	4.28	0.54	4.61	0.50	+0.35	2.912	0.008
2c. I have a well-developed understanding of Appalachian culture.	4.16	0.75	4.78	0.42	+0.57	4.092	0.000
2d. I appreciate and understand culture when working or interacting with people from rural Appalachia.	4.00	0.65	4.78	0.42	+0.74	5.725	0.000

SD, standard deviation.

American. That love for the land, commitment to family and community, resistance to oppression, and fierce freedom appeal to our sense of who we are as a nation. To serve well in Appalachian communities requires moving beyond stereotypes and systematic oppression to the development of an appreciation of the rich culture of Appalachia through study, community experiences, and immersion in regional service.

Training for Services in Appalachia

Developing training experiences that resulted in service providers who appreciated and could skillfully negotiate mountain culture was also a focus of development within PRISYM. The following didactic, experiential, and formal assignments were used within the PRISYM program of study. Focused study of Appalachian culture, history, impacts of poverty, economic issues, communication patterns, and health care services and beliefs occurred in the course, OTS 520/720 Providing Health Services in Appalachia. In the class, students also observed an Appalachian, grassroots organized, community health clinic. PRISYM Seminar I included cohort outings to community mountain festivals, brief observation site visits to anticipated regional training sites, and presentations by state agencies and the Kentucky Partnership for Families and Children. Their service provision experiences in mountain communities were from 4 to 16 weeks in duration, depending on discipline.

We used the same pre- and posttest method of assessment of cultural competence as we did to examine the trainee's development of team skills (Table 23-3). Four of the five items had a statistically significant increase between

Table 23-4. Site Supervisors' Perceptions Regarding Students' Cultural Competence

Supervisor Perceptions	Strongly Agree
Understood the beliefs that clients may have about their mental health.	30%
Understood that his/her culture might be different from the culture of clients' families.	65%
Treated clients with respect.	96%
Understood that people from the clients' culture are not all alike.	83%
Understood clients' needs.	74%

pre- and posttest. The greatest degree of change was with the item, "I have insights into how my own cultural background shapes my interactions with others on a daily basis."

Table 23-4 provides data regarding site supervisors' perceptions regarding the cultural competence of the students at their sites. Ninety-six percent of the supervisors strongly agreed that students treated their clients with respect, and 83% strongly agreed with the statement that students understood basic differences among different cultures.

LESSON THREE: THE CHALLENGES OF SERVING AN UNDERSERVED RURAL AREA

Getting Comfortable with Challenge

One of the greatest challenges for both staff and trainees in PRISYM was in understanding, accepting, and working effectively within a severely underserved rural area. Without such an understanding and acceptance, burnout was not far behind. The tension this continual challenge caused could be seen in how new trainees regarded the less than luxurious surroundings of rural clinics, could not understand why their inquiring calls could not be promptly returned by overburdened rural service coordinators, or struggled with the demanding drive to their service sites. For the staff, it was seen in the relationship between the university-based project and its collaborating rural mental health regions, which had to be handled with great sensitivity and egalitarian decision making, and in feelings that no matter how hard we worked we could never overcome such resource issues. Still, with mutual support, acceptance, and openness, this issue could be managed and the positive aspects of rural practice could be displayed to the trainees for their consideration as a part of their future careers. Many of the trainees were from rural Kentucky and wanted very much to develop good professional relationships in their home counties that might lead to that treasured rural accomplishment, a good local job.

Systemic Economic, Service, and Education Challenges

In 1965 Congress created the Appalachian Regional Commission (ARC) to advocate for a 13-state impoverished, mountainous area of the eastern United States, including Kentucky. The poverty rate in the designated 51-county region of Appalachian Kentucky is 24%, almost double the U.S. average.[4] Eighty-eight percent of the counties in Appalachian Kentucky are classified by the ARC as economically distressed or at-risk.[5] Both service regions of PRISYM, the Cumberland River and Kentucky River Community Care, have lower median income; greater levels of child, youth, and household poverty; fewer adults who have completed high school; and higher levels of unemployment than the state as a whole.

Services to adolescents with mental health needs are made more complex by the fact that their needs seem to be the responsibility of several systems and yet of no particular system. Adolescents with mental health needs are legally mandated to receive educationally related services through school systems under the Individuals with Disabilities Education Act (2005 IDEA Amendments) but often have unmet needs. Health care systems often do not give care coverage for mental health disorders to the degree that they do other medical diagnoses. Community-based mental health services attempt to address these needs but are often short of resources. Adolescents with emotional and behavioral disorders enter the juvenile justice and court systems at high rates. This multiplicity of systems and the difficulties in coordinating between them make services to adolescents with mental health needs especially challenging.

In the Kentucky school system from 1992 to 2002, there was a 78% increase in the number of students identified with emotional and behavioral disabilities.[6] Although 16% of students in Kentucky's public schools are identified as having a disability, 46% of youth in state-administered, nontraditional educational settings in Kentucky have disabilities.[7] Most of the adolescents who received services through PRISYM are in nontraditional educational settings. Youth with disabilities are overrepresented in nontraditional educational settings for several reasons. One reason is because the actions of teenagers with emotional and behavioral disorders are frequently misinterpreted as delinquent and criminal acts. This leads to higher arrest rates and higher placement rates in alternative facilities for adolescents with mental health disorders.[8,9] Some have argued that budgetary pressures on Kentucky schools to show rapid improvements under Kentucky Education Reform Act have increased the numbers of youth moved to alternative settings to remove the scores of less successful students from school accountability data.

Challenges of Distance, Weather, and Technology

By its very nature, rural practice occurs in distant and underserved communities. During their training, students spent a great deal of time traveling between their homes and their placement sites. Several of the students at both campuses also spent up to 2 hours each way traveling to the university to attend classes each week. Because the service experiences began in January, this meant dealing with eastern Kentucky winter weather—icy roads and frequent school closures. Rural roads are not typically plowed, so transportation during the winter months is treacherous. Many of the students were placed in nontraditional, alternative, and secure educational settings.

PRISYM trainees were enrolled at two different campuses that were a 2-hour drive apart. For this reason, most of the PRISYM plan of study was taught over the KTLN, a real-time video instruction system that covers the state. Although this technology allows rural students access to classes they would otherwise not have, it also presented some barriers for these classes. Usually, the university instructors preferred to stay in the college town for instruction rather than teach from the distant site. This put the more rural campus students at a disadvantage and displayed a power differential. Many times, facial expressions, body language, and voice inflection was lost over the video connection. Comments were often misconstrued because the speaker's intent or intended audience was not clear to the students in the distant site. In several cases, there were problems with the audio reception. Many strategies were tried to ameliorate these technology challenges, including instructor travel, starting each semester with face-to-face sessions, local cluster meetings instead of KTLN meetings, and gathering the students at a single site periodically for potlucks.

Site Development Challenges

Site development emerged as a focus early in the action research cycles. A lack of qualified supervisors for the students in their placements was a significant problem at several sites. PRISYM had specifically targeted Mental Health Professions Shortage Area (MHPSA) counties, which meant there were few advanced-level clinicians available to supervise students on a day-to-day basis. This challenge was partially overcome by using weekly supervision by an additional regional professional for social work students, a paid itinerant weekly supervisor for psychology students, and employing a full-time supervisor for occupational therapy students.

There was an additional challenge in finding placements that provided services in a way that affirmed conceptualizations of quality care in all three disciplines. Because of lack of staff, limited budgets, and few community resources, some rural agencies were not operating in a way that was appropriate for student placement. Biweekly cluster meetings were held for all PRISYM trainees during the second semester in which they completed their field placements. In the clusters, students could discuss the complex situations of providing best quality care within constrained resources and the different ways in which each team resolved those challenges.

The leadership team focused on developing key sites that promised variety and potential for exemplary care to at-risk adolescents in rural Kentucky. This resulted in many innovative demonstration models for training in the two regions. They provided excellent rural experiences for the PRISYM trainees. Many of them have been incorporated into the social work and occupational therapy educational programs. The sites included both traditional models such as residential facilities, crisis stabilization units, drug treatment clinics, youth and family outpatient centers, alternative schools, juvenile detention centers, and also a variety of nontraditional sites. The nontraditional sites included Building Bridges of Support Project, a multidisciplinary wraparound team model providing mental health services to youth within the school system; Creating Opportunities for Parents Everywhere, an advocacy facility run by parents; Reclaiming Mountain Futures, a Robert Wood Johnson Foundation systems change grant focusing on youth with substance abuse problems concurrently involved with the juvenile justice system; and Community Collaborations for Children, a public nonprofit organization mobilizing community supports for youth.

Learning Experiences Focused on Considering a Rural Practice Career

A primary objective of PRISYM was to prepare graduates more likely to enter rural practice and to deliver health care services to youth in rural regions of Kentucky, where a significant shortage of mental health care professionals exists. To increase this likelihood, PRISYM trainee selection occurred through application and interview. An essay describing rural background and experiences and degree of interest in a career in rural practice was required and scored. The coordinators and project director developed a scoring system for the essay that indicates strength of interest in rural practice. A Likert scale questionnaire was also used to assess comfort and familiarity with Appalachian culture, rural experiences, and desire to practice in a rural setting. The project was successful in seeing many trainees take positions in rural practice after graduation, often in their previous training placements.

Table 23-5. Student Data Related to Rural Employment

Items	Pretest		Posttest		Paired Samples t-Test		
	Mean	SD	Mean	SD	Mean	t Score	Significance
3. Trainees will examine the advantages and disadvantages of rural practice as a personal career choice.							
3a. I am well prepared to work in a rural, underserved area.	3.72	0.84	4.61	0.50	+0.83	5.527	0.000
3b. I am planning to work in a rural Appalachian area upon graduation.	3.96	0.89	4.05	1.21	+0.05	0.188	0.853
3c. I understand the many advantages and disadvantages of working in a rural area.	3.92	0.76	4.7	0.47	+0.74	4.101	0.000
3d. I am confident that strategies can be learned to manage any disadvantages of working in a rural area.	4.08	0.40	4.43	0.73	+0.39	2.598	0.016
3e. My internship experience assisted me in understanding the advantages and disadvantages of working in a rural area.	3.72	0.84	4.52	0.59	+0.78	4.413	0.000

SD, standard deviation.

The primary learning experience in regard to rural practice was, of course, service provision in a rural site. PRISYM trainees spent 4 to 16 weeks in a rural immersion experience of interprofessional service provision for adolescents with mental health needs. The trainees engaged in a number of additional learning experiences concerning the advantages and disadvantages of rural practice, including observation of diverse rural service sites in OTS 520/720 Providing Health Services in Appalachia, in PRISYM Seminars I and II, and in the service placement; cohort outings to community mountain festivals; qualitative interviews of practitioners regarding their perspective on rural practice; sharing of experiences in different rural settings in seminars and cluster meetings; and reflective journaling on personal choice of rural practice.

Again, we assessed cohort 2 perceptions regarding employment in rural areas using a pre- and posttest assessment. Data regarding student perceptions about rural employment are shown in Table 23-5. Four of the five items had a statistically significant increase between pre- and posttest. The greatest degree of change was with the item, "I am well prepared to work in a rural, underserved area." At the same time, there was little, if any, change in student responses regarding actually working in a rural environment. This was likely influenced by many decisions, especially the psychology students' commitment to completing PhD programs after graduation.

Only 35% of site supervisors perceived students to be well prepared at the beginning of the field experience. When asked to what degree did site supervisors agree with the statement that students "developed sufficient strategies to work successfully in a rural area," 83% strongly agreed. These data suggest significant growth in student skills. Several students described their discovery of the realities of working in rural Appalachia, such as the limited opportunities for children to receive psychiatric services because of the severe shortage of health care professionals and high turnover as well as the stigmatizing effects of mental illness in children.

LESSON FOUR: ADDRESSING JUSTICE AND POWER AT MANY LEVELS

Deal Openly with Justice and Power

Working in a region with a history of exploitation and an appropriately skeptical view of new service programs, it is best to deal openly and very consciously with issues of power and justice. This can be done through education of project personnel and trainees about and public acknowledgements of the history of the region. Open relationships between the university and its regional service providers and between the university and state agencies are also critical when operating within such a region. Ensuring egalitarian relations and full input for all within the management team, between co-instructors, within student teams, and in service sites helps to demonstrate and make real the values of the project within all its operations. In PRISYM, there was also a very direct advocacy of the values of social justice and occupational justice in the students' training.

Social justice is the view that everyone deserves equal economic, political, and social rights and opportunities. Armed with the long-term goal of empowering their clients, social workers use knowledge of existing legal principles and organizational structure to suggest changes to protect their clients, who are often powerless and underserved. This is particularly true in rural areas, where clients are statistically most likely to live in poverty and experience a lack of services in the areas of human service. Occupational justice is the right of all individuals to daily opportunities for action that are meaningful and satisfying to them.

PRISYM's use of an action research approach was a primary way of keeping justice and power issues fully in focus. Action research uses an ongoing cycle of data collection, analysis, and action to develop useful knowledge.[10] Action research has long been used as a method of professional development in nursing[11] and in teaching[12,13] as well as for program development and evaluation.[14,15] The ability of PRISYM to meet its objectives was continually reevaluated and improved through the action research cycle. In this way, PRISYM was methodologically responsive to the needs of trainees, clients, rural partners, and the university. The action research cycle repeats: establishment of a research question during a leadership team meeting, data collection, data analysis, data review by the leadership team, and recommendations for improvement. Initially, the program objectives and training competencies were the focus of the action research process. This focus gradually shifted, however, to hone in on key challenges to PRISYM objectives, such as those reported here as "lessons." Use of the leadership team to establish questions ensured that the voices of the rural partners, the client advocates, and the three training disciplines are all heard in the selection of areas of development. Although the team would have preferred a more participatory action research approach that directly included data from the adolescents, the barriers of human subjects review for this population could not

Table 23-6. Student Data Related to Participatory Action Research

Items	Pretest		Posttest		Paired Samples t-Test		
	Mean	SD	Mean	SD	Mean	t Score	Significance
4. Trainees will collaborate within an action research approach to training and service program development.							
4a. I have studied and understand action research.	3.4	0.71	4.22	0.52	+0.78	4.159	0.000
4b. I have observed the action 4c. research cycle.	3.32	0.85	4.13	0.76	+0.78	3.332	0.003
4c. I have participated in data collection in action research.	3.08	0.95	4.13	0.87	+1.05	4.219	0.000
4d. I understand the process of action research in the continued improvement of research projects.	3.48	0.82	4.35	0.57	+0.87	4.800	0.000
4e. I would consider using action research in my own clinical practice or direct service position.	3.76	0.72	4.39	0.66	+0.57	3.214	0.004

SD, standard deviation.

be surmounted. Action research data included scheduled audio-taped reflective responses to questions periodically revised by the leadership team, student interviews of rural service site practitioners, and more traditional collection of indicators of PRISYM's effectiveness in meeting its objectives.

Training in Justice, Power, and Participatory Action Research

The operation and values of PRISYM were kept fully transparent to the trainees. In the course, "Health Care Services in Appalachia," the regional history of exploitation and injustice was explored as a part of learning the culture within which trainees would be providing services. Seminars I and II included guest speakers who described the resource constraints in various rural care sites, interview and observation assignments to generate date for the development of PRISYM, and study of the action research process itself.

Once again, we used the pre- and posttest assessment to gauge changes in student perceptions regarding participatory action research (Table 23-6). All five items had a statistically significant increase between pre- and posttest. The greatest degree of change was with the item, "I have participated in data collection in action research," as would be expected after participating in the intervention. The second largest change was the item regarding an understanding of the process of action research in the continued improvement of research projects.

CONCLUSIONS: A SUCCESS AND TAKE HOME LESSONS

A Success in Training for Team Service to Appalachian At-Risk Youth

Everyone involved with PRISYM considers it a strong success. Despite the defunding of the third year of the project due to congressional budget cuts, PRISYM provided in-depth preparation to 46 new graduates in occupational therapy, psychology, and social work to provide services to at-risk Appalachian youth that were culturally effective and used a family-driven and student-centered team model. Items from each of the training objectives were aggregated and analyzed at the objective level. The resulting data for each objective are listed in Table 23-7. Statistically significant growth ($p < 0.05$) was observed for three of the four objectives, and strong support ($p = 0.066$) was found for the fourth objective. These data suggest that stu-

Table 23-7.   Student Data Related to Successful Completion of the Four PRISYM Training Objectives

Expected Areas of Impact	Mean Difference Between Pre and Post	t Score	Significance
1. Trainees will be competent in interdisciplinary collaboration.	+0.557	4.774	0.000
2. Trainees will be prepared to provide culturally sensitive services to rural Appalachian clients.	+0.522	5.509	0.000
3. Trainees will examine the advantages and disadvantages of rural practice as a personal career choice.	+0.559	4.465	0.000
4. Trainees will collaborate within an action research approach to training and service program development.	+0.548	1.936	0.066

dents experienced significant growth throughout their field experience in the areas of team collaboration, cultural competence, rural employment, and action research.

As displayed in Table 23-8, supervisors were also satisfied with the growth of PRISYM students. Ninety-one percent of the site supervisors strongly agreed with the statement, "I would hire this person after my experience working with her/him." Less support was shown for students' knowledge of content necessary to complete their assigned work, but 74% of the site supervisors strongly agreed with the statement, "I am satisfied with their knowledge of content necessary to complete the work assigned to her/him."

PRISYM students provided qualitative feedback regarding short-term outcomes and ideas for future program improvement:

- The program provided the opportunity to work and practice skills hands-on with at-risk youth at their agencies.
- Fieldwork sites gave students a level of competence that the classroom didn't provide.

Table 23-8. Site Supervisors' Overall Impression of PRISYM Student Performance

Supervisor Perceptions	Strongly Agree
I am satisfied with their overall performance in their field experience during the spring of 2006.	87%
I am satisfied with their knowledge of content necessary to complete the work assigned to her/him.	74%
I would hire this person after my experience working with her/him.	91%

- Several students mentioned that this was their first opportunity to work with at-risk adolescents, and after this experience they would choose to work with this population.

Take Home Lessons

The lessons described here are those that seemed most intriguing to us as PRISYM unfolded. We developed many good training strategies that may serve to spur ideas in other training teams, though certainly all projects are considerably different and require custom design. At this point, our strongest recommendations to those serving at-risk youth or rural areas are as follows:

- Open up your conceptualization of your service team to put children and families in charge of their services and to include key players in the lives of your clients who can positively impact client outcomes. Connect more inclusively to communities and agencies in all levels of your operations.
- Use sophisticated, in-depth, and multistrategy preparation to improve service providers' negotiation of client cultures. They can never understand too much about the culture of the communities they serve. This will also go far in reducing the power differential between providers and clients that can be so debilitating to team effectiveness.
- Get comfortable with the permanent challenge of underresourced rural services. Help young service providers get comfortable with this. The issue is too large to be corrected by an individual or team. Therefore, it must be acknowledged, accepted, and managed as a stressor and as a

unique facet of service provision. Get very good at prioritizing, flexibility, and collaboration to stretch resources further.

- Examine and share the advantages of rural practice within teams. Too often we speak about the difficulties and not often enough about the things we treasure about rural practice: driving through beauty, working in communities where people know each other, living affordably or in nature, and flexible, self-directed, and variety-filled work lives.
- Deal with justice and power at all levels and at all times by acknowledging permanent injustices publicly, seeking open and collaborative work styles within all teams, using advocacy when opportunities arise, and using program development strategies such as action research to keep services responsive to all stakeholders.

REFERENCES

1. Shapiro H. *Appalachia on Our Mind: The Southern Mountains and Mountaineers in the American Consciousness, 1870–1920*. Chapel Hill, NC: University of North Carolina Press; 1978.
2. Eller RD. Foreword. In: Billings DB, Norman G, Ledford K, eds. *Confronting Appalachian Stereotypes: Back Talk From an American Region*. Lexington, KY: University Press of Kentucky; 1999:ix–xi.
3. Cole L, Siegel E. *2000–2001 State of Kentucky's Environment: A Report of Environmental Trends and Conditions*. Frankfort, KY: Kentucky Environmental Quality Commission; 2001.
4. Appalachian Regional Commission. Poverty rates, 2000. Available at: http://www.arc.gov/index.do?nodeId=58. Accessed January 10, 2007.
5. Appalachian Regional Commission. County economic status: Fiscal year 2006. Available at: http://www.arc.gov/index.do?nodeId=58#econ. Accessed January 10, 2007.
6. Kentucky Department of Education. Students with disabilities in the educational setting: 2001–02 school year. Available at: http://www.kde.state.ky.us/osis/children/Data2001-02/2001Disability.XLS. Accessed January 10, 2003.
7. Kentucky Department of Juvenile Justice. *Annual Report: Fiscal Year 2002*. Frankfort, KY: Kentucky Department of Juvenile Justice; 2002.
8. Leone P, Rutherford R, Nelson C. *Special Education in Juvenile Corrections: Working With Behavioral Disorders*. Reston, VA: Council for Exceptional Children; 1991.
9. Winters CA. Learning disabilities, crime, delinquency, and special education placement. *Adolescence*. 1997;32:451–462.
10. Stringer ET. *Action Research*, 2nd ed. Thousand Oaks, CA: Sage Publications; 1999.
11. Taylor B. Identifying and transforming dysfunctional nurse-nurse relationships through reflective practice and action research. *Intl J Nurs Pract*. 2001; 7:406–413.

12. Lloyd C. Developing and changing practice in special education needs through critically reflective action research: a case study. *Eur J Spec Needs Educ.* 2002;17: 109–127.
13. Rock T, Levin B. Collaborative action research: enhancing preservice teacher development in professional schools. *Teach Educ Quart.* 2002;29:7–21.
14. Letts L. Occupational therapy and participatory action research: a partnership worth pursuing. *Am J Occup Ther.* 2003;57:77–87.
15. Roth LM, Esdaile SA. Action research: a dynamic discipline for advancing professional goals. *Br J Occup Ther.* 1999;62:498–506.

The Forgotten Population: Health Communication with Rural Racial/Ethnic Communities

Shirley A. Wells, MPH, OT, FAOTA

INTRODUCTION

Creative and innovative communication materials and strategies are needed to address the determinants of health and life expectancy among rural (nonmetropolitan) racial/ethnic communities. The nonmetropolitan racial/ethnic minorities most affected by health gaps are African-Americans, Hispanics, and Native Americans. Yet, most health promotion and communication methods frequently use a cultural surface approach to racial/ethnic groups. This is matching messages and communication strategies to observable social and behavioral characteristics of a culture such as familiar and stereotypical people, foods, music, language, and places.[1] How can effective communication occur within a community that is neither linguistically nor culturally homogeneous? How can specific strategies and approaches be identified to reach a population that includes subgroups with cultural, racial, religious, ethnic, linguistic, educational, geographical, and socioeconomic differences?

This chapter provides information to help health care providers and students meet the challenges of communicating effectively with racial/ethnic communities. Understanding the audience, drawing on community-based values and traditions, and working with knowledgeable persons from the community or population to develop strategies, messages, and health promotion materials are paramount to effecting lifelong changes. Students must be trained to use culturally appropriate communication strategies and approaches aimed at effecting individual, community, organizational, and policy change. Cultural interventions can effectively address multiple determinants of health that underline disparities.

Public perception of rural America is often of a white, poor, elderly population. In reality, a high concentration of African-Americans, Hispanics, and Native Americans live in rural areas. They are more likely to be poor but also more likely to live in communities that have close cultural practices, limited access to health care, low educational attainment, and tighter constraints on total economic resources.[2] Understanding this combination of individual and regional poverty is absolutely critical if we are to create innovative communication materials and strategies to address the determinants of health among rural racial/ethnic communities.

Identifying communication strategies that positively influence basic lifestyle behaviors has become increasingly important for improving the health of all Americans. Health communication is defined as the study and use of communication strategies to inform and influence individual and community decisions that enhance health.[3] Making health communication programs work in rural areas requires the active participation of both affected individuals and communities in the creation of health communication interventions and the consideration of culture in crafting the message. If these requirements are not met, health communication ventures can reflect a lack of commitment to speak up for racial and socioeconomic equality and fail to reduce inequalities.

Let's examine the communication approach used by Forest Hill Family Outreach Agency (a fictitious organization):

> *Forest Hill Family Outreach agency designed a program to provide mental health services to those who are low to moderate income, uninsured, and ineligible for Medicaid. To reach their predominately rural Hispanic population, the agency decided to advertise their program through brochures translated into Spanish placed throughout the community and ads placed in Spanish in the local community newspapers. After 6 months, the agency reported that the number of participants in their program who were Hispanic had not improved.*

When the Forest Hill Family Outreach agency did not achieve an increased number of Hispanics attending their program, they should ask a series of questions: How well have we informed or not informed this population about our services? Have we taken into account the literacy level of the targeted population? What are the cultural beliefs surrounding this type of health service? Is the written form the best media or culturally appropriate for this group?

Communicating about health is an everyday part of life. Mass media coverage, entertainment programming, and public policy debates are important places for public communication. Complex text is very common in health information from insurance forms, informed consents, and privacy notices to advertisements. Some families and individuals may lack the literacy skills in both Spanish and English to benefit from written information. People with limited literacy skills may not use the written word as their method of communication. Accordingly, all types of media should be considered to increase health communication.

Health communicators must consider literacy and all its facets when developing health materials and communication strategies for a range of diverse audiences—each with differing abilities, experiences, levels of knowledge, cultural beliefs and practices, and communication expectations. A person who has finished high school and knows how to read may still not be able to navigate the health system. Valuable health communication comes from a convergence of education, culture, social factors, and health services.[4] Training and practice in health communication, particularly in the areas of public information campaigns, community and patient education, and provider–patient communication, are essential for designing effective health intervention for rural racial/ethnic populations.

LITERACY

Issues related to literacy can undermine an agency's, community's, individual's, or family's ability to care for and support their health needs. Forms, discharge plans, medication instructions, information about health plans and programs, and other materials are key to using the health system. Yet, millions of Americans have difficulty reading these texts and also understanding them. Even people with strong literacy have trouble obtaining, understanding, and using complex health information: A physician may have trouble helping a family member with Medicare forms, a science teacher may not understand information sent by a pharmacist about a pain medication, and an accountant may not know when to get a mammogram.[4,5,6]

The education system of the United States is charged with the development of literacy and numeracy skills in English, which form the foundation for more complex skills involving comprehension and application. Adult education programs provide opportunities for individuals who dropped out, for those who did not acquire strong skills, for elders who did not have access to schooling opportunities, and for immigrants who may never have access to education and/or wish to learn to speak, read, and write English.[4] Yet, in 2003 the National Assessment of Adult Literacy reported that 14% of adults in the United States demonstrated skills at the lowest levels of reading prose literature. An additional 29% were at only the basic level. A disproportionate percentage of Black and Hispanic adults in their sample were at the below-basic level. Adults over age 65, those with less than a high school education, and those with multiple disabilities were also overrepresented in those adults with below-basic skills. Approximately 5% of their sample had no literacy skills in English (Table 24-1).[7,8,9]

Basic print literacy ability means the ability to read, write, and understand written language that is familiar and for which one has the requisite amount of background knowledge regardless of the language (i.e., English or

Table 24-1. Literacy Scales

Prose literacy	The knowledge and skills needed to perform prose tasks (i.e., to search, comprehend, and use information from continuous texts). Examples include editorials, news stories, brochures, and instructional materials.
Document literacy	The knowledge and skills needed to perform document tasks (i.e., to search, comprehend, and use information from noncontinuous texts in various formats). Examples include job applications, payroll forms, transportation schedules, maps, tables, and drug and food labels.
Quantitative literacy	The knowledge and skills required to perform quantitative tasks (i.e., to identify and perform computations, either alone or sequentially, using numbers embedded in printed materials). Examples include balancing a checkbook, figuring out a trip, completing an order form, and determining the amount of interest on a loan from an advertisement.

Source: Kutner M, Greenberg E, Jin Y, Boyle B, Hsu Y, and Dunleavy E. *Literacy in Everyday Life: Results From the 2003 National Assessment of Adult Literacy* (NCES 2007-480). Washington, DC: U.S. Department of Education; 2007.

Spanish).[7,10] Some people with limited skills may be able to decode letters into sounds and pronounce words but may not be able to understand the meaning of a sentence formed by these words. Individuals who are considered "low literate" or "limited" reading have difficulty with reading and comprehending materials written beyond very simple levels. Those who are referred to as "illiterate" have few if any of the skills needed for basic print literacy.[4,7] Possessing the skills needed for basic literacy does not guarantee that one can read and comprehend all types of written text regardless of the language (Table 24-2).

An individual's ability to apply his or her literacy skills changes with the challenges of the task.[8] For example, the text of the following letter captures a very complicated message even for someone who holds a graduate degree.

Table 24-2. Literacy Levels

	Levels	NAEP Literacy Levels	U.S. Grade Levels	Adult Levels
People with very poor skills	1	Rudimentary	1–2	Below basic
People who can deal only with simple material	2	Basic	3–6	Basic
Roughly the skill level required for successful secondary school completion and college entry	3	Intermediate	7–11	Intermediate
People who demonstrate command of higher-order information processing skills	4	Adept	12–15	Proficient
People who demonstrate command of higher-order information processing skills	5	Advanced	16+	Proficient

Naep, National Assessment of Educational Progress.
Source: Kutner M, Greenberg E, Jin Y, Boyle B, Hsu Y, and Dunleavy E. (2007). *Literacy in Everyday Life: Results From the 2003 National Assessment of Adult Literacy* (NCES 2007-480), Washington, DC: U.S. Department of Education; 2007. National Center for Education Statistics. *Plain Language At Work Newsletter,* October 10, 2005.

The patient anxiety would be greatly increased as a result of a confusing message, as follows:

> *Mr. Jones,*
>
> *The results of your recent thermography and evaluation indicate that you are suffering from Complex Regional Pain Syndrome, type II (formally Reflex Sympathetic Dystrophy). I suggest that you increase the NSAID from bid to tid. You should schedule an appointment with the PM&R department for OT & PT as soon as possible for myofascial release and trigger point manipulation as well as electrical stimulation. If this approach does not relieve your pain then we will consider a Cervicothoracic Stellate Ganglion Block.*
>
> *Two weeks after starting your therapy sessions, please see me for a consultative office visit.*
>
> *Sincerely,*
> *John Doe, MD*

Whether about self-care procedures or medications, medical instructions are often hard for patients and caregivers to learn, remember, and follow when they have to change lifelong habits and behaviors. This is in part because the instructions may be complicated and explained in unfamiliar words and with lots of numbers. And patients may not be at their learning best when they are overwhelmed with new diagnoses or scared, sick, or in pain.

HEALTH LITERACY

Health literacy is about communication and understanding. People have difficulty understanding health information for a range of reasons, including literacy, age, disability, language, culture, and emotion. It affects how people participate in health promotion and prevention activities, weigh decisions about treatment, take medications, and follow self-care instructions.[9] The Institute of Medicine (IOM) described health literacy as a critical issue affecting the U.S. population. They defined health literacy as the "degree to which individuals can obtain, process, and understand basic health information and services they need to make appropriate health decisions."[3] Studies have shown that people with poor health literacy understand health information less, get less preventive health care, have a higher rate of hospitalization, and use expensive health services such as emergency room care more frequently.[4]

Although reading, writing, and math skills are the basic components of health literacy, many other skills and abilities are also important—speaking, listening, having adequate background information, and being able to advocate for oneself and family in the health system. Health literacy is not just a problem for recent immigrants or those with little education. The arcane language physicians, therapists, pharmacies, hospital personnel, and others use to communicate both verbally and in writing causes problems for many patients. And patients living in rural areas are no exception. Research shows that health literacy must be improved to reduce the negative effects of limited health knowledge as well as racial/ethnic health disparities.[4,5,6]

Efforts to reach all segments of the population with needed health information have become more important—and more challenging. A complex array of health literacy skills is needed for functioning in a variety of health contexts. Rural racial/ethnic populations should be able to read, listen to, and understand and act on complex medical and health information. Yet, many lack the basic health literacy skills needed to deal with such care. The challenge is clear: How do we communicate the language of good health so that it is uniformly received—and accepted—by rural racial/ethnic populations?

IMPACT OF CULTURE

Culture is a strong part of people's lives. It influences how people understand and make sense of their lives, their values, their humor, their hopes, their loyalties, and their fears. Culture is a learned set of beliefs, values, and norms that are shared by a group of people; it is a design for how to live.[11] It influences a wide range of behaviors, including dietary choices, hygiene practices, sexual practices, and illness behaviors. Through such behaviors, culture has an effect on health and thus is relevant to health programs and health messages. For example, if your message is about daily consumption of meats and fresh vegetables and how they are prepared, it is also important to be able to identify your audience as an African-American from New York versus Mississippi. In such a case both African-Americans have strong cultural identities and specific dietary choices related to daily food consumption and preparation that present an opportunity for health care providers to build cultural identity into their health programs and communications. The strong cultural identity can also create conflicts and miscommunications if the program or message is perceived as threatening to their culture or being inconsistent with their cultural beliefs.[12] The interaction of culture and illness lends credence to the theory that illness is at least in part socially and culturally constructed. This interaction can be seen in both physical and mental illnesses.

Health literacy relies on cultural and conceptual knowledge. Culture gives significance to health information and messages. Perceptions and definitions of health and illness, preferences, languages and cultural barriers, care process barriers, and stereotypes are all strongly influenced by culture and can have an influence on health literacy and health outcomes.[4] Understanding cultures helps to overcome and prevent racial and ethnic as well as geographical divisions, which can result in loss of opportunities and miscommunication.[12,13]

Cultures also influence styles of communication, in meaning of words and gestures, and in what can be discussed regarding the body, health, and illness. Effective health communication requires a mutual understanding between patients and their families and health care providers and staff. Differing cultural and educational backgrounds among providers and patients, as well as those who create health information and those who use it, can contribute to communication problems.[12] People bring individual experiences, values, customs, and logic to each situation. Today's families and communities consist of people with multiple cultural backgrounds and experiences who cannot be put into rigid "boxes" by using racial, ethnic, or geographical labels. Thus culture and health literacy both influence the content and outcomes of health care encounters.

Rural Racial/Ethnic Culture

When working with people and building relationships with them, it helps to have some perspective and understanding of their culture. To work within rural communities we need to understand and appreciate their culture, establish relationships with people from these cultures, and build strong alliance with their different cultural groups. The rural culture has it own health-related behaviors. According to the National Rural Health Association, rural residents smoke more, exercise less, have less nutritional diets, and are more likely to be obese than suburban residents. Chronic illnesses are more prevalent in rural areas. Rural communities represent about 20% of America's population; however, less than 10% of physicians practice in those communities.[14,15]

Information regarding racial/ethnic populations in rural areas is sparse. Rural racial/ethnic populations are geographically concentrated in historic regions: African-Americans in the southern states (70%), Hispanics in south-western states (73%), and Native Americans in the western states (57%).[16] Poverty is a more prevalent problem for these groups. Seven of every 10 African-American young children (77.2%) and 57.8% of adolescents living in rural areas live in poverty, and 6 of every 10 Hispanic young children (61%) and 51% of adolescents live in poverty.[17] Nearly 3 of every 10 rural African-Americans and Native Americans and about one in every four rural Hispanics live in poverty. Sixty-eight percent of rural African-Americans, 62% of rural Hispanics, and 48% of rural Native Americans hold high-poverty job classifications.[18] In counties where racial/ethnic populations make up more than half the population, the proportion of poor is higher and the total community economic resources are more constrained.[19]

Rural racial/ethnic populations are more likely to have less than a high school education; 39% of African-American working-age adults and 50% of Hispanic working-age adults had not completed high school.[18] Rural racial/ethnic children disproportionately live in households characterized by low maternal education and poverty.[17] Rural racial/ethnic elders are severely handicapped in education, income, and health status as compared with Whites. Over three-fourths of African-American (76%) and Hispanic (81%) elders have less than a high school education, over three-fourths of African-Americans (77%) and Hispanics (76%) have a total household income of less than $20,000, and over three-fourths of African-American (52%) and Hispanic (44%) elders describe their health as poor or fair.[20] Low education and poverty translate into lack of health insurance and poor health.

Many factors, including rural residence, region of the country, age, sex, family size, and health status, combine to influence whether or not an individual is insured. Low income and low education levels in rural areas convert into jobs that do not offer health insurance.[15,18] Rural racial/ethnic residents are generally less likely to be insured if aged younger than 65 years and less likely to have supplemental insurance if Medicare eligible.[20] Rates of uninsured or underinsured ranging from 47% among Hispanic rural population and 30% among African-Americans place these working adults at a disadvantage.[16] Seventy-seven percent of rural Hispanics are less likely to have an ongoing source of care. An estimated 20% of Hispanics and 33% of African-Americans have fewer primary care visits than Whites.[15,20]

Access to care requires providers. Shortages are more common in counties where racial/ethnic minorities represent more than half the population. Sixty-five percent of rural counties are whole or partial health professional shortage areas (HPSAs)—81% of rural counties in which Hispanics are the majority of population, 83% of counties with an African-American majority, and 92% of counties with a Native American/Alaska Native majority.[16,19] Rural racial/ethnic residents have reduced odds of receiving preventive care and cancer screening services, inadequate prenatal care, and limited emergency medical services.[16,17,19,20]

Rural racial/ethnic populations are linked to rural America through ties of land and history, and it is critical that we understand their lives as well as their health. Effective communication must also be based on rural regional and geographical differences. In some rural communities, water quality, agricultural methods, forestry, or mining complicate the effect of place on residence. Type of landscape can affect health by creating real or perceived isolation.[21]

Rural racial/ethnic populations have the following in common: geographical and informational isolation, fragmentation of services, limitations regarding transportation, educational limitations, and disproportionate poverty. They also experience cultural differences: differences regarding health beliefs, language barriers, and migratory patterns. The reduction and elimination of health disparities among rural racial/ethnic populations requires culturally based population approaches that are sensitive to local variations in physical and cultural realities. Health care services need to be provided in areas of need. All rural racial/ethnic residents need to be made aware of health risks through better education. Hence, communication goes beyond words to encompass the meaning behind the words, a meaning that is affected by culture, knowledge, experience, and location.

COMMUNICATION STRATEGIES

Health communication encompasses the study and use of communication strategies to inform and influence individual and community decisions that enhance health. It can contribute to all aspects of disease prevention and health promotion. It is relevant in a number of contexts, such as (a) health professional–patient relations; (b) individuals' exposure to, search for, and use of health information; (c) individuals' adherence to clinical recommendations and regimens; (d) the construction of health messages and campaigns; (e) the dissemination of individual and population health risk information; (f) images of health in the mass media and the culture at large; (g) the education of consumers about how to gain access to the public and health care systems; and (h) the development of telehealth applications.[3,22]

Effective health communication can increase the intended audience's knowledge and awareness of a health issue, problem, or solution; influence their perceptions, beliefs, and attitudes; and raise awareness of health risks and solutions. Effective health communication is the degree to which improvements in health are, in fact, attained. It can prompt people to action, show the benefit of behavior changes, and increase the demands for health services. It can increase participation in treatment decisions, consent (or not) to procedures, follow self-care instructions, and recognize and take appropriate action in medical emergencies.[3,6,10] Health communication can be used to influence public agenda, advocate for policies and programs, promote positive changes in the socioeconomic and physical environments, improve the delivery of care, and encourage social norms that benefit health and quality of life.[23] Health communication alone, however, without cultural and environmental support and language is not effective at sustaining behavior changes at the individual or community level. Health communication may not be effective in communicating very complex messages, and it cannot compensate for lack of access to health care or healthy environments.[1]

Based on an analysis of 18 large-scale campaigns on shaping the health behavior of diverse population, the IOM[23] found that current data do not effectively address whether there is any added benefit in addressing health disparities by using communication that takes diversity into account. They recommend that more research should be undertaken to evaluate the comparative effectiveness of communication programs designed to influence diverse populations with programs using a generic or traditional approach. Further theories of communications and health behaviors should be considered in a more consistent and aggressive way during the development and implementation of communication programs for diverse population. Effective health communication campaigns use various methods to reach intended audiences:[1,24,25,26] Some of these are described as follows:

1. *Education–entertainment:* Seeks to include health-promoting messages and storylines into entertainment and news programs or to eliminate messages that counter health messages. This is the exposure of health information and behaviors through entertainment media such as television. More than half of regular prime time and daytime drama viewers reported that they learned something about a disease or how to prevent it from a television show. This method has the capacity to reach significant proportions of rural racial/ethnic populations.[1]

2. *Media advocacy:* Uses mass media and their tools, in combination with community organizing, for the purpose of advancing healthy public policies through influencing the mass media's selection of topics and shaping debate on these issues. It seeks to change the social and political environment in which decisions on health and health resources are made.

3. *Interactive health communication:* Uses computer-based media that allows users to access information and services of interest via the Internet. This method allows users to tailor and personalize content to better suit their needs, to access as often as they wish, and to engage around their own schedule.

4. *Interpersonal communication:* Focuses on the provider–client interaction, the role of social support (real or virtual) in health, and the ways in which interpersonal relationships influence health behaviors and decision making.

5. *Media literacy:* Teaches an intended audience to analyze media messages to identify the sponsor's motives. It teaches communicators how to create messages geared to the intended audience's point of view.

6. *Advertising:* Paid or public service messages placed in the media or in public spaces to increase awareness of and support for a product, service, or behavior.

7. *Public relations:* Promotes the inclusion of messages about a health issue or behavior in the mass media, using earned media strategies rather than paid advertising.

Traditional health communication approaches are aimed at stimulating individual behavior changes and are often channeled to print text and face-to-face communication. In the past strategies to promote health-related behavior change have relied on educational messages in pamphlets, brochures, and direct mail and mass communication methods such as public service announcements on billboards, radio, and television. These methods can reach a large number of people, and the time investment is for the development of the material only. On the other hand, they are expensive and have a fixed message. It is difficult to evaluate whether the message reached the intended audience as well as customer reactions and effectiveness of the message. Social marketing has also been used. Other common forms of media include telephone solicitations and seminars.[24,26,27]

These approaches remain just as valid and useful now as in the past. New communication technologies have the potential to support important innovations in program delivery (Table 24-3). Increasingly, digital technologies such as video cassette recorders, digital video disks, compact disks, the Internet, mobile telephone with enhanced capacities, and wireless communication options such as instant messaging are replacing traditional communication methods. These methods are highly interactive and have the capacity to both gather data from users and provide personalized feedback. They eliminate time restrictions on access to material, allow more open responses to sensitive questions and more willingness to explore sensitive issues, and the use of multimedia interfaces reduces the literacy requirements for material. These approaches are proving to be interactive, appealing, and engaging.[24]

The uses of new communication technology capacities are in early stages of development. There are significant obstacles to the use of these technologies to enhance health. The "digital divide" between those who have access and those who do not have access to information technology continues to be a major barrier for disadvantaged groups. According to Owen et al.,[24] the cost of developing, disseminating, and accessing health-related applications are prohibitive for many groups, especially those living in rural communities. Culturally appropriate content still lags behind need. There is also the problem of information overload that new communication media creates, but the

Table 24-3. Communication Methods

Traditional Communication Media	Emerging Communication Media
Self-help books and booklets	Multimedia CD-ROM, DVD programs
Television and radio broadcasting programs	Websites
	Interactive e-mail advice
Public service announcements	Automated telephone messages
Videotapes	Tailored print communications
Mailouts/brochures	Interactive websites
Targeted print communications	Mobile telephones with enhanced capacities
	Personal digital assistant
	Web television

formidable quantity and variable quality of such information can themselves be barriers.

When working with rural racial/ethnic communities, there are multiple dimensions to consider when creating a health communication campaign, ranging from economic contexts and community resources to commonly held attitudes, norms, efficacy, beliefs, and practices pertinent to health.[28,29] Understanding cultural backgrounds and life experiences of communities and its individuals enhances the current knowledge base for designing and evaluating communication strategies. It is more important to go beyond the culture surface and address deep structures that reflects the cultural, social, psychological, environmental, and historical factors that affect health for a diverse community.[1]

To design effective health intervention, we must understand the complexity of culture and integrate cultural factors into our health communication efforts. We must work collaboratively with rural racial/ethnic communities experiencing disparities to overcome historical context of distrust and create meaningful, effective health communication interventions.

COMMUNITY HEALTH COMMUNICATION PROJECT: HEALTH LITERACY EDUCATIONAL SYMPOSIUM

In 2006, Health Communities of Brownsville, Inc. (HCB) Health TrendBender group initiated a plan to identify, address, and improve the health literacy of the community. HCB is a nonprofit, grassroots community organization dedicated to improving the quality of life in Brownsville, Texas. It was founded in 2001 and organized into three committees known as TrendBender groups to focus on the community areas of concern: education, health, and environment. Its members come from local hospitals, schools, universities, churches, businesses, and service agencies. They are doctors, nurses, therapists, university professors, teachers, clergy, retired elderly, "promotoras 32" (lay community people who receive training and instruction in the art and ways of promoting health and safety), and business owners. They are high school students, health care professionals (i.e., pharmacy, occupational therapy, medicine, nurse, and public health), and university students. They are all different but all share a common vision—to build a healthier, cleaner, and more beautiful Brownsville.[30]

Brownsville is the largest city in the lower Rio Grande Valley, positioned at the southernmost point of Texas on the United States–Mexico border, and is about 25 miles inland from the Gulf of Mexico. (See Figures 24-1 and 24-2.)

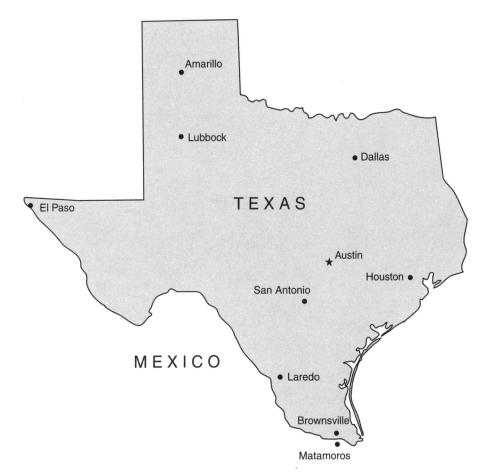

Figure 24-1
Location of Brownsville, Texas on a state map.

According to the U.S. Census Bureau,[31] Brownsville has a population of 171,528 that is 81% White, 0.2% African-American, 0.4% Native American, and 0.3% Asian. In terms of ethnicity it is 91% Hispanic. It has a young population with a median age of 26, and 63% of the population is below 34 years of age. Forty-three percent of the population live below the poverty level, and more than 50% of high school students never graduate. The median income in Brownsville is $24,207. The city industries include agriculture, shrimping, metal fabrication, electronics, food processing, and much more.

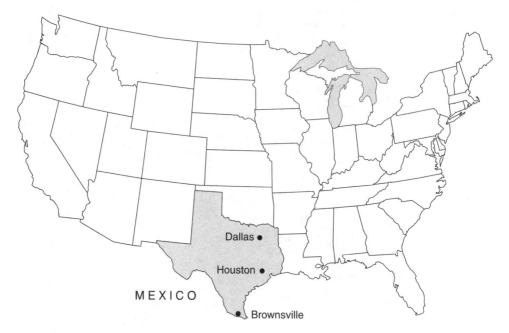

Figure 24-2
Location of Brownsville, Texas on U.S. map.

With its proximity to Mexico, it is the gateway for U.S.–Mexico commerce. Brownsville/Matamoros is the third largest border employment center, better known as the "Maquiladora Program."

Brownsville is served by three hospitals, one free-standing rehabilitation facility, four nursing homes, and several outpatient rehabilitation centers serving children and adults. The health problems are shaped by many factors such as language and cultural barriers, lack of access to care and health insurance, and a shortage of health professionals. It has been designated as an HPSA and a medically underserved area. Brownsville has one of the highest incidences of tuberculosis and obesity-related type 2 diabetes. Sexually transmitted disease and AIDS are also high. The leading causes of illness and deaths include heart disease, cancer, diabetes, and unintentional injury/ accidents.[32]

The needs are massive, but there are concerned local people who are willing to dedicate time and resources to address issues crucial to the healthy development of the community. Using proven principles of health communication, cultural diversity, and cultural competence, the Health

TrendBender group began a six-stage process to increase the health literacy of its community.[28,32]

1. *Planning and researching the problem:* Identify the health problem and determine whether communication should be part of the intervention.
2. *Selecting the message, materials, and channel:* Identify the audience and determine the best way to reach them.
3. *Developing materials and pretesting:* Develop and test communication concepts, messages, and materials with representatives of the target audiences.
4. *Implementing the plan:* Implement the health communication program based on the results of the testing.
5. *Assessing its effectiveness:* Assess how effectively the message reached the target audience.
6. *Refining the program:* Modify the communication program if necessary.

The committee reviewed national, regional, and local studies related to literacy and health literacy for Hispanics and low-education populations. They also assessed local anecdotal information. By partnering with the Parental Involvement Program of the Brownsville Independent School District and the City of Brownsville Public Health Department, they discovered that there were no solid data about the health literacy of the Brownsville community. Thus they began the pilot demonstration project—a Health Literacy Educational Symposium on Risky Behaviors of Youth—to assess the current level of health literacy among the parents of the school children and to test a culturally appropriate approach to educating them on health issues related to youth and children.

The planning committee consisted of community leaders, educators, health professional students, and representatives from several health agencies that met on a monthly basis for approximately a year. The local health professional students—medical, nursing, occupational therapy, and public health—were instrumental throughout the planning and implementation of the project. They attended all the planning sessions; participated in discussion related to the communication message, concepts, and materials; and recommended speakers and presenters. They also assisted with the setup and cleanup of the event.

Grant funding along with donations were obtained for the project. A pre- and postsurvey (both English and Spanish in one document) was designed to assess health literacy levels as well as knowledge about the risky behaviors of youth and children. The presurvey was disseminated through the school parent involvement program as part of their preregistration packet for the symposium. About 600 parents registered for the event, and approximately 540 actually attended.

The event was held entirely in Spanish with English translators for non–Spanish-speaking attendees. All handouts and powerpoints were presented in both languages. Local health agencies and organizations were onsite to share and disseminate information. A hot meal was served to everyone, and numerous door prizes were given away. To ensure return of the postsurvey, water bottles were given to each attendee as they exited the event and turned in a survey. These components are common for parent-focused gatherings and expected by the local culture.

HEALTH COMMUNICATION STRATEGIES

Health communication training and practice should be an established part of all health disciplines. Effective communication strategies combine theories, frameworks, and approaches from behavioral sciences, communication, social marketing, and health education. Research indicates that effective health promotion and communication initiatives adopt an audience-centered perspective that reflects audiences' preferred formats, channels, and contexts. These considerations are relevant for rural racial/ethnic populations who may have different languages and sources of information. Communication initiatives must be conceptualized and developed by individuals with specific knowledge of the cultural characteristics, medical habits, and language preferences of the intended audiences.[27,28]

Even the most carefully designed communication programs have limited impact if the underserved communities lack access to crucial health professionals, services, and communication channels. Even with access to information and services, disparities may still exist if people lack the health literacy to navigate the health care system and better manage their own health.

What Works?

Health service providers and students must be knowledgeable, aware, and responsive to the health literacy of patients, clients, and consumers. A health care provider's ability to use common words and to perceive whether a patient or consumer is understanding a discussion (or not) must be considered. "The message is clear: plain, straightforward language trumps fancy works and medical jargon when it comes to communicating with your patients" (p. 71).[27]

To be effective in successfully promoting changes in people's behaviors, communication needs to be strategic. It has to be participatory and collaborative, and a concrete vision is needed and should be shared with all stakeholders. Also, it has to be results oriented. The people targeted should also clearly perceive the benefit they will gain from taking the action being promoted. The communication program should be cost effective, sustainable over the long term, and flexible enough to be adapted effectively to changing circumstances.[22]

The following recommendations reflect lessons learned from national and local campaigns and communication programs that have targeted diverse populations.[9,25,26,28,32]

1. Work with partners who can add their resources to your own.
2. Patients should be asked to repeat back their care instructions.
3. Always avoid stereotypes.
4. Facilitate sharing and discussion on experiences.
5. Build on the strengths of the rural racial/ethnic community and its cultural values.
6. Promote respect from elders and promote interest in disappearing traditions.
7. All health materials should be written at a fifth-grade level, using graphics where appropriate. Form should not be considered secondary to content. An appealing form enhances the content of messages.
8. Visual images offer a good opportunity to reverse stereotypes. Identify appropriate visual images and cultural symbols.
9. Develop and write text in both English and Spanish for bilingual material. Consider providing both texts in one document.
10. Direct translation of English health information or health promotion materials should be avoided. Do not rely on just translating the English text into the other language.
11. Look for alternatives to print materials; use oral messages in all involved languages whenever possible. Television and radio serving specific racial and ethnic populations can be effective means to deliver health messages.
12. Develop materials at the appropriate literacy level of the audience. Make written material as brief and clear as possible. Keep the use of technical jargon a minimum. Use a type size (12 font or larger) large enough to be easily read.

Health care providers and students need to provide help in increasing health literacy skills and in adapting communications to ensure that rural racial/ethnic populations have the information they need to care for themselves and their families.

CONCLUSIONS

Rural communities are rich in cultural diversity. Yet living in a rural area is itself a health risk for those from racial/ethnic groups. To start reducing the negative effects of living in a rural area and being a member of a minority racial/ethnic group, students and health care providers must be knowledgeable and responsive to the cultural differences and similarities. It requires a willingness and ability to draw on community-based values and traditions and to work with knowledgeable persons from the targeted community or population in developing strategies, messages, and materials.

Effective communication is the backbone of health promotion and disease prevention. People need to understand health information to apply it to their own behavior. Communicating about health is an intellectual framework, a scientific endeavor, and a set of processes and interventions as well as an art for health improvement. To get their message across and to promote and distribute their material successfully, the Forest Hill agency should make good use of the positive family and communal values that are central to rural racial/ethnic populations. Their strategies should include an awareness of local and generational characteristics, with special emphasis on promoting those basic historical and cultural foundations that untie all rural populations. They should take advantage of the links that bind the individual to the family, the family to the community, and the community to the country. The ability to pique the target population's interest is not proof that the materials are successful. To be effective, the communication message not only must be presented in an appealing fashion, but it must also be understood. Above all, it has to elicit some kind of action.

REFERENCES

1. Freimuth VS, Quinn SC. The contributions of health communication to eliminating health disparities. *Am J Public Health*. 2004;94:2053–2055.
2. Samuels ME, Probst J, Glover S. *Rural Research Focus: Minorities in Rural America*. Available at: http://ruralhealth.hrsa.gov/pub/MinoritiesinRuralAm.htm. Retrieved February 20, 2007.

3. Healthy People 2010 (2000). Health communication. Available at: http://www. healthypeople.gov/document/HTML/Volume1/11HealthCom.htm. Retrieved February 18, 2007.

4. Institute of Medicine. *Health Literacy: A Prescription to End Confusion.* Washington, DC: National Academies Press; 2004.

5. Lindau ST, Tomori C, Lyons T, et al. The association of health literacy with cervical cancer prevention knowledge and health behaviors in a multiethnic cohort of women. *Am J Obstet Gynecol.* 2002;186:938–943.

6. Williams MV, Parker RM, Baker DW, et al. Inadequate functional health literacy among patients at two public hospitals. *JAMA.* 1995;274:1677–1682.

7. Kutner M, Greenberg E, Baer J. *A First Look at the Literacy of America's Adults in the 21st Century.* Washington, DC: U.S. Department of Education, National Center for Education Statistics; 2005.

8. Kirsch IS, Jungelbut A, Jenkins L, Kolstad A. *Adult Literacy in America: A First Look at the Results of the National Adult Literacy Survey (NALS).* Washington, DC: National Center for Education Statistics, U.S. Department of Education; 1993.

9. Kutner M, Greenberg E, Jin Y, Boyle B, Hsu Y, Dunleavy E. *Literacy in Everyday Life: Results From the 2003 National Assessment of Adult Literacy.* (NCES 2007–480). U.S. Department of Education. Washington, DC: National Center for Education Statistics; 2007.

10. Osborne H. *Health Literacy from A to Z: Practical Ways to Communicate Your Health Message.* Sudbury, MA: Jones and Bartlett Publishers; 2005.

11. Spector RE. *Cultural Diversity in Health and Illness,* 3rd ed. Norwalk, CT: Appleton & Lang; 1991.

12. Issel LM. *Health Program Planning and Evaluation.* Sudbury, MA: Jones and Bartlett Publishers; 2004.

13. Wells SA, Black R. *Cultural Competency for Health Professionals.* Bethesda, MD: The American Occupational Therapy Association, Inc.; 2000.

14. NRHA Policy Brief. *Health Disparities in Rural Populations: An Introduction.* Available at: http://www.HRHArural.org. Retrieved August 17, 2006.

15. Gamm LD, Hutchison LL, Dabney BJ, Dorsey AM, eds. *Rural Healthy People 2010: A Companion Document to Healthy People 2010, Vol. 1.* School of Rural Public Health, Southwest Rural Health Research Center; 2003. College Station, TX: Texas A&M University Health Science Center, School of Rural Public Health Southwest Rural Health Research Center; 2003.

16. Probst JC, Samuels ME, Jespersen KP, Willert K, Swann RS, Duffie JA. *Minorities in Rural America: An Overview of Population Characteristics.* Columbia, SC: South Carolina Rural Health Research Center; 2002.

17. Probst JC, Moore C, Roof KW, et al. *Access to Care Among Rural Minorities: Children.* Columbia, SC: South Carolina Rural Health Research Center; 2002.

18. Probst J, Samuels M, Moore CG. *Access to Care Among Rural Minorities: Working Age Adults.* Columbia, SC: South Carolina Rural Health Research Center; 2003.

19. Pobst JC, Moore CG, Glover SH, Samuels ME. Person and place: the compounding effects of race/ethnicity and rurality on health. *Am J Public Health.* 2004;94: 1695–1703.

20. Probst JC, Samuels ME, Moore CG, Gdovin J. *Access to Care Among Rural Minorities: Older Adults.* Columbia, SC: South Carolina Rural Health Research Center; 2002.

21. Hartley D. Rural health disparities, population health, and rural culture. *Am J Public Health.* 2004;94:1675–1678.

22. U.S. Department of Health and Human Services. *Health People 2010,* 2nd ed. *With Understanding and Improving Health and Objectives for Improving Health.* 2 vols. Washington, DC: U.S. Government Printing Office; 2000.

23. Institute of Medicine. *Speaking of Health: Assessing Health Communication Strategies for Diverse Populations.* Washington, DC: National Academies Press; 2002.

24. Owen N, Fotheringham MJ, Marcus B. Communication technology and health behavior change. In Glanz K, Rimer BK, Lewis FM, eds. *Health Behavior and Health Education: Theory, Research, and Practice,* 3rd ed. San Francisco: Jossey-Bass; 2002:510–529.

25. Hargroves M. Elevating the voices of rural minority women. *Am J Public Health.* 2002;92:514–515.

26. Plimptom S, Root J. Materials and strategies that work in low literacy health communication. *Public Health Rep.* 1994;109:86–92.

27. Thrall TH. Dump the mumbo-jumbo. *Hosp Health Netw.,* Health Forum, 71–74.

28. National Prevention Information Network. *Health Communication Strategies.* Available at: http://www.cdcnpin.org/scripts/campaign/strategy.asp. Retrieved February 18, 2007.

29. Center for Substance Abuse Prevention. *Developing Effective Messages and Materials for Hispanic/Latino Audiences.* Rockville, MD: National Clearinghouse for Alcohol and Drug Information; 1997.

30. Healthy Communities of Brownsville. *Working Together to Build a Better Brownsville.* Available at: http://www.healthybrownsville.org. 2006.

31. U.S. Census Bureau. *The 2005 American Community Survey, 2005.* Available at: http://factfinder.census.gov. Retrieved January 26, 2007.

32. Center for Health Statistics. *Texas Selected Health Facts Data Sources, 2002.* Department of State Health Services. Available at: http://www.dshs.state.tx.us/chs/. Retrieved January 15, 2007.

CHAPTER 25

Health Report Card Project: Building Community Capacity

Marlene Wilken, RN, PhD

INTRODUCTION

The U.S. government made a promise to provide health care to Native Americans over 150 years ago. The tribes paid for their health care by giving up their land to the federal government for the promise of health care. The U.S. Congress, however, has yet to keep its promise. Government funding for Native American health care has never been at the level that other Americans receive. Significant health disparities exist for Native Americans in health status, quality of health care, and available resources. According to Dixon and Roubideaux, "raising the health status of American Indians to the highest level is one of the most significant public health challenges facing our nation today."[1]

One significant disparity for Native Americans is diabetes, which has reached epidemic levels. The Omaha Tribe of Nebraska is an example of a Native American tribe that has recognized the increased prevalence of diabetes and is focusing efforts on building diabetes prevention for their youth. One of the first steps in this effort has been collection of regular school health screening data in the community schools. The community was now in a position to engage in a process that would identify the diabetes risk factors for their youth and plan next steps in prevention program development. In this chapter, the interdisciplinary process used to work with a rural, Native American community for building community capacity to address diabetes prevention is discussed. Key participants in this interdisciplinary process include Creighton School of Nursing, the Creighton University Office of Interprofessional Scholarship, Service, and Education (OISSE), and the

Omaha Tribe. In this chapter we discuss a conceptual framework, the need for community capacity building, the groups involved in the process, the process involved in making the health report card, and the findings.

BUILDING COMMUNITY CAPACITY

The conceptual model used for the Health Report Card Project was a community capacity building wheel (Figure 25-1). The model consists of four dimensions within the wheel that provide a foundation for building and strengthening community action. The outside of the wheel is surrounded by all the groups that participated in the process of community capacity building. The four dimensions necessary to build and strengthen community capacity include a (a) a sense of community, (b) commitment, (c) ability to problem solve, and (d) access to resources. The sense of community is about connectedness and mutual recognition of shared values, norms, and vision among community members. Commitment refers to the willingness of community members to actively participate in the collective well-being of their community. Out of this active participation to commitment comes the ability to solve problems. Solving problems involves access to resources within and outside the community.[2] Each of the groups involved in the health report card

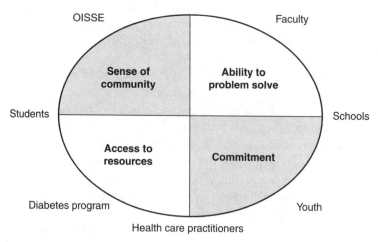

Figure 25-1
Community capacity building wheel.

project exhibited varying levels of commuity-building capacity. The groups encompassing the community capacity building wheel included health professionals, the tribal diabetes program, two K–12 schools, tribal community leaders, the OISSE, nursing faculty, and graduate nursing students. In Christiansen's discussion of the connection between the health or well-being of the community and the responsibilities of health professionals, he writes that the trust and goodwill that can come from people working together is essential to the well-being of a community.[3] Everyone involved in the project viewed this invitation as a starting point to begin to address the public health challenges related to diabetes for the Omaha Tribe. The Health Report Card is one example of how the well-being of each community was strengthened.

NEED FOR BUILDING COMMUNITY CAPACITY

The key to working with any community is to let the community identify their needs. Other participants must be willing to listen as community members describe what they believe are the problems and allow the community members to reach consensus on what needs to be done to help solve the problem. Once the community has identified their needs and found participating groups willing to help them problem solve, a sense of energy is generated, fueled by commitment and access to resources. The wheel of capacity building has momentum and the process is engaged.

The need for analyzing years of school health screening data via a health report card was evident. The sources included federal level documents, national organizations, university mission, and tribal information. The Healthy People 2010 goals of increasing quality and years of healthy life and eliminating health disparities served as an overarching call to action for the health professionals. More specifically, the health report card data provided a starting point to address the Nebraska Healthy People Goals of reducing diabetes prevalence and decreasing the number of children who are overweight and obese. In 2006, over 700 adults, about 14%, of the Omaha Tribe, had been diagnosed with diabetes, but the community believed there were many others with diabetes who have not been diagnosed. This prevalence rate is much higher than the state Healthy People 2010 goal, which is to reduce the prevalence of diagnosed diabetes to no more than 2.5% (25 per 100,000 population) for Nebraska adults.[4]

The 2003 Institute of Medicine (IOM) report included the challenges of thinking more strategically, planning more collectively, and performing more effectively. These challenges offered opportunities for schools of health professions to expand their participation to include working with communities through planning and partnerships to help meet identified needs.[5] In addition to the IOM challenges, the call to action provided faculty and students at Creighton University the opportunity to be exemplars of living out the mission. The mission's focus on core values of service to others, an appreciation of cultural diversity, and social justice added importance and significant relevance to the health report card project. Being a health professional implies obligations to contribute to a community's well-being. Curricula for the health professions that include service learning provide students the opportunity to engage in fulfilling their social and professional obligations to communities and carry out the mission of the university.

The National Rural Health Association and other national organizations, including the American Nurses Association, Agency for Healthcare Quality and Research, and the American Association of Colleges of Nursing, identified the need for action to address rural health issues. The proposed policy recommendations and strategies included knowing how to form and sustain community partnerships, practicing cultural competency, making necessary adjustments to accommodate rural social structures and their impact on practice, and capitalizing on scarce resources and engaging the community. The Health Report Card Project addressed in this chapter served as one venue for addressing health care delivery in rural America.[6]

In 2000 the American Diabetes Association recommended that children be tested for insulin resistance who are 10 years of age or older with a body mass index (BMI) more than the 85th percentile for age and evidence of the acanthosis nigricans marker, a skin pigmentation found on the back of the neck.[7] The rationale for these two measures is as follows: BMI is a calculation that identifies individuals who are overweight or obese and BMI is one potential indicator of developing type 2 diabetes mellitus; research indicates a relationship between acanthosis nigricans and diabetes. Copeland et al. concluded that among Native American children at high risk for developing type 2 diabetes, acanthosis nigricans is an independent marker of insulin resistance and may be useful as an early indicator of high risk for diabetes.[8]

The evidence for the need to reduce the burden of diabetes was compelling. Each group's commitment to the project was supported by the information above. The yearly school health screenings for the Omaha Tribe youth provided these necessary data used for analysis in the Health Report Card Project.

GROUPS INVOLVED IN THE PROCESS

Omaha Tribe Community

Located in rural northeastern Nebraska, the Omaha Indian Reservation is home to 5,227 Native Americans. The reservation covers five counties and comprises just over 31,100 acres, with 50% designated as agricultural and grazing land. There are two towns, Macy and Walthill, which are 12 miles apart. Macy has a population of 956 individuals of whom 96.4% are Native American, 49.4% are under the age of 18 years, and almost 50% live below the poverty level. Walthill has a population of 909 individuals of whom 68% are Native American, 41.3% are under the age of 18, and 23% of the total population is considered to be below the poverty level. Nearly 50% of the individuals do not complete high school.[9] The Omaha Tribe exhibits the rural characteristics of a higher percentage of children, more unemployment and underemployment, and more poverty than urban counterparts.[6]

The Omaha Tribe has limited access to healthy foods such as fresh fruits and vegetables, which are important in diabetes prevention and control. In Macy, there is only a small convenience store where minimal fruits and vegetables are sold, most often onions and lemons. In Walthill, the convenience/grocery store has a somewhat larger selection of fresh fruits and vegetables. When transportation is available, most drive the 30 miles to shop in South Sioux City at the Hy-Vee or new Super Wal-mart. Other food sources include the Women, Infant and Children program and food stamps. The monthly government food commodities program at Macy does offer fresh fruits and vegetables on a regular basis, for instance, a bag of apples and oranges mixed or perhaps grapefruit when available. The vegetables include onions, baby carrots, and potatoes on a regular basis and green peppers and cucumbers on a seasonal basis. Many households are quite large, however, and it is not known how long these items last.[10]

Omaha Tribe Diabetes Program

Macy is the only tribal health care center to serve the reservation. The health center's outpatient clinics and services include primary care, mental health, dental, home health nursing, long-term skilled care, a renal dialysis unit, and the Diabetes Program. The clinic has over 700 individuals diagnosed with diabetes who receive health care services at the clinic. The nine-bed renal dialysis unit, opened 2 years ago, added an additional shift to accommodate the needs of the tribal population. The director of the Carl T.

Curtis Health Education Center has been an instrumental community member in a number of health promotion and disease prevention projects involving Creighton University, the OISSE, and the Omaha Tribe. The Omaha Tribe Diabetes Program has one full-time diabetes educator who is responsible for developing programs and services to help meet the needs of community members across the lifespan in the areas of diabetes prevention and treatment. A variety of diabetes prevention programs is offered in collaboration with the Four Hills of Life Wellness Center and the Valentine Parker Jr. Youth Prevention Center in Macy. In Walthill, the school and senior center have provided some education on diabetes and prevention, and a building to house a youth prevention center is being renovated. The Diabetes Program includes the yearly school screenings to help target which youth need additional education to promote diabetes prevention.

School Communities

Both Macy and Walthill have a school for K–12 grades and share a school health nurse who has served the community for several years. Every year the school health nurse, teachers, health professionals, and volunteers perform the school health screenings at both schools. Between the two schools, a total of 1,010 students participated in the screenings at least once during the last 5 years of data collection. The school health screenings include the mandated measurements for height, weight, blood pressure, vision, and the presence of the acanthosis nigricans skin marker. The same physician has been screening students for the acanthosis nigricans marker for over 15 years. The acanthosis nigricans marker is identified through visual examination of the back of the neck. A photograph is taken of every student who shows signs of the marker. The acanthosis nigricans assessment results in a quantitative number between zero and four for each student, with zero being the absence of discoloration and four being the most marked discoloration. The school community has found acanthosis nigricans to be an educational tool regarding diabetes prevention. Some students identified with the acanthosis nigricans marker have been known to show their marker to adults and tell them what it means.

OISSE Community

The relationship between the Omaha Tribe and Creighton University started over 15 years ago when the Departments of Physical Therapy and Occupational

Therapy formed a partnership with the tribe to provide services. Several Health Resources and Services Administration grants were received that expanded the interprofessional group at Creighton to include the schools of pharmacy and nursing. The OISSE was formed to support, plan, organize, and implement the School of Pharmacy and Health Professions' interprofessional education and scholarship initiatives related to community engagement.

Faculty Community

A faculty member from the School of Nursing and Core Faculty of the OISSE received a vFellowship from the Creighton Cardoner program to explore vocation. Vocational fellowship—the purpose is to build a community of faculty who directly incorporate their developing understanding of vocation-as-calling in their work as teachers, scholars, and their service to Creighton University and the broader communities. Cardoner at Creighton is named after the Cardoner River in Spain where St. Ignatius found guidance for his personal calling in life. The vFellowship is a Cardoner program designed for faculty to cultivate a deliberate exploration of life purpose, vocation-as-calling, and well-being. The faculty member identified her vocation-as-calling as a desire to bring more involvement from the School of Nursing to the work already being done with the Omaha Tribe and engage students in the meaning of vocation in a Jesuit institution. During a faculty retreat, the faculty member identified her commitment to continue working with health care needs identified by the tribe. A new graduate faculty member expressed interest in the idea and was invited to participate in the process. The two faculty members met to identify the role that selected graduate students could play in the project.

Graduate Student Community

Graduate students who have an interest in community are required to take two courses. The two community courses require identification and development of a community health project and 48 hours of direct community clinical experience. After discussions with the faculty member teaching the two classes, it was decided that the Health Report Card Project would be a benefit to the Omaha Tribe and provide the graduate students with many opportunities. These opportunities included meeting course objectives, having a hands-on experience at the community level, and living the mission of the university, which includes service to others. In addition, graduate students have the advantage of professional autonomy as registered nurses and a more flexible schedule that allowed for making the 150-mile roundtrip drive to participate in school health screening and attend community meetings.

The students were involved in all aspects of the project, which included community assessment, planning, intervention, and evaluation. The community assessment included the school health screening data and analysis as well as the information obtained from the face-to-face planning meetings and other written materials obtained by the students about the tribe. Planning was done formally at the face-to-face meetings and in the classroom and informally outside the classroom via discussions on the drive up and back from the reservation with faculty members and students meeting separately outside of class. The interventions included participation in the school screening, data entry and analysis, development of the school health report card, and dissemination of the findings. The findings were disseminated with face-to-face meetings with teachers, administrators, and community members; a written report given to the schools and diabetes program director; and giving out individual student health report cards at published school events. In addition, the students and faculty were actively engaged in fulfilling professional societal obligations and living the mission of service to others.

THE PROCESS

The project spanned the course of 10 months. There were numerous face-to-face meetings that occurred on the reservation with community stakeholders. The 150-mile roundtrip drive provided faculty, graduate students, and the OISSE coordinator time together in a van with the chance for discussion before the meetings and for debriefing and planning for the next steps on the trip back. At these meetings faculty, students, and the OISSE coordinator discussed with community stakeholders how the health report card should look, what it should say, who else to contact in the community for input, and what events would be held to best maximize family attendance so that the health report card could be discussed with students and families. Cultural leaders in the community provided their expertise to make the health report card a culturally sensitive and relevant tool for families regarding their child's health status.

Data Collection

In the fall of 2006, four graduate students and three faculty members joined the school nurse, diabetes educator, physician, and volunteers to perform school health screenings for over 700 youths in the Omaha Tribe. The indicators chosen for the health report card were those available from the annual school health screenings at the two K–12 schools: year of screening, birth date/age, gender, school name and grade, height, weight, blood pressure, vision screening, waist and hip measurements, and grading for acanthosis nigricans. The parent/guardian name and address were also recorded for contact purposes.

Height and weight were measured by typical means, with tape measures and straight edges used to determine inches of height and floor scales to measure pounds of weight. Measurements were casual, with several students wearing their school clothes and shoes. Using guidelines of the Centers for Disease Control and Prevention, BMI classification for weight status was identified as overweight, at risk for overweight, healthy weight, or underweight. Overweight is defined as a BMI equal to or greater than the 95th percentile for children of the same age and gender. The primary focus of this health indicator was to promote the understanding of healthy weight, not to label a child as obese from a single BMI reading. A child's BMI changes from year to year, and the trend of these changes can identify children who would benefit most from health improvement interventions.

Blood pressure readings were taken by nurses and other trained personnel with students in a sitting position. Blood pressure percentiles were calculated according to Centers for Disease Control and Prevention guidelines using age and gender and were reported as "normal," "needs monitoring," or "needs referral."

Vision was screened using the standard symbols or letters on Snellen eye charts at the prescribed distance. Children were asked to cover their right eye for the left-eye test and vice versa. Children with prescription lenses were requested to screen using the lenses, although a large proportion of students with corrective lenses did not have them available for the screening event.

Assessment for acanthosis nigricans was consistently done by the same physician who has participated in the school screenings for over 15 years. The hairline at the back of the neck was observed for a characteristic darkened or discolored skin. Marker presence was recorded using a scale of 0 to 4, with "0" indicating the absence of the marker and "4" indicating the most severe presence.

Generation of the Health Report Card

Handwritten data from 2002 through 2006 were entered by community volunteers and Creighton School of Nursing graduate students and faculty. The electronic entry of data for the calculation of health-related risk categories based on age and gender percentiles occurred in an efficient manner. To provide a framework for such data evaluation as well as dissemination, a relational database management system (using Microsoft Access) was developed. All students were assigned an individual nonrepeating record number to relate the database table of demographic data to the table of yearly screening data. Data cleaning was completed by graduate nursing students and faculty. A mail-merged health report card was created for each of the 540 students who participated in the 2006–2007 school health screening. Some students had up to 5 years of school health screening data on their report card. The design of the health report card was approved by the Omaha Tribe community to ensure a culturally appropriate document.

Dissemination of Information

A written report of the school health screening 2006–2007 analysis was prepared by one of the faculty members and the graduate students. The findings of the report were discussed at a face-to-face meeting at the Carl T. Curtis Health Center in Macy. The meeting was attended by the physician who performs the acanthosis nigricans screening, the school nurse, two diabetes educators, three graduate students, three nursing faculty and the OISSE coordinator and one codirector. On two different days, a 15-minute Power Point presentation was given by the graduate students to the teachers and staff of each school. The presentation covered the significant findings of the school screening. The written report was given to each school administrator, the school nurse, and the Diabetes Program director.

Written information to announce the availability of the students' health report card was sent to families from each school with an invitation to discuss each child's results with a health care professional before, after, or during several scheduled school functions. Dissemination of the health report card was done face-to-face with family members who attended the annual school-sing program and graduation ceremonies. The health report card provided the focus for the opportunity to inform parents about their child's annual school health screening results and to provide appropriate education and interventions, if necessary, for prevention of potential health problems such as obesity and diabetes. Health professionals, including the graduate nursing students, were present to discuss the health report card with the family if requested. The health professional team contacted high-risk students for further evaluation and implementation of behavior change for health promotion and disease prevention. A total of 254 health report cards was distributed using this approach. The remaining health report cards were mailed to the child's parent or guardian.

Dissemination of information regarding the process and product of the health report card has begun. Faculty and students have presented at local and international conferences. An article for publication is near completion. The authorship is shared among graduate students, the school nurse, diabetes educator, OISSE coordinator, and nursing faculty. Each of the communities involved has shared in telling their story of the project to others. Hopefully, the Health Report Card Project will serve as an exemplar for other communities.

FINDINGS

The data analysis performed by the graduate students and faculty indicated that the acanthosis nigricans marker was present in 20% to 30% of the students screened in 2003–2006. The BMI analysis of each student for the years 2001–2006 revealed that in each year the percentage of students with BMIs that warranted monitoring or referral to a health professional exceeded 50% of the total number of students screened. The analysis of the BMI data provided the specific information needed for the Omaha Tribal communities to take actions that might help decrease the number of students identified as being overweight or obese and help address the Nebraska Healthy People 2010 goal to reduce the proportion of children who are overweight or obese to no more than 3% for youth 12–19 years of age. The information provided direction for the communities in their work on building community capacity to decrease the burden of diabetes.

OUTCOMES

The Health Report Card Project had many positive outcomes at the individual, family, group, and community levels: (a) addressing Healthy People 2010 objectives, (b) service to a rural Native American community with a focus on health promotion and disease prevention, (c) experience for students to meet essential competencies for interdisciplinary health professional education, (d) addressing some of the issues posed by the National Rural Health Association, and (e) the active participation of engaging in the work of building community capacity and partnerships.

The health report card made visible to the tribe, the school health screening indicators, and the overall health status of their children, at an individual and community level. Each group involved in the Health Report Card Project exhibited their own sense of community and all had commitment, problem-solving abilities, and resources. Working together, each community contributed actively to the process and outcome and in so doing each improved their own and each other's well-being.

The invitation provided a wealth of opportunities for collaboration among the communities involved in the project, such as exploration of issues related to rural health, elements of health promotion and disease prevention, interdisciplinary collaboration, nursing education, and building community capacity and partnerships. In the process of working together, each community's sense of self, commitment, ability to problem solve, and access to resources was strengthened.

The Health Report Card Project has helped make the nursing faculty and administration aware of the rich potential for other clinical experiences in rural communities. One graduate student continues to work on the project. She has conducted focus groups with parents who received the health report card so that their input can be used to make necessary changes for next year. Reflections of the project given by the graduate students indicate evidence of personal and professional growth.

WHERE DO WE GO FROM HERE?

Follow-up work has started to make changes in the health report card for next year based on input from the communities involved. Discussions have already taken place regarding ways to improve the school health screenings, data collection, and health report card dissemination. Although work between the university and the tribe will continue, the goal is that the health report card will become a project done completely by the tribal community. OISSE and interested faculty continue to look for sources of funding through grants and foundations that can be used to address diabetes prevention and health promotion. Regardless of funding, implementation of community-based health promotion and disease prevention programs are under way and will continue. The university has been asked to work on data analysis from programs already in place that address health promotion and disease prevention.

CONCLUSIONS

The Health Report Card Project provided a rich experience on several levels. First, the project involved each community sharing and actively using their capacity-building skills to enhance the well-being for all. Dissemination of the health report card served to start the dialogue among individuals, families, and communities about health promotion and disease prevention education for diabetes. Interventions that could be implemented to address Healthy People 2010 goals and objectives for prevention of diabetes and obesity were identified, and some were implemented. The health report card provided tangible evidence and direction for the tribe in addressing interventions for diabetes prevention. The project was one way in which the faculty and students at Creighton could engage in meeting the mission of the university through service to others, recognizing the inalienable worth of each individual, and the appreciation of ethnic and cultural diversity as core values. The project provided the opportunity to take moral action to honor the words and promises made to Native Americans by our country. The hope is that the project will be a springboard for more opportunities and further the work with the community on the implementation of specific health promotion and disease prevention interventions for diabetes.

REFERENCES

1. Dixon M, Roubideaux Y, eds. *Promises to Keep*. Washington, DC: American Public Health Association; 2001.
2. Chaskin RJ. *Building Community Capacity*. New York: A deGruyter; 2001.
3. Christiansen C. Creating Community: An essay on the social responsibility of Health Professionals. In Purtillo R, Jensen G, Royeen C. *Educating for Moral Action*. Philadelphia: FA Davis; 2005.
4. *Rural 2010 Health Goals and Objectives for Nebraska*. Nebraska Health and Human Services System: Department of Regulation and Licensure and Department of Finance and Support, November 2004.
5. Institute of Medicine. *Health Professions Education: A Bridge to Quality*. Washington, DC: National Academy Press; 2003.
6. National Rural Health Association Issue Paper: Recruitment and Retention of a Quality Health Workforce in Rural Areas, No. 6. Available at: http://www.nrharural.org/advocacy/sbu/issuepapers/nursing/2006workforceNo.6.pdf
7. http://www.diabetes.org/type-2-diabetes/skin-complications.jsp
8. Copeland K, Pankratz K, Cathev V, et al. Acanthosis nigricans, insulin resistance (HOMA) and dyslipidemia among Native American children. *J Okl State Med Assoc*. 2006;99.
9. http://ehealth.creighton.edu/commres_history.htm, http://www.mnisose.org/profiles/omaha.htm
10. Personal communication on February 5, 2007 with Judy Held, Nutritionist for Diabetes Education Program, Macy, NE.

Future Directors

CHAPTER 26

Next Steps in Rural Health Interprofessional Education and Practice

Kevin J. Lyons, MA, PhD

INTRODUCTION

As we move past the middle of the first decade of the 21st century, we are faced with what many believe is a crisis in rural health care. Most rural areas suffer shortages in health professionals as well as health care facilities.[1] Attracting health professionals to these areas is not an easy task because they are often isolated, and positions in these areas do not pay as well as those in affluent communities. Compounding this problem is the fact that, generally, rural residents are older and less wealthy than those living in urban or suburban areas.[2] Health problems of this group tend to be more complex than those of younger individuals. The federal government has further exacerbated the problem as it continues to cut funds for rural and other underserved areas. One such case is the removal of funding for the Quentin N. Burdick Interdisciplinary Rural Health Program, which funded the working conference from which this book developed. Finally, lack of health insurance poses an extreme burden on those seeking medical care.[1] Some estimates put the number of individuals in the country without health insurance at 45 million, many of whom live in rural areas. This is a situation that should be an embarrassment for the richest country in the world.

All the problems noted above represent restraining forces, hindering attempts to provide comprehensive, affordable, and quality health care to residents in rural areas. There are few driving forces available to overcome these restraining forces, other than the motivation on the part of health professionals to "do good." Besides this motivation, however, advances in technology and team approaches to care may offer some hope in addressing the problem.

Before these three driving forces can be used to improve practice, there are at least three things that will need to occur: revising our approach to education, addressing the needs of practice, and applying a leadership model to the situation. Each of these is discussed separately.

APPROACH TO EDUCATION

In viewing the need to change the way health professionals are educated, one needs to look at the changing nature of the health care system. The complex nature of health problems in underserved communities suggests that health professionals need a different mix of skills than they currently have. The Institute of Medicine drafted a vision statement that, "All health care professionals should be educated to deliver patient-centered care as members of an interdisciplinary team, emphasizing evidenced-based practice, quality improvement approaches and informatics."[3] They identified five core competencies required of future professionals:

1. Provide patient-centered care
2. Work in interdisciplinary teams
3. Use evidence-based practice
4. Apply quality improvement
5. Utilize informatics

Three of these, the need to work in interdisciplinary teams, use of evidence-based practice, and the use of informatics seem particularly germane to rural health practice. To realize this vision, educators will be required to reconsider the way in which future health care professionals are educated.

Interprofessional Teams

Over the years there have been claims that interprofessional teams may be effective approaches to providing care, especially in dealing with complex medical conditions.[4] Intuitively, interprofessional practice would seem to be one approach to alleviate the disparities of health across the country, particularly in rural areas. Unfortunately, the promise of interprofessional education and practice seems to be unfulfilled for the following reasons. Barriers to curricular change to reflect interprofessional education include professional programs designed to educate students in isolation, learning the skills of their profession at the expense of understanding others, the existence of a cultural hierarchy that fosters individual responsibility and decision making, and the lack of support by many accrediting agencies. There is also a lack of substantive research on either the effectiveness or the cost-effectiveness of this approach. Although cuts in federal spending for health professions education programs and in state spending for higher education pose significant problems, the way in which interprofessional education is introduced seems to be a bigger problem. Many approaches assume that involving students in purely didactic courses with students in other disciplines are sufficient to prepare them for interprofessional practice. What is needed are true interdisciplinary courses were students have opportunities to interact in meaningful ways and that involve the teaching of the process skills needed to work on collaborative teams. Some of these skills include communication, conflict resolution, negotiation, shared leadership, and decision making. What is also needed is opportunities for students to have experiences in underserved settings along with courses designed to increase awareness of cultural and ethnic differences. Without the above opportunities, students will continue to be unprepared to engage in any kind of meaningful interprofessional practice.

Evidence-Based Practice

Most health professions educational programs are now attempting to include a focus on evidence-based practice in their curriculum. Evidence-based practice is defined as the "integrations of the best research evidence with clinical expertise and patient values."[5] Although this is a promising step, problems exist with its implementation. One significant problem is that although programs may train students in the process of evidence-based practice, it is not part of the culture of many practice sites.[6] Novice clinicians tend to adopt the practice patterns of the clinical site rather than work to incorporate the best research evidence in their practice. Among other problems are that clinicians also report a lack of time to conduct literature searches, a lack of access to electronic databases, perceptions of the lack of available research evidence focused on individual patient needs, and limited skill in using electronic databases and in doing critical appraisals of the research.[6] To overcome these barriers, educational programs need to become more focused on the use of information technology and on developing critical thinking and research skills in addition to the principles of evidence-based practice in their curriculum.

Uses of Informatics

Given the shortage of health care practitioners, anticipated for the immediate future what new approaches must be implemented to overcome these shortages? One approach is to take advantage of emerging technology. Information technology is fast becoming a significant addition to the practice of many health professionals. One use of this technology is through e-Health, which is defined as, "The use of emerging information and communication technology, especially the internet, to improve or enable health and health care."[7] This is a broad, flexible approach that includes telemedicine, which is defined as "The use of electronic information and communication technologies to provide clinical care across distance."[8] Educating students in using e-Health as well as taking advantage of available technology to critically appraise the literature is critical for future health professionals.

ADDRESSING THE NEEDS OF PRACTICE IN RURAL AREAS

Changing the way health professionals are educated is one step in approving care delivery in the next decade. Given the nature of the problems facing those in rural underserved areas, professionals should be able to use new skill sets emerging from training in interprofessional approaches to care, evidence-based practice, and competence in using new technology in addressing the health issues facing the rural poor. Although the e-Health approach is a flexible one, rural communities, generally, are not currently organized to take advantage of the approach. Rural residents as a group are older, less wealthy, and have lower levels of educational attainment than those in urban and suburban areas.[2] Also, senior citizens and low-income people in rural areas are less likely to be on-line than their counterparts in suburban or urban areas. However, this situation is beginning to change. The Pew Internet and American Life Project, conducted in 2004, reported that in 2000, 41% of rural residents were on-line, but by 2003 the percentage rose to 52% as compared with 66% of suburban and 67% of urban residents. They also found that rural communities hold larger portions of relative Internet newcomers who are more enthusiastic adopters. They also found that rural users on-line for 3 or more years are more likely to seek health information on-line. "Almost three quarters of experienced rural users have done so, while 68% of similarly experienced suburban users and 64% of similarly experienced urban users have sought health information online."[2]

Although the situation is improving, there are still some issues that must be addressed before e-Health can be a viable option in rural settings. The first is the digital divide, which is simply the divide between people who have access to computers and the Internet and those who do not.[8] This still exists, although according to the Pew committee, the divide appears to be lessening. The second is health literacy, "the degree to which individuals have the capacity to obtain, process and understand basic health information and services needed to make appropriate health decisions."[3] The third is computer literacy, defined as "Competence in basic mouse and keyboarding sills, use of email, and skill in locating resources on the Internet."[9] And, finally, the implementation of an e-Health infrastructure, "(which) includes computer and Internet access plus computer and Internet literacy."[9]

Although these barriers are formidable, they can be overcome. One mechanism, already in place, is the Area Health Education Centers (AHEC), funded by the Health Resources and Services Administration of the U.S. Department of Health and Human Services. Two of the goals of the AHEC system are to provide needed health consultation services to the regional AHEC offices and, through them, to the professional communities they serve and to make the resources of the system more readily accessible to medically underserved communities in frontier, rural, and urban regions through their programs.[10]

A second important approach is through interprofessional collaboration and collaboration with the community. Interprofessional collaboration has received much attention in the literature in recent years. Claims for the value of interprofessional teams are many. They are thought to make better use of scarce resources, particularly by taking advantage of the complementary skills of participants. By taking advantage of the skills of participants, they have the ability to address more complex problems.[4] This is critically important in rural and other underserved communities. The problems in underserved communities are multiple and complex, and there needs to be the meaningful involvement of those who understand these problems. Members of communities, therefore, have important contributions to make and true collaborative partnerships provide the opportunity for gaining these contributions. It is also through these partnerships that health professionals can begin to understand the needs, values, and goals of those in the community.

Nature of Collaboration

For teams to be successful, particularly those that are interprofessional, they must also be collaborative. There are a number of definitions of collaboration that can be found in the literature. One that seems appropriate for this discussion is the following:

In effective collaborative teams, experts from the same or different disciplines are linked in such a way that they build on each other's strengths, backgrounds and experiences and together develop an integrative approach to resolve a research or educational problem. Problem formulation and solutions reflect a perspective that is more than the sum of each participant's contribution.[4]

One key term in this definition is "expert," where each member of the team is considered to be an expert in some facet of the task at hand. As an expert, each member of the team, whether it be a community member or a health care professional, has something of importance to contribute to the solution of the problem. To take advantage of the potential contributions of each team member, certain things must exist. Participants must learn about other team members' expertise, background, knowledge, and values. They must be able to demonstrate group skills, including communication, negotiation, delegation, time management, and others related to group dynamics, and they must ensure that accurate and timely information reaches those who need it at the appropriate time.[4]

If members engage in a concerted effort to work closely in an open environment, a "culture of collaboration" should emerge over time. This culture is defined by a number of characteristics. The first of these is agreement on the goals of the group, and these must be clear and understandable. Unless all group members agree on what the goals are, the danger exists that they will be working at cross purposes with one another. A lack of agreement, or a misunderstanding on what the goals of a group are, can also result in unnecessary conflict within the group.

The second characteristic is open communication. A pattern of open communication allows members to understand what is expected of them, and it brings ideas to the table so that they can be evaluated and, if necessary, debated in an open atmosphere.

The third characteristic is a climate of mutual trust. This is probably one of the most important of the characteristics. This climate allows for open communication in that members not only feel free to express opinions about an issue, but also know that each member of the groups can be trusted to carry out his or her assignment.

The fourth is a norm of cooperation, in which it is expected that all group members agree to work with one another toward attainment of the agreed upon goals of the group and in which individual interests are subordinated to these goals if they are in conflict. If this norm is present, then it is much easier to achieve the fifth characteristic, which is a process of consensual decision making. This does not mean that all decisions are unanimous, it means that in making any major decision, all viewpoints are taken into consideration and members agree to a course of action.

The sixth characteristic is one of shared leadership. Leadership comes about when one member of a group influences the actions of the group. Because each member, according to the definition, is an expert in some aspect of the group's task, it is reasonable to assume that the use of this expertise, given the other characteristics of trust, open communication and cooperation, will be accepted by other members of the group and acted upon.

APPLYING A LEADERSHIP MODEL

A critical component in collaboration within community settings is the concept of leadership. This is particularly true in understanding how one might work in the community setting to improve the health of the community. As described earlier, a culture of collaboration has a number of characteristics, all designed to accomplish a particular goal or set of goals. Understanding the process of leadership is critical to the success of this endeavor. Two questions arise. The first is why would members of a community want to collaborate on a project? To answer that question, it is necessary to ask the second question: Why do individuals join groups in general? There are quite a few theories of leadership in the literature, but for this purpose, one that appears to fit are the transactional theories.[11] In their simplest form, these theories suggest that individuals join groups because of the benefits available to them as a result of group membership, because groups provide opportunities for attaining these benefits. Depending on the type of group, these benefits could vary considerably. Groups, however, expect members to reciprocate and contribute skills and knowledge to attain the group goals. This then has the potential to become a continual process of exchange, where individuals contribute needed skills in exchange for receiving the desired benefits. The relationship becomes a mutually beneficial one. In the case of a community, improving the health status of the community is one benefit that would result from successful group functioning.

In working with community groups it is necessary to show the group that the benefits of membership outweigh the benefits of nonmembership. An assumption that must be changed is that community groups, particularly those in underserved communities, do not have a valuable contribution. To achieve success, it is necessary to understand the values and goals of the community. Helping a group understand these is one critical contribution. Community members have the expertise and the knowledge about the community to determine what strategies will work and what will not. They also know with which interventions people will comply. The issue that must be dealt with is convincing community members or other participants that a benefit will be received through satisfying group requirements, that the individual members can satisfy the requirements if they try, and that the benefit is worth the effort. This will partially depend on developing the characteristics of collaboration, because this climate of trust can result in improved communication, an atmosphere that fosters creative thinking and risk taking, and a sense by community members that their contributions are valuable. The climate of trust has one other positive outcome: At the beginning of a relationship, the benefits expected by members may not be readily available. Because of that, they must trust that the benefits will be forthcoming.

CONCLUSIONS

The major problems facing health care are formidable. Given the lack of resources available from the federal government to address the major issues, health care professionals need to assume responsibility to take the steps necessary to provide care to some of the more vulnerable individuals in our society. Three areas seem to be promising ones in improving this situation. The first is making better use of technology through implementing programs in the community, such as e-Health programs, based on evidence to allow individuals to take more control over their health issues. The second is to develop more interprofessional approaches to care, using collaborative models, to take advantage of the skills of health professionals from different disciplines. The third critical area is to take an active leadership role, with community members as integral participants, in the identification, planning, and implementation of programs to address community needs.

REFERENCES

1. Ricketts T. The changing nature of rural health care. *Annu Rev Public Health*. 2000;21:639–657.
2. Bell P, Reddy P, Rainei L. *Rural Areas and the Internet*. Washington, DC: Pew Internet and American Life Project; 2004.
3. *Health People 2010: Understanding and Improving Health*. Washington, DC: U.S. Department of Health and Human Services; 2000.
4. Gitlin L, Lyons K, Kolodner E. A model to build collaborative research or educational teams of health professionals in gerontology. *Educ Gerontol*. 1994;20:15–34.
5. Sackett D, Straus SE, Richardson WS, Rosenberg W, Haynes RB. *Evidence-Based Medicine: How to Practice and Teach EBM*, 2nd ed. Edinburgh, Scotland: Churchill Livingstone; 2000.

6. Swenson-Miller K. Creating and Sustaining Environments for Evidence-based Practice. Grant proposal submitted to the U.S. Department of Health and Human Services, Bureau of Health Professions; 2004.

7. Eng TR. *The eHealth Landscape: A Terrain Map of Emerging Information and Communication Technologies in Health and Health Care.* Princeton, NJ: The Robert Wood Johnson Foundation; 2001.

8. U.S. Department of Commerce. *Falling Through the Net: Defining the Digital Divide.* Washington, DC: National Telecommunications and Information Administrations, 1999. Available at: http://www.ntia.doc.gov/ntiahome/digitaldivide/. Retrieved July 29, 1999.

9. Swenson-Miller K, Cornman-Levy D, Lyons KJ. Presentation to eHealth Training Institute of the Allied Health Center for Excellence in eHealth Promotion Programs for Underserved Populations. A funded project by the Bureau of Health Professions in the U.S. Department of Health and Human Services, Allied Health Project Grant D37 HP 00898 01.

10. Harvan RA, Westfall J. The National AHEC Bulletin (2006), Colorado Rural Health Center Issue Paper, June 2003, Colorado AHEC System Annual Reports.

11. Jacobs TO. *Leadership and Exchange in Formal Organizations.* Alexandria, VA: Human Resources Research Organization; 1970.

CHAPTER 27

Interprofessional Education: Themes and Next Steps

Charlotte Brasic Royeen, PhD, OT, FAOTA
Gail M. Jensen, PhD, PT, FAPTA
Robin Ann Harvan, EdD

INTRODUCTION

In preparation of this last chapter of this book, it is appropriate to reflect on the setting in which the "think tank" conference* leading to this book was held. We met in the Nighthorse Campbell Building of the University of Colorado Medical Sciences Center, a rotunda representing love, honor, respect, and courage as foundations for honesty and reciprocity of relations among people, especially family. This building opens from the east so the sun greets you in the morning. The building is based on the concept of the circle, including the four seasonal solstices, depicting the cycle of life and the connection of all things.

The purpose of this, the last chapter in the book, is to help provide a connection of all things in this book for your "take-home" reflection, contemplation, and use. The Nighthorse Campbell Building succeeds in its goal—the building is an awesome homage to the heritage of Native American culture. Only time will tell if our goal—to facilitate change in health professions education in the United States and thus change the future of health care delivery in United States—is facilitated. Regardless of the eventual outcome,

*Leadership in Rural Health Interprofessional Education & Practice: A Working Conference for Leaders in Rural Health Care. Funded in part by a Health Resources Services Administration (HRSA) grant no. 1D36HP03168, Circles of Learning: Community and Clinic as Interdisciplinary Classroom, a Quentin N. Burdick Interdisciplinary Training Project.

however, is the fact that we all had the opportunity to participate in what Dr. Ruth Purtilo called "sacred space of the conference."[1] We hope that some aspects of this sacred space came across to you in the chapters of this book.

GESTALT OF THE CONFERENCE

Many swirling images of concepts remain long past the conference and the operationalization of these concepts in these book chapters. Key images constructed by participants during the conference, heard floating through the air amid discussions, are presented in Table 27-1.

In turn, each of these concepts are briefly discussed. We need to collaborate with those outside of health care to promote and provide best services in an interprofessional manner. This might mean reaching out to those not typically considered to be in the health care arena, such as public school teachers, local, regional, and state governments and associations, and to implement academic–community partnerships wherever we are able.

The concept of social and occupational justice for all, though not explicitly addressed in these chapters, is a recurring current underpinning action depicted by the authors or envisioned for the future. All people are entitled to quality health care delivered in an interdisciplinary or interprofessional manner. Health care as a justice for all is not just for the U.S. Congress, not just for those of us gainfully employed with employee health benefits, but for all who are human and in need. That is not the case currently. Compared with suburban areas, rural settings (having less than 10,000 people) and inner-city urban areas are more likely (a) to have residents in poverty, (b) have higher mortality rates, and (c) have poorer health status.[2] Thus there is a strange similarity between urban and rural settings in terms of health!

Table 27-1. Conceptual Images From the Interprofessional Conference

1. Collaborate outside of health care

2. Justice for all

3. Practice as change agents

4. Reaching across the mountains

5. Reaching across agencies

We are challenged to practice as change agents in that interprofessional practice extends beyond those who we immediately touch and affect. Good interprofessional practice also identifies system limitations and challenges each practitioner to serve as a change agent to effect change where and when needed. This concept of service not just as a practitioner but also as a change agent is a relatively new concept for health care practitioners: To implement this concept, our health professions' educational programs need to provide students the skills and abilities to serve as effective change agents.

Reaching across the mountains refers to the geographical location of the conference held in Denver and how we hope this book reaches out to others. That is, for any of us to be optimally effective, we need to reach out to those with whom we typically do not speak, interact, or socialize. By reaching across, we can forge new bonds and liaisons that will allow for continued work as agents of change and social justice.

Reaching across agencies refers to the need not just to work in an interprofessional manner but to also work across agencies for the good of the people involved. This would mean coordination of case care across boundaries of first dollar payment, across social institutions, across agencies, and across groups.

At the conference which led to this book, one of the key note speakers, Dr. Ruth Purtilo, presented a discussion of "What is goodness?"[1] She hypothesized that, in part, when anyone participates in something all together—as the participants did in this conference—the heart can be grabbed in a way that is deep and transforming and that, in this case, we have been touched by goodness. Collectively, it is our sincere hope that some aspects of this book reflect the spirit of the conference, that you as a reader have been transformed in some way by what you have read, and that you have been touched by "goodness." If so, a more immediate goal than changing health professions education and practice has been met. For first, we must change ourselves to change others and systems.

Also as part of the think tank conference, Dr. Amy Haddad presented an additional keynote.[3] In her talk, she presented a model of facts of understanding based on the work of Lee Shulman. We use an adaptation of her model of facts of understanding as a way for the reader to contemplate the vast scope of information, understanding, and wisdom the participants have presented in this book.

The first fact of understanding is explanation, or what happened. In this case, the federal government funded an innovative grant that spawned a think tank conference that led to this book.

The second fact of understanding is interpretation, or what does this mean? We believe that these events, with the outcome of this book, mean that a certain level of appreciation for interprofessional education in health professions education has been achieved and distilled. We believe that it is the first of its kind in the United States and hope that it serves as a turning point for recruitment of others into the "pedagological cause."

The third fact of understanding is application, or how to respond in real life. It is our dearest hope that what the authors of this book have shared in their chapters provides you tools and means of application of dimensions of interprofessional education in health professions' education.

The fourth fact of understanding is perspective, or to see and hear others' points of view. Again, we hope that this book has provided you with perspective different from your own, or at least new ways of seeing possibilities as a way to expand thinking and understanding.

The fifth fact of understanding is empathy, or the ability to empathize with others. Let us empathize with how our current educational systems educate bright and talented students into parochial disciplinary silos and how this hinders efficient and effective teamwork needed for real-life practice in the complex world of health care.

The sixth and final fact of understanding is self-knowledge, or reflection of "what did this experience mean?" We urge you to consider what this book of collective wisdom of practitioners and educators has meant to you and how your actions can move our collective understanding and move us forward.

Given these "facts of understanding," we now address themes emerging from this book. Much of the focus of this book is on rural health, reflecting the shared belief of authors that good practice in rural health can lead the way to quality health care in all areas.

THEMES

A strong interpretative theme from the conference as reflected across many of the chapters of this book is that interprofessional education opens up a lens that can transform health professions education. This transformation depends on three core ingredients: people, programs, and partnerships. Each of these core ingredients or themes is described here.

People: Committed to Promoting the Good

The people involved in interprofessional education share similar core values. They are like-minded faculty who are committed to promoting social justice in underserved communities. They believe that health professionals have a social contract with society and therefore an obligation to provide health care to those in greatest need. Furthermore, they are committed to making authentic learning experiences in these communities an essential element in professional education. They frequently are the faculty who have practiced in communities where there is limited access to health care services. In many ways, they find themselves called to serve in these communities. When one is working in underserved communities, resources are scarce and require work across the disciplines. Interprofessional work is necessary if one wants to address the health care needs of the medially underserved. One of the ways to extend the clinical service delivery is by integrating experiences into the professional curriculum. They find creative ways to link their clinical service commitment to student teaching and learning, often with few resources or rewards. These faculty are often maverick leaders in their educational institutions because they are committed to finding ways to meet these community needs. The funding frequently provides far less status and support than "research funding," yet the work is central to community and society.

Students, much like faculty role models, are also drawn to the interprofessional education and work in underserved communities. The community partners too are leaders in their communities, finding ways to maximize the scarce health care resources in their communities. The bridge between the academic community and the communities where much of the interprofessional work takes place is built through the relationship and trust building between the people involved. Flexibility, patience, and a high tolerance for uncertainty are shared characteristics of all involved.

Programs: Flexible Pedagogy and Preparation

Interprofessional education programs must be creative, engaging, and flexible to meet community needs and student needs. Successful programs must find the right balance of preparing students for the challenges of sharing and collaborating across disciplines and within communities. Students must move from a learning environment that is often only student-centered to an other-centered and community-centered model. It is not the student needs that are first and foremost, but it is the needs of others. For some students this is a tremendous challenge, whereas other students are well suited to this altruistic environment. Interprofessional learning experiences are most successful if they are based on sound pedagogy. Faculty understand that interprofessional learning experiences need to engage learner's in active problem solving that has all members of the team contributing and collaborating. Moving the interprofessional learning experiences and clinical practice into the community requires skillful faculty guidance, strong partnership with the community, and good student preparation.

Partnerships: Presence and Patience

The partnership built between institutions and communities are essential for interprofessional education. These partnerships are built on the trusting relationships developed by faculty and community leaders over years of interaction and collaborative work. Underserved communities generally have had prior experience with some institutions that are only present when there is funding and gone when the funding is gone. Both sustained presence and patience are key ingredients in these partnerships. The best partnerships evolve to where there is collaboration between institutions and communities toward a common goal. Long-lasting partnerships develop from a sustained presence of the institution. Institutional missions that support core values such as civic engagement, social justice, or other community work are excellent environments to build such programs. Institutions, however, must not only have civic mission statements but must also have other institutional roles and reward structures that support such efforts for faculty and students.

Given this review of themes uncovered in the content of these book chapters, we now address the next steps in the implementation of interprofessional education in the United States.

NEXT STEPS

We challenge the reader to think about what you can do to promote good, interprofessional work in difficult times. Recall the overarching challenge from the Institute of Medicine: All health professionals should be educated to deliver patient-centered care as members of interdisciplinary teams, emphasizing evidence-based practice, quality improvement approaches, and informatics.[4] In this book we have focused on interprofessional education, yet the other competencies called for by the Institute of Medicine may also remain as underdeveloped in implementation as interprofessional education. Future work should continue to address not just interprofessional education, but also quality improvement approaches and informatics.

Many of the health professions are engaged in discussions about how to best promote professionalism among students and the professional community. We believe that interprofessional education and practice in underserved communities must be an essential aspect of all health professions education.

William Sullivan argues that professionals must renew their social contract with society and that educational institutions must focus more on teamwork and flexibility in efforts to respond to the problems of society.[5]

A professional model of work requires that specialization be integrated more by teamwork than by centralized direction. The desirable change is from stiff organizational hierarchy bolstered by amassed credentials toward a partnership network in which a demonstrated competence confers authority. A more permeable and flexible organization of the professions is the logical extension of these developments and the university's need to be a critical participant in them. Real expertise is never entirely separable from a community or practice, it is never fully purified of social and moral engagement.[5] As a way of closing out this chapter, let us look at the final challenges.

FINAL CHALLENGES

We challenge the reader to think about what you can do to promote good, interprofessional work in difficult times. Again referring to the keynote by Dr. Purtilo, she urged us all to participate in goodness and to participate in something larger than oneself. We leave you, our reader, with the challenge to participate in interprofessional education in some way and in a manner that transcends just you.

Specific and immediate actions that need to be taken to facilitate interprofessional education across health professions education serves as our final comments and challenges (Table 27-2).

Table 27-2.   Immediate Actions to Foster Interprofessional Education

1. Infuse interprofessional education competencies within profession-specific accreditation requirements.

2. Spread the word about the need for interprofessional education; communicate and present your work within your institution and national and international conferences.

3. Recognize that interprofessional education comes in many shapes and forms and that it needs to be tailored to the context of any particular setting.

4. Expose students early in their health professions educational career to interprofessional education, while also providing a strong disciplinary identity.

The steps put forth in Table 27-2 are our best judgments of what needs to happen next to further foster and implement interprofessional education in the United States. We, the editors, leave you with these actions as a call to arms for what you can do, now.

Of course, the constant challenge of assessment and documentation of outcomes is with us. Consequently, as we move forward in these next steps, we should pay attention to the outcomes of our work. Barr et al.[6] expanded on Kirkpatrick's[7] four-point typology into a six-point typology to capture the following outcomes for interprofessional education:

1. Learner reactions
2. Modification of learners' attitudes/perceptions
3. Learners' acquisition of knowledge and skills
4. Learners' behavioral change
5. Change in organizational practice
6. Benefits to patients/clients

CONCLUSIONS

All involved in this project have labored to "get it right." Yet, we fully recognize our inherent limits to getting it right. Thus we ask for your cooperation where we have fallen short, and ask that you take up the challenge to correct or complete what we may not have been able to do conceptually, operationally, or in full scope. We are all striving toward the culture of interprofessionalism[8] or interprofessionality[9] and appreciate your interest in traveling this road with us.

REFERENCES

1. Purtilo R. Ethical foundations for healthcare in rural underserved communities: A goodness curriculum. Key note presentation at Leadership in Rural Health Interprofessional Education & Practice: A working conference Leaders in Rural Health Care; 2006.
2. Blumenthal SJ, Kagen J. The effects of socioeconomic status on health in rural and urban America. *JAMA*. 2002;287:109.
3. Haddad A. Teaching and learning in interprofessional education. Key note presentation at Leadership in Rural Health Interprofessional Education & Practice: A working conference Leaders in Rural Health Care; 2006.
4. Institute of Medicine. *Health Professions Education: A Bridge to Quality*. Washington, DC: National Academy Press; 2003.

5. Sullivan W. *Work and Integrity: The Crisis and Promise of Professionalism in America,* 2nd ed. San Francisco: Jossey-Bass; 2005:256.
6. Barr H, Koppel I, Reeves S, Hammick M, Freeth D. *Effective Interprofessional Education: Argument, Assumptions and Evidence.* Oxford, UK: Blackwell; 2005.
7. Kirkpatrick DL. Evaluation of training. In Craig R, Bittel L, eds. *Training and Development Handbook.* New York: McGraw-Hill; 1967:87–112.
8. Mitchell PH, Belza B, Schaad DC, et al. Working across the boundaries of health professions disciplines in education, research, and service: The University of Washington Experience. *Acad Med.* 2006;81:891–897.
9. D'amour D, Oandasan I. Interprofessionality as the field of interprofessional practice and interprofessional education: an emerging concept. *J Interprof Care.* 2005;(19(2)):8–20.

Content of the Interdisciplinary Education Perception Scale

Factor	Items
Professional competence and autonomy	• Individuals in my profession are well trained. • Individuals in my profession demonstrate a great deal of autonomy. • Individuals in other professions respect the work done by my profession. • Individuals in my profession are very positive about their goals and objectives. • Individuals in my profession are very positive about their contributions and accomplishments. • Individuals in other professions think highly of my profession. • Individuals in my profession trust each other's professional judgment. • Individuals in my profession are extremely competent.
Perceived need of professional cooperation	• Individuals in my profession need to cooperate more with other professions. • Individuals in my profession must depend on the work of people in other professions.

Factor	Items
Perception of actual cooperation and resource sharing within and across professions	• Individuals in my profession are able to work closely with individuals in other professions. • Individuals in my profession are willing to share information and resources with other professionals. • Individuals in my profession have good relations with people in other professions. • Individuals in my profession think highly of other related professions. • Individuals in my profession work well with each other.
Understanding the value and contributions of other professions/professionals	• Individuals in my profession have a higher status than individuals in other professions. • Individuals in my profession make every effort to understand the capabilities and contributions of other professions. • Individuals in other professions seek the advice of people in my profession.

Source: Luecht RM, Madsen MK, Taugher MP, et al. Assessing professional perceptions: Design and validation of an interdisciplinary education perception scale. *J Allied Health.* 1990;19:181–191. Used with permission

Proposed Cultural Proficiency Elective for Health Care Professions Schools

COURSE DESCRIPTION

This course will explore cultural diversity and health disparities globally and locally. Through a cultural self-assessment, students will explore how their own culture influences their worldview. Selected components of complex cultural environments that relate to health disparities will be analyzed. Students will examine existing health disparities, systems, and potential solutions. Because this course recognizes cultural competency as a basic requirement of any health care system and its constituents, students will determine the importance of responding respectfully to and preserving the dignity of people of all cultures both within and outside of health and social systems.

COURSE GOALS

Students will have the opportunity, through independent inquiry of a racial group other than their own, to investigate the following:

- Who is experiencing the health disparity?
- What is the nature of the disparity?
- Why is the disparity occurring?
- How can the disparity be effectively reduced?

LEARNING OBJECTIVES

Understand and describe how culture creates differences in disease explanations.

Identify and describe the distribution of health inequalities and their contributing factors across population groups and disease outcomes.

Investigate interactions among culture, class, demographics, and health care providers.

Explore strengths of different populations to improve health.

Describe and critique current medical care and social interactions of the chosen group.

TEXT

Creighton University Center of Excellence website http://medicine.creighton.edu/coe/

Community Healthcare Challenges (4 VCR Tape Series)

Additional reports and/or articles may be supplied.

EVALUATIVE TECHNIQUES

The course director will complete an evaluation report on the research project.

Each student will research and produce a critical evaluation of a selected culture, which will be graded for credit and published on the Creighton Multicultural Health Information Resource Center website as a resource for physicians and patients.

STUDENT RESPONSIBILITIES/CLINICAL SCHEDULES

Meet with course director or designee once a week.

Interview practitioners, representatives of a racial group in the community, different from the student's race.

Author a website and/or a six-page paper on the subject.

EXAMPLES OF QUESTIONS THAT WILL GUIDE THE STUDENT'S INQUIRY

What significant aspects of the culture (being studied) are different from or similar to other racial and ethnic groups?

What health concerns are specific to or significantly impact individuals from this culture in the United States?

What other obstacles do individuals from this culture face when it comes to quality health care?

How does one begin to step out of their own worldview to approach the issues and social challenges that people of different races may face daily?

GRADING POLICY

Successful completion of the elective course with at least 98% participation in class discussions and attendance and submission of a term paper translates to a "Pass" grade.

Index

A

Academic–community
   partnerships
   benefits of, with community-
      based nonprofit organiza-
      tions, 223–224
   older adults and, 98–99
Academic health centers, integrating AHEC programs into, 223
Academic research, community-
   based research *vs.*, 172–173*t*
Academic settings
   best practices for, 105–106
   medical librarians in, 121–122
Acanthosis nigricans, 258
   assessment for, 418, 421, 423
   diabetes and, 416
Access to care
   in Brownsville, Texas, 406
   rural racial/ethnic culture and,
      399–400
Accomplishments, sharing credit
   for, sustainable community
   partnerships and, 178
Accountability, 63
   ethics and, 16
   for interprofessional education,
      37
Accreditation, of health professions and interprofessional
   education, 21, 36–37
Accreditation Council for
   Occupational Therapy
   Education, 40*t*
Accreditation Council for
   Pharmacy Education, 41*t*
Accreditation Review
   Commission on Education
   for the Physician Assistant,
   Inc., 41*t*

Accreditation standards, review
   summaries of, across nine
   health-related professions
   related to interprofessional
   education, 38–41*t*
Acquired immunodeficiency syn-
   drome, 32, 406
Action research, 386
   participatory
      student data related to, 385*t*
      training in justice, power
         and, 386
   PRISYM and, 384
Activities of daily living, older
   adults and, 97
ADA. *See* American Diabetes
   Association
Administration, interprofessional
   education and, 33
Administration on Aging, 96
Administrators, leadership competencies for, 19
Advertising, effective health communication campaigns and,
   402
Advocacy, as theme within Doisy
   College of Health Sciences
   curriculum, 319, 320*t*
African Americans, 201
   disparities in health care for,
      202
   in four health care professions,
      203*t*
   geographical concentration of,
      in rural areas, 398
   as healthcare providers in six
      healthcare professions, 204*t*
   infant mortality and, 202
   land ownership and, 191
   literacy and, 394

low education levels and, 399
low income and poor quality
   care for, 158
New Deal and, 192
in New Mexico, 205
nurse practitioner graduate
   program and recruitment
   of, 207
rural, health gaps experienced
   by, 391
in rural America, 392
sharecroppers, 191
type 2 diabetes in, 265
After-school programs, 167
Agencies, reaching across, 441
Agency for Healthcare Research
   and Quality, 50, 52, 58, 416
   health care teamwork report
      by, 55
   key conclusions from literature
      of, 51 (box 4–1)
Aging in place, 97
AHECs. *See* Area Health
   Education Centers
AHRQ. *See* Agency for Healthcare
   Research and Quality
AIDS. *See* Acquired immunodeficiency syndrome
Alaska Natives, 201
   in four health care professions,
      203*t*
   as healthcare providers in six
      healthcare professions,
      204*t*
Albuquerque Public Schools, 211,
   212
Alcohol abuse, Omaha Tribe and
   prevention of, 256, 257
Alcoholics Anonymous, 257
Alcoholism, Native Americans
   and, 250

Alinsky, Saul, 141, 142, 145, 155,
    156, 163
Amaro, D. J., 211
American Association of Colleges
    of Nursing, 416
American Association of Medical
    Colleges, 80
American Bar Association, 36
American Diabetes Association,
    265, 267, 416
American Geriatrics Society Task
    Force on the Future of
    Geriatric Medicine, health
    care goals stated by, 98
American Nurses Association,
    416
American Society of Addiction
    Medicines, 257
America's Health Rankings,
    Minnesota ranking within,
    350
Andrews, J. E., 114
Andrus, M. R., 267
Appalachia
    challenges of serving in,
        378–383
    distance, weather, and tech-
        nology challenges,
        379–380
    getting comfortable with,
        378
    site development challenges,
        380–381
    systemic economic, service
        and education chal-
        lenges, 378–379
    dealing openly with justice and
        power in, 383–384, 386
    training for services in, 377–378
Appalachian at-risk youth
    defining a strong service team
        for, 370–373
    success in training for team ser-
        vice to, 386–388
Appalachian culture
    appreciating and providing ser-
        vices within, 375, 377–378

site supervisors' perceptions re-
    garding students' cultural
    competence, 377t
student data related to compe-
    tencies in, 376t
Appalachian families, strength of,
    129–130
Appalachian people
    building trust with, 131–132
    stereotyping of, 375
Appalachian region
    building rural health network
        in, 133–137
    building trust in, 131–132
    corporate culture and climate
        in, 132–133
    link to interprofessional educa-
        tion and leadership devel-
        opment in, 137–138
Appalachian Regional
    Commission, 378–379
Application, 181, 442
APS. See Albuquerque Public
    Schools
Aragon, L., 214
ARC. See Appalachian Regional
    Commission
Area Health Education Centers,
    433
    added value of services pro-
        vided by trainees of, 228
    campus-community partner-
        ships, 222–224
    collaborations in Colorado,
        230–233
    community health education
        and development,
        229–230
    creation of, 219
    defined, 219
    federal-state-local partnership
        funding model for, 221
    functions provided by, 226
    funding model for, 221
    health care workforce resources
        improved through, 225
    impact of, 221–222

locations of, 220
reforming rural health care and
    role of, 233–236
retention of health profession-
    als and, 228–229
in rural America, 224–226
Area Wide Health Committee
    (Tillery, North Carolina),
    194
Arthritis, older adults and, 96,
    102
Asian Americans, 201
    in four health care professions,
        203t
    as healthcare providers in six
        healthcare professions,
        204t
    in New Mexico, 205
Assessment tools, future direc-
    tions with, 72–73
Association of Academic Health
    Centers, 49
Asynchronous communication
    networks, 329, 332
Asynchronous video presenta-
    tions, 341
Atkins, J., 99
At-risk youth, PRISYM and rec-
    ommendations for those in
    service to, 388–389
Attitude competencies, primary
    teamwork competencies
    and, 57t
Attitudes, service learning con-
    structs measures and, 69t
Attitudes Toward Community
    Health Scale, 71
Audiologists, ethnic/gender di-
    versity among, 204t
Australian Capital Territory (ACT)
    Department of Health, 50
Autonomy, 35t
    paradox of: mutual autonomy
        and interprofessional col-
        laboration, 244–245
AWHC. See Area Wide Health
    Committee

B

"Baby Ben" paper case, 209
Baby boomers, 97
Barr, H., 52, 446
Barriers to health care, in rural
    setting, 112
Barriers to information access,
    rural professionals and, 114
Behaviorism, 52
Bell, R. A., 268
Benner, P., 238, 241, 245
Bernal, C., 214
Best Evidence in Medical
    Education, 50
Best practices, for academic set-
    tings, 105–106
Bias
    cultural, 308
    provider, 202
Billboards, promoting health-
    related behavior change
    via, 402
Bingo Palace, The (Erdrich), 306
Biomedical model, sociomedical
    model vs., 281–284
Blacks. See African Americans
Bligh, J., 32
Blood pressure, diabetes out-
    comes and, 268
BMI. See Body mass index
Bodenheimer, T., 268
Body mass index, 416, 421
Bolivian story, 143–145, 156
Bond, Kit, 154
Bonuses, underserved communi-
    ties and, 79
Bower, P., 277
Boyer, E. L., 64, 181, 286
Boys and Girls Clubs of Omaha,
    Nebraska, 302
Bradley, P., 32
Bray, P., 275
"Bridging" teachers, 211
"Bringing Health Information to
    the Community" web log,
    119
Bringle, R. G., 68

Brochures, promoting health-
    related behavior change
    via, 402
Brooks, R. G., 78
Brownsville, Texas
    demographics in, 405
    location of, 405
    TrendBender groups in, 404
Brownsville Independent School
    District, Parental
    Involvement Program of,
    407
Brownsville Independent School
    District (Texas), 407
Brownsville/Matamoros, Texas,
    406
Brukardt, M. J., 181
Buduburam Refugee Camp
    (Ghana), 120
Building Bridges of Support
    Project, 381
Bureau of Health Professions, 303
Butters, J., 284

C

CAIPE. See Centre for the
    Advancement of
    Interprofessional Education
California Achievement Test,
    302
Cambodian enclaves, in
    Minnesota, 353
Campus–community partnerships
    Area Health Education Centers
        and, 219–236
    benefits with, 287
    University of Minnesota
        Medical School and next
        generation of, 356–358,
        361, 363
Cancer, older adults and, 96
Cannon-Bowers, J. A., 58
Care. See also Ethics of care
    redesigned systems of, 268–269,
    277
Caring Communities program
    (Missouri), 153

Carl T. Curtis Health Education
    Center (Omaha Tribe), 118,
    251, 253, 256, 417–418,
    422
    long-term care services at,
        254–255
    outpatient primary care ser-
        vices at, 258
Carl T. Curtis Health Education
    System, history of, 258–259
Carnegie Foundation for the
    Advancement of Teaching,
    37
Case studies, 314
CDSAs. See Child development
    service agencies
Cedar burning, 251–252
Center for Collaborative Research
    (Thomas Jefferson
    University), 119
Center for Healthy Aging, 98
Center for Interprofessional
    Education and Research,
    315
Center for Interprofessional
    Education (Minnesota),
    364–365
Center for Research Strategies,
    231
Centers for Disease Control and
    Prevention, 250, 421
Centre for the Advancement of
    Interprofessional Education,
    47, 52
Certification, cultural diversity
    and, 215
Change agents, 441
Charles, G., 283
Charles Drew Health Center
    (Nebraska), 302, 306, 307
Charleston Area Senior Citizens
    Center (South Carolina), 101
Chat rooms, 341
CHCs. See Community health
    centers
Child death rate, 202
Child development service agen-
    cies, 341

Child mental health arena, 126–127

Child mortality rates, 142

Children with disabilities, evaluating UNM graduates' impact on outcomes in, 213

Chinle community (Navajo Nation), 86, 87

Christiansen, C., 415

Chronic care model, 277
  eastern North Carolina chronic care pilot project and, 275
  fundamental areas identified by, 270–272

Chronic illness, 15
  older population with, 95–96, 97
  rural population and, 281

City of Brownsville Public Health Department, 407

Clan system, Omaha Tribe and, 252

Clark, P. G., 34t, 48, 53

Classrooms, sharing, 287

Cleary, K. K., 284

Client safety/risk reduction, as theme within Doisy College of Health Sciences curriculum, 320, 321t

Clifford, J., 194

Clinical education, reforming, 6

Clinical information system, chronic care model and, 271

Clinical laboratory science, accreditation standards in, 38t

Cochrane Collaboration, 50, 269

Cognitive development, 53

Cognitivism, 53

Collaboration, 35t, 50
  defined, 433–434
  medical librarians and, 116–117
  nature of, 433–435
  systems integration and, 127–128
  theoretical frameworks of, 59

Collaboration in interprofessional practice, defined, 319

Collaborative community partnerships, 176, 177

Collaborative health care practice
  competencies for, 314
  interprofessional education and, 22
  older adults and, 99

Collectivism, Tillery, North Carolina and, 194

Colorado
  Area Health Education Centers collaborations in, 230–233
  health care workforce development pipeline in, 233
  partnerships between health professions education schools and community partners in, 233
  strategies for strengthening health professions training infrastructure in, 232

Colorado Occupational Employment Outlook, 230

Colorado Rural Health Center, 231

Colorado Trust's Health Professions Initiative, 230, 232

Commission on Accreditation for Dietetics Education, 39t

Commission on Accreditation for Health Informatics and Information Management Education, 36, 38t

Commission on Accreditation in Physical Therapy Education, 41t

Commission on Community-Engaged Scholarship in the Health Professions, 180

Committee on the Future of Rural Health Care (IOM), 225, 233

Committee on the Health Professions Education Summit, establishment of, 6

Committee on the Quality of Health Care in America (IOM), 4–5, 272

Common good
  possible "competing" elements underlying concept of, in communities and health care, 25
  promoting, 18, 23
  rethinking learning for IPE and, 24–25

Communicating with Strangers: An Approach to Intercultural Communication (Gudykunst and Kim), 307

Communication, 35t
  health care team efficacy and, 284
  sustainable community partnerships and, 178
  as theme within Doisy College of Health Sciences curriculum, 319, 320t

Communication methods, traditional vs. emerging, 403t

Communication style, culture and, 398

Communities of practice, electronic communication and, 329

Community, 35t
  human and community needs defined by, 167

Community assessment, 144

Community-based care, geriatric care and, 98

Community-based health professional competencies, 283t

Community-based health professions education, statewide campus-community partnership for, 222

Community-based participatory research
  Appalachian culture and, 130
  defined, 171

Community-based research, 171–174
  academic research vs., 172–173t
  interdisciplinary nature of, 171
  outcomes and products of, 171

Community-Campus
    Partnerships for Health, 99,
    167, 168, 177, 180
Community capacity building
    need for, 415–416
    Omaha Tribe and, 260, 414–415
Community capacity building
    wheel, four dimensions
    within, 414, *414*
Community coalitions, 141
Community Collaborations for
    Children, 381
Community development
    Area Health Education Centers
        and facilitation of, 230
    functional governance struc-
        tures and, 155
    methods, 141
    principles, use of, 142
Community dwelling elders,
    97–99
Community-engaged scholarship
    products, disseminating, 183
Community engagement
    characteristic principles of,
        180
    community-based research
        and, 171, 173–174
    context of, 168–176
    health care skills enhanced
        through, 288*t*
    interprofessional education and
        service-learning common
        teaching strategies,
        174–176
    service learning and, 169–171
Community health centers, 228
    AHECs partnerships with,
        224
Community health workers, in
    Washington County,
    Missouri, 149–150
Community-identified needs, ed-
    ucational experiences
    molded around, 286
Community intervention, 141
Community linkages, chronic care
    model and, 271–272

Community of practice, Wenger's
    definition of and members
    of, 330
Community partnerships, sus-
    tainable, principles for,
    177–179
Community Partnerships in
    Health Professions
    Education, 103, 104
Community service, service learn-
    ing *vs.*, 169
Compact disks, promoting health-
    related behavior change via,
    403
Competencies
    for collaborative health care
        practice, 314
    for community-based and in-
        terprofessional related
        health professionals, 283*t*
    primary teamwork, 56–57*t*
Competency-based educational
    models, 55
Competency-based education sys-
    tem, 9
Computer literacy, defined, 433
Conceptual model, defined, 45
Concerned Citizens of Tillery
    (North Carolina), 192, 193
Conferencing software, 89
Congress (U.S.), 440
    Area Health Education Centers
        and, 219, 221
    interprofessional student train-
        ing grants cuts by, 286
Conley, D., 190
Constructivism, 53
Contract health services, 256
Coon, P., 267
Cooperation, 434
Cooperative learning, 53
Cooperatives, 142
Coordination, 35*t*
Copeland, K., 416
Corporate culture, in Appalachian
    region, 131, 132–133, 375
Cost-effective practice, promot-
    ing, 42

Costs for health care, rising, 32
Council for Higher Education
    Accreditation, mission state-
    ment for, 36
County health departments, 228
Cox, D., 181
Crandall, L. A., 78
Creating Opportunities for
    Parents Everywhere, 381
Creighton Health Sciences
    Library/Learning Resource
    Center, 118, 122
Creighton University, 80, 119, 288,
    416, 418
    Cardoner program, 419
    cultural competency training
        for postbaccalaureate stu-
        dents at, 306–307
    founding and philosophy of,
        297–298
    Health Careers Opportunity
        Program at, 302, 306
    health professions partnership
        initiative at, 303
    Health Sciences
        Library/Learning
        Resource Center, 118, 122
    Health Sciences Schools, 298
    Office of Health Sciences
        Multicultural and
        Community Affairs, 81,
        298
    Office of Interprofessional
        Scholarship, Service, and
        Education, 9, 84, 118, 119,
        413
    Omaha Tribe and partnership
        with, 260, 418–419
    online pathway to Doctor of
        Pharmacy degree at, 88
    Pre-Matriculation Program at,
        303, 306
    School of Dentistry, 298
    School of Medicine, 298
        Center of Excellence, 303
    School of Nursing, 298, 413
    School of Pharmacy and Health
        Professions, 289, 298

Creighton University Center of
  Excellence web site, 452
Creighton University Medical
  Center, 122
Critical Access Hospitals, 116
Critical self-reflection, importance
  of, for students, 20–21
Critical thinking
  service learning constructs
    measures and, 70*t*
  student proficiency in, 65
*Crossing the Quality Chasm: A New
  Health System for the 21st
  Century*, 4, 126
  key skills addressed in, 7
  recommendations of, 5–6
Cross-professional education,
  practice, and research, 49
Cross-professions analysis, 37, 42
CU. *See* Creighton University
Cullen, T. J., 79
Cultural awareness, Omaha Tribe
  health care needs and,
  259–260
Cultural beliefs, identifying conflicts in traditional curriculum content with, 209–210
Cultural bias, 308
Cultural collaboration, 434, 435
Cultural competency training, for
  postbaccalaureate students
  at Creighton University,
  306–307
Cultural considerations, students
  and, 284
Cultural diversity, 201, 215, 307
  adjusting curriculum to student
    lifestyles, 208–209
  financial aid and, 214–215
  identifying conflicts in tradi-
    tional curriculum content
    with cultural beliefs,
    209–210
  incorporating faculty mentor-
    ship for educational sup-
    port, 210–211
  integrating experiences into
    curricula, 209

Project ESCUELA, 211–213
  respecting cultural responsibili-
    ties and rituals, 210
  workforce and, 202
Cultural experiences, integration
  of, into curricula, 209
Cultural immersions, interprofessional structured, in
  rural/underserved communities, 84
Culturally competent care, critical
  nature of, 307
Cultural proficiency training,
  Health Sciences
  Multicultural and
  Community Affairs and experience in, 303, 306–307
Cultural responsibilities and rituals, respecting, 210
Culture, rural racial/ethnic populations and impact of,
  397–400
"Curin' House" (Tillery, North
  Carolina), 193, 194
Curriculum
  adjusting to student lifestyles,
    208–209
  cultural experiences integrated
    into, 209
  identifying conflicts with cul-
    tural beliefs in, 209–210
  interprofessional, 312–313
  interprofessional education and
    design of, 21–22
Curtis, Carl T., 258, 259
Cutchin, M. P., 190, 191

D

D'Amour, D., 50, 58, 312
Danisiewicz, T. J., 243
Dansky, K. H., 266
Decision making
  community development and
    community involvement
    in
  HOPE, Great Mines Health
    Center and, 145–156

James House Health Center
  and, 156–162
La Paz, Bolivia and, 143–145,
  156
Decision support, chronic care
  model and, 271
Dee, C., 114
Delivery system design, chronic
  care model and, 270–271
Delta Regional Authority, 154
Demographics, health care work
  shortages and, 63
Dental health, elderly and health
  conditions related to,
  159
Dental health services
  HOPE consortium and, 148
  James House Health Center
    and, 159
Department of Health and
  Human Services, 282, 303,
  433
Deprofessionalization, 244
Devereux Plantation, 191
Dewey, John, 16, 25
Diabetes, 202. *See also* Health
  Report Card Project
  among youth, 3, 15
  body mass index and, 416
  comparison of outcomes in
    rural and urban patients,
    267*t*
  complications and mortality as-
    sociated with, 265
  Native Americans and, 250, 413
  Nebraska Healthy People
    Goals and reduction of,
    415
  new model of care delivery for,
    270–272
  older adults and, 96
  Omaha Tribe and
    screenings/care for, 258
  outcomes, 267–268
  in rural America, 266–267
  type 2, 265, 266, 267, 269, 274
    among Omaha people, 255
    in Brownsville, Texas, 406

Diabetes care team members, in rural areas, 274
Diabetes mellitus, 272
    eastern North Carolina chronic care pilot project and, 274–277
    prevalence of, in United States, 265
Diabetic retinopathy, screening for, 269
Dialysis, Omaha people and need for, 255
Diet, diabetes prevention and, 417
Differentiated fees, underserved communities and, 79
Digital divide, 114, 119, 403
Digital technologies, promoting health-related behavior change via, 403
Digital video disks, promoting health-related behavior change via, 403
Dirani, R., 266
Direct mail, promoting health-related behavior change via, 402
Discovery, scholarship and, 181
Discrimination, 195
Discussion boards, 341
Disparities in health care, 142, 202–203, 205
    building community capacity and, 415–416
    cultural diversity and, 201
    National AHEC Organization and, 235
    for Native Americans, 250, 251
    racial, 158
    rural areas and, 189
    seeking elimination of, 127
    in urban vs. rural Minnesota, 351
Dissemination products, community-based research and, 171
Distance challenges, in Appalachia, 379–380
Distance education, 88–91

Diverse populations, effective communication programs and, 409
Diversity, recruitment and, 207–208
Doctor of Occupational Therapy (OTD) degree, 91
Doctor of Pharmacy degree, at Creighton University, web-based education and, 88–91
Document literacy scale, 394t
Donne, John, 156
Dorsch, J., 113, 114
Drinka, T., 48
Drug abuse, Omaha Tribe and prevention of, 256
Ducanis, A., 47
Dugan, Máire, 144
Duke Endowment, The, 332

E

East Carolina University, 192
Eastern Kentucky University, Center for Appalachian Studies, 371
Eccles Health Sciences Library (University of Utah), 117, 118
Economic challenges, in Appalachia, 131, 378–379
Education. See also Interprofessional education
    approach to, 430–432
        evidence-based practice, 431
        informatics, 431–432
        interprofessional teams, 430–431
Educational content, ethics of justice vs. ethics of care and, 246
Educational design, 284–293
    benefits with, 287
    exemplar, 284–285, 288–289, 291, 293
    obstacles to, 285–287
Educational organization, interprofessional education and, 21–22

Educational outcomes, Kirkpatrick's model of, 66, 66t
Educational Testing Service, 65
Educational theory, IPE assessment and, 65
Education challenges, in Appalachia, 378–379
Education-entertainment, effective health communication campaigns and, 401
Education leaders, motivating and supporting, 9
Education level, rural racial/ethnic culture and, 399
Education-to-practice, as two-way street, 60
Edward and Margaret Doisy College of Health Sciences (St. Louis University), 157, 160, 161, 312
    courses, 322–324
        criteria for interprofessional course, 322t
        evidence-based health care, 323
        health care ethics, 323
        health care system and health promotion, 323
        integrative interprofessional practicum experience, 323–324
        interprofessional, criteria for, 322t
        introduction to interprofessional health care, 323
    curriculum
        integration of learning activities within, 324–325
        interprofessional education themes in, 320–321t
    curriculum plan, 317–322
        competencies, 320–321
        definitions, 318–319
        principles of course development, 321–322
        purpose, 319
        themes, 319–320

evaluation of interprofessional
    education program,
    325–326, 326*t*
formation of, 312, 316
interprofessional curriculum,
    312–317
    institutional factors,
        315–317
    learner, 313–314
    learning activities, 314–315
Edwards, J., 71
Effective Interprofessional Education:
    Argument, Assumption, &
    Evidence, 53
e-Health, 432, 436
Elderly population, community-
    dwelling, 97–99
Elders, of Omaha Tribe, 254–255
e-learning, 88–91
Electronic study groups, 90
e-mail, 331
Emancipation, 191
Empathy, 442
Empowerment praxis, 141
e-NC Authority, 331
End-of-life health care, ethics of
    justice and ethics of care re-
    lated to, 242–243
Engagement, value of, in rural
    communities, 195–196
Environmental justice, rural areas
    and, 190, 191
Epistemology, of interdisciplinary
    learning, 53
Erdrich, Louise, 306
Errors, reducing, 42
Ethical development, 53
Ethics of care
    autonomy and, 244
    creating interprofessional
        moral community and,
        245
    educational content and activi-
        ties associated with, 246
    end-of-life health care and,
        242–243
    ethics of justice *vs.,* 239–240*t*

interprofessional moral com-
    munity and, 246
professionalization and,
    237–247
strengths and limitations with,
    241–242*t*
Ethics of justice
    barriers to interprofessional
        practice and, 246
    creating interprofessional
        moral community and,
        245
    educational content and activi-
        ties associated with, 246
    end-of-life health care and,
        242–243
    ethics of care *vs.,* 239–240*t*
    professional autonomy and, 244
    strengths and limitations with,
        241–242*t*
Ethiopian enclaves, in Minnesota,
    353
Ethnic communities, rural, health
    communication with,
    391–410
Ethnic diversity, of students in
    four health care professions,
    203*t*
Ethnicity. *See also* Race
    disparities in health care and,
        202
    of health professionals in
        Nebraska, 301*t*
    type 2 diabetes and, 265
Evaluation, of Doisy College of
    Health Sciences interprofes-
    sional education program,
    325, 326*t*
Evidence based medicine, infor-
    mation-seeking and, 113–114
Evidence-based practice, 430, 431
    employing, 7*t*
    as theme within Doisy College
        of Health Sciences cur-
        riculum, 319, 320*t*
Experiential learning, 53
Experts, team members and, 434

F

Facilitators, 175
Faculty
    community-engaged scholar-
        ship opportunity for, in
        interprofessional educa-
        tion, 180–182
    cultural diversity issues and,
        203
    incentives and recognition of,
        286
    as role models, 18
    social justice and, 442–443
Faculty attitudes, interprofes-
    sional education and, 33
Faculty development
    approaches to, in interprofes-
        sional education, 20*t*
    in geriatrics, 102–104, 105
    interprofessional education
        promotion and, 19
Faculty Leadership Council,
    Minnesota Area Health
    Education Center, 358–359,
    360
Faculty mentorship, incorporat-
    ing for additional educa-
    tional support, 210–211
Faculty resources, sharing, 287
Faculty scholarship, recognizing
    diverse products and dissem-
    ination pathways of commu-
    nity-engaged research as
    products for, 182–184
Fairview Mesaba Clinics/Range
    Regional Health Services
    (Hibbing, Minnesota),
    359
Family ties, in Appalachian cul-
    ture, 129–130
Feedback process, sustainable
    community partnerships
    and, 178
Females, as healthcare providers
    in six healthcare professions,
    204*t*

Fergus Falls, Minnesota, Central Minnesota Area Health Education Center, 359
Fertman, C. I., 67
Financial aid, Project ESCUELA and individual student experiences with, 214–215
Fiscella, K., 202
Food stamps, 417
Foot lesions, diabetes and screening for, 269
Ford, V. B., 120
Forsyth, B. F., 243
Four Hills of Life Wellness Center (Omaha Tribe), 118, 119, 253, 418
    community services at, 256–257
    diabetes management and, 258
Freeth, D., 47, 66
    model of outcomes of interprofessional education, 67t
Freyer, P. J., 179
Fruits and vegetables, diabetes prevention and, 417
Funding
    community-based work and, 286–287
    for community partnerships, 103–104
    inadequate, for interprofessional education, 33

G

Gahimer, J., 282
Gannon University Physical Therapy Program, 173
Gashytewa, Carrie, 205–206, 213
GECs. See Geriatric education centers
Gelmon, S. B., 169
Gender diversity, of healthcare providers in six healthcare professions, 204t
General Congregation of Society of Jesus (34th), conclusions of, 315

Geriatric education centers, 100
Geriatric models, current, 100–102
Geriatric population, as underserved population, 96–97, 105
Geriatrics, faculty development in, 102–104, 105
Geriatrics Task Force, 105
Gerontology, 31
Gilligan, Carol, 238
Glycemic control, diabetes and, 267, 273
Goals, sustainable community partnerships and, 177
Golin, A., 47
Good, promotion of, 442–443
Goodness, 441
Graduation, cultural diversity and, 215
Grand rounds sessions, interprofessional, 314
Grant, Gary, 192
Grants, interdisciplinary rural health training, 288–293
Grant-writing workshops, in Appalachian region, 135
"Greater Minnesota Strategy," 355–356
Great Mines Health Center (Missouri)
    factors related to success of, 155–156
    formation of, 154, 162
Great Spirits, traditional Omaha ways and, 251
Green, J., 16
Group processes, organizational theory and, 54
Group projects, 314
Gudykunst, William, 306
Gupta, J., 174, 175, 176

H

Habits of mind, developing, 24
Haddad, Amy, 441
Hamilton, C., 284
Harris, D. L., 103

Haskey, Glennita, 206, 210, 215
Hayward, K. S., 70
HbA$_{1c}$ tests, diabetes screening and, 267, 272, 275, 276
HCB. See Health Communities of Brownsville, Inc.
Heady, Hilda, 179
Healing, Omaha Tribe and traditional ways of, 251–252
Health Canada, 50, 312
Health care, changing and challenging landscape of, 12, 15
Health care clinics, 167
Health care costs
    escalating, 3, 15
    rising, 32
Health care delivery system, changing, 42
Health care disparities. See Disparities in health care
Health careers, Area Health Education Centers and recruitment and preparation in, 226–227
Health Careers Exploration Club (Creighton University), 302, 306
Health Careers Opportunity Program (Creighton University), 302, 306
Health care ethics/professionalism, as theme within Doisy College of Health Sciences curriculum, 320, 320t
Health care goods, interdependence of health professions and, 23–24
Health care organization, chronic care model and, 271
Health care practitioner shortages. See Shortages of health care practitioners
Health care professional programs, lack of cultural diversity and enrollment in, 203

Health care professions schools
  ethnic diversity of students in,
    203t
  proposed cultural proficiency
    elective for, 307–308,
    451–453
    course description, 451
    course goals, 451
    evaluative techniques, 452
    examples of questions for
      student's inquiry,
      452–453
    grading policy, 453
    learning objectives, 451–452
    student responsibilities/
      clinical schedules, 452
    text, 452
"Health Care Services in
  Appalachia," PRISYM and,
  386
Health care team training, assumptions about, 55, 58
Health care teamwork, global interest in, 50
Health communication
  effective, 401
  health literacy, 396–397
  literacy, 392, 393–396
  with rural racial/ethnic com-
    munities, 391–410
  strategies for, 400–404
Health Communities of
  Brownsville, Inc., Health
  TrendBender group, 404
Health delivery system, transforming, 126
Health informatics, accreditation
  standards in, 38t
Health Information Portability
  and Accountability Act,
  343
Health insurance
  Americans without, 429
  older adults without, 95
Health interventions, effective,
  designing, 404
Health literacy, 396–397
  in Brownsville, Texas, 407

Health Literacy Educational
  Symposium on Risky
  Behaviors of Youth
  (Brownsville, Texas), 407
Health on the Net Code of
  Conduct, 337
Health outcomes, interprofes-
  sional education and, 71–72
Health Outreach and Preventive
  Education. See HOPE
Health professional education,
  disparities in, 202–203, 205
Health professionals
  21 competencies for, for the
    21st century, 282, 283t
  core competencies in, 7t
Health professions, accreditation
  of, 36–37
Health professions administra-
  tors, influence of, on faculty
  and students, 19
Health professions education
  reform of, five cross-cutting
    strategies for, 8t
  vision for transformation of, 8–9
Health Professions Education: A
  Bridge to Quality, 4
  recommendations of, 6
  two core competencies from,
    19–20
  vision developed in, 8–9
Health Professions Education
  Summit, 6–8
Health promotion, effective, 408
Health providers, disparities in,
  202–203, 205
Health Report Card Project
  (Omaha Tribe), 413–425, 419
  background, 413–414
  building community capacity,
    414, 414–415
  conceptual model for, 414,
    414–415
  dissemination of information
    related to, 422–423
  findings, 423
  follow-up work, 424
  generation of, 418, 421–422

groups involved in, 417–420
  faculty community, 419
  graduate student commu-
    nity, 419–420
  OISSE community, 418–419
  Omaha Tribe Community, 417
  Omaha Tribe Diabetes
    Program, 417–418
  school communities, 418
health care delivery in rural
  America and, 416
need for building community
  capacity, 415–416
outcomes, 423–424
process for, 420–423
  data collection, 420–421
  dissemination of informa-
    tion, 422–423
  generation of Report Card,
    421–422
Health Resources and Services Administration, 80, 128, 303, 433
  grants, 9, 288–289
  Title VII programs, 100
Health Sciences Multicultural and
  Community Affairs
  (Creighton University), 308
  creation of, 298
  experience in cultural profi-
    ciency training, 303,
    306–307
  health disparities addressed by
    programs of, 300, 302
  success of, 299
  summary of pipeline activities
    of, in rural and urban
    poor Nebraska, 304–305t
Healthy Internet café, at Wellness
  Center for Omaha Tribe, 119
Healthy People 2010, 98, 282, 351,
  357, 415, 425
Heart disease, older adults and,
  96
Held, Virginia, 238, 239, 244
Hemmelgarn, A. L., 132
Hibbing, Minnesota, Northeast
  Minnesota Area Health
  Education Center, 359

Higher Learning Commission of the North Central Association of Schools and Colleges, 36
Hilton, R. W., 315
Hilton, S., 32
Hirokawa, R., 49
Hispanics, 201
    disparities in health care for, 202
    in four health care professions, 203t
    geographical concentration of, in rural areas, 398–399
    as healthcare providers in six healthcare professions, 204t
    literacy and, 394
    low education levels and, 399
    in New Mexico, 205
    rural, health gaps experienced by, 391
    in rural America, 392
Historical trauma, Native Americans and, 250
Hmong enclaves, in Minnesota, 353
Homeless clinics, 228
HOPE consortium (Missouri), 145–156, 162
    community health workers and, 149–150
    community involvement with, 147–148
    leadership and, 148–149
    outcomes of, 150–152
    population-based assessment and, 145–147
    services provided through, 148
    setting of, 145
    sustainability challenge and change, 152–156
Hornby, S., 99
Housing, 286
Housing Authority of Erie, Pennsylvania, 173
Howell, D. M., 284

HRSA. See Health Resources and Services Administration
HS-MACA. See Health Sciences Multicultural and Community Affairs (Creighton University)
Hudson, M., 68
Humanistic care, increasing, 42
Human rights, 195
Human solidarity movement, 156
Huthuga (sacred circle), 252
Hypertension, 96, 102, 202

I

Idaho State University Senior Health Mobile program, 101
IEPS. See Interdisciplinary Education Perception Scale
Ignatius (saint), 419
IHS. See Indian Health Services
Immigrants, diversification of, in Minnesota, 353
Income disparities
    health care racial disparities and, 158
    older adults and, 95, 96
Indenture models, 79
Independent, 35t
Indian-Chicano Health Center (Nebraska), 302, 306, 307
Indian Health Services, 87, 88, 255
Individual level, within organizational framework for ethics, 17, 17
Individual processes, organizational theory and, 54
Individuals, societal level and, 17, 17, 18
Individuals with Disabilities Education Act, 212, 379
Infant mortality rates, 142, 202
Informatics
    as theme within Doisy College of Health Sciences curriculum, 320, 321t
    utilizing, 7t, 430, 431–432

Information technology, rural professionals and, 115
Instant messaging, 89, 403
Institute for Family Medicine, 157, 159, 161
Institute of Medicine, 4, 42, 126, 202, 282, 311, 349, 401, 415, 444
    Committee on Quality of Health Care in America, 272
    Committee on the Future of Rural Health Care, 225, 233
    core competencies for future professionals identified by, 430
    "Education for the Health Team" conference (1972), 30
    health literacy described by, 396
    Workshop on Disability in America, 96
Institutional resources, 168
Instructional design models, grounding of, in theory, 45–54
Integration, scholarship and, 181
Integrative Interprofessional Practicum Experience (Saint Louis University), 161
Integrative power, 145
Interactive health communication, effective health communication campaigns and, 402
Interdependency, collaboration and, 59
Interdisciplinary, 35t
    defined, 48
    use of term, 283
Interdisciplinary education, defined, 47
Interdisciplinary Education Perception Scale, 70
    components within, 101
    content of, 449–450

Interdisciplinary health care team, defined, 47, 48
Interdisciplinary integration, in Appalachian region, 136
Interdisciplinary learning, epistemology and ontology of, 53
Interdisciplinary rural health training grants, 288–293
Interdisciplinary teaching and learning, Pellegrino's definitions for, 31t
Interdisciplinary teams, 430–431
   ability to work well in, 29
   learning outcomes for students and, 20
   working in, 7t
Internet
   Omaha Tribe members and access to, 119
   promoting health-related behavior change via, 403
   rural setting and, 114
Interpersonal communication, effective health communication campaigns and, 402
Interpretation, 442
Interprofessional, 35t
   defined, 48
Interprofessional collaboration, 3–4, 433
   faculty development in geriatrics and, 103
   mutual autonomy and, 244–245
   rural population and, 272–274
Interprofessional competencies, effective teaching of, 313
Interprofessional conceptual model, 68t
Interprofessional curriculum, 312–313
Interprofessional definitions, basic, by Clark, 34t
Interprofessional education, 3–4, 12, 15, 16, 34t
   accreditation of, 36–37
   assessment quandary, 64–66
   barriers to, 237

collaborative practice settings and, 167
community-engaged scholarship opportunity for faculty in, 180–182
defined, 35t, 47, 48
ethics framework for, 16–18
five barriers to, 33–34
flexible pedagogy and preparation, 443–444
Freeth and colleagues' model of outcomes for, 67t
growth in programs for, 30–31
health outcomes and, 71–72
immediate actions related to fostering of, 445t
importance of, 25
inadequate funding for, 33
individuals and, 18–19
language of, 34–35
leadership linked to, in Appalachian region, 137–138
measurement and, 66–67
nonthreatening environment for, 177
organizations and, 21–22
outcomes for, 446
partnership processes and, 184
primary goal of, 174
recommendations for, 42
rethinking learning for common good and, 24–25
   individuals in, 19–21
   organizations in, 22–23
review summaries of accreditation standards across nine health-related professions related to, 38–41t
roots of, 141
scholarship of engagement and, 64, 73
service-learning common teaching strategies and, 174–176
seven approaches for faculty development in, 20t
society and, 23–24

in United States, key events in, 4–6
Interprofessional education and practice, conceptual model for, 10
Interprofessional education assessment, future directions for, 72–73
Interprofessional Education for Collaborative Patient-Centered Practice, 312
Interprofessional education literature, glossary of current terms in, 35t
Interprofessional education programs
   effective, criteria based on Parsell, Spalding, and Bligh, 32t
   goals of, 313
   professional identity and, 30
Interprofessional experiences, benefits with, 287
Interprofessional health care, Simpson's definition of, 251
Interprofessional health care education, theoretical models for, 52–54
Interprofessional health care practice, theoretical models for, 54–55
Interprofessional health care teamwork, evidence base and rationale for, 50–52
Interprofessionality, 35t, 312
Interprofessional models of health care delivery, assumptions related to, 283
Interprofessional moral community, development of, 247
Interprofessional practice, defined, 319
Interprofessional pre-matriculation program (Creighton University), 80–84
Interprofessional related health professional competencies, 283t

Interprofessional rural health training, 85–86
Interprofessional short-term immersions (Creighton University), 84–85
Interprofessional teams, 3
ability to work in, 311–312
Interprofessional teamwork model, 67
Interprofessional telehealth training plan, 334–336t
IOM. *See* Institute of Medicine
IPE. *See* Interprofessional education
Irvine, R., 237

J

James House Health Center (Missouri), 156–162
community involvement and, 158–159
delineation of services at, 159–161
outcomes for, 161–162
population-based assessment and, 157–158
setting of, 157
sustainability of, 162
Jensen, G. M., 72
Jesuit mission, philosophy of, 315
Jewish holidays, 210
John Paul II (pope), 156
John Rex Foundation, 342
Johnson, M., 181
Johnson Plantation, 191
Joint Commission on Accreditation of Healthcare Organizations, 114
Joint Review Committee on Educational Programs in Nuclear Medicine Technology, 36, 39t
Journaling, students and, 284, 291
Justice. *See also* Ethics of justice; Social justice
care and, 238–242
dealing openly with, 383–384, 386, 389

K

Kaplan, R., 135
Karges, Joy, 284
Kember, D., 65
Kentucky Bridges Project, 372
Kentucky Department of Mental Health and Mental Retardation, 371
Kentucky Education Reform Act, 379
Kentucky IMPACT, 370, 372
Kentucky Partnership for Families and Children, 371, 377
Kentucky River Community Care, 379
Kentucky Tele-Link Network, 371
Ker, J., 32
Kim, Young Yun, 307
King, Martin Luther, Jr., 156
Kinsinger, L., 268
Kirkpatrick, D. L., 446
model of educational outcomes, 66, 66t
Klein, J., 49
Knowledge-based information resources, critical role of, 115
Knowledge competencies, primary teamwork competencies and, 56t
Kohlberg, Lawrence, 238
KTLN. *See* Kentucky Tele-Link Network

L

Land ownership, cultural-specific meaning of, 190–191
Laotian enclaves, in Minnesota, 353
La Paz, Bolivia, Tembladurani community in, 143–145
Last Buffalo Hunt Walking Program, 252, 253
Latinos, 201
in Minnesota, 353
type 2 diabetes in, 265

Lay health advisors, 274
Lead Belt, Missouri, 145
Leadership
effective, debate over, 126
leveraging benefits of Area Health Education Centers and, 233–236
native, 155–156
shared, 35t, 435
telehealth endeavors and, 343
Leadership competencies, for administrators, 19
Leadership development, interprofessional education linked to, in Appalachian region, 137–138
Leadership in Rural Health Interprofessional Education & Practice Conference, 9, 439–445
conceptual images from, 440t
gestalt of, 440–442
next steps, 444–445
themes, 442–444
partnerships: presence and patience, 444
people: committed to promoting the good, 442–443
programs: flexible pedagogy and preparation, 443–444
Leadership model, applying, 435–436
Learners, in interprofessional education experience, 313–314
Learning
rethinking, for individuals in interprofessional education, 19–21
rethinking, for interprofessional education and the common good, 24–25
Learning activities, integration of, within Doisy College of Health Sciences curriculum, 324–325

Learning and Teaching Support Network Centre for Health Sciences and Practice (UK), 66

Learning organizations, defined, 22

Learning Together to Work Together, 31

Lefever, G., 181

Liason Committee on Medical Education, 36

Librarian, role of, in rural health outreach, 111–122

Library services, lack of, rural professionals and, 114

Licensure standards, interprofessional education and, 22

Lipid control, diabetes outcomes and, 267, 268

Listservs, 341

Litaker, D., 276

Literacy
computer, 433
diverse populations, health communication and, 409
health, 396–397
health communication and, 392, 393–396
media, 402
rural populations and low levels of, 249

Literacy levels, 395*t*

Literacy scales, 394*t*

Liverman, C. T., 112

Loansome Doc, 116

Long-term care, 97

Luecht, R. M., 70

Luke, A., 16

M

Macrosystems, 55

Macy, Nebraska, Omaha Tribe community in, 417

Mainous, A. G., 267

Making Health Care Safer: A Critical Analysis of Patient Safety Practices, 52

Males, as healthcare providers in six healthcare professions, 204*t*

"Maquiladora Program" (Brownsville/Matamoros, Texas), 406

Maritz, C., 181

Market forces, collaborative, interprofessional care and, 272

Massing, M. W., 268

McGoogan Library of Medicine, 121

McNair, R., 176

McRoberts, J., 70

McWhirter, G., 207, 208, 210

Measure of Service Learning, The: Research Scales to Assess Student Experiences (Bringle, Phillips, and Hudson), 68

Measures, of service learning constructs, 69–70*t*

Media advocacy, effective health communication campaigns and, 402

Media literacy, effective health communication campaigns and, 402

Medicaid, 159, 202, 281, 343
grant funding for HOPE (Missouri) and, 152, 153
Omaha Tribe services and, 255
rural settings and reimbursement through, 79

Medical errors, reducing, 5

Medical instructions, understanding, literacy skills and, 396

Medical librarians
in academic settings, 121–122
access to, 116
collaboration and, 116–117
expanded example on rural outreach and interprofessional practice, 117–119
global reach and, 120–122
roles and responsibilities of, 111, 114–115

Medical Library Association, 111
Hospital Libraries Section of, 116

Medical profession, ethnic diversity of students in, 203*t*

Medical University of South Carolina, College of Health Professions, 101

Medicare, 96
diabetes mellitus, services use patterns and, 266
rural settings and reimbursement through, 79

Medicare Direct Access legislation, for physical therapists, 174

MedlinePlus, 120, 121

Mental health services, HOPE consortium and, 148

Mental illness, PRISYM team member's experience with, 369–370

Mentoring, 245

Mentors, 84, 89

Mentorships, successful, 210–211

Mercy Circle of Care initiative (Philadelphia), 181, 182

Meredith College (Raleigh, North Carolina), 333

Mexican medicine, 209

Mezirow, J., 65

Microsystems, 55

Mining industry, corporate abuse in Appalachia and, 375

Mining politics, Appalachian region and, 131

Minnesota
America's Health Rankings rating of, 350
changing demographics in, 351, 353–354
distribution of health professionals
metropolitan, micropolitan, and rural, 352*t*
urban and rural, 352*t*
health professions trainee exit survey: 2001-2003, 353*t*
health professions workforce shortages in, 351

international immigration and refugees in, 353
moving toward healthier state of, 364–365
rural, changing demographics and health disparities, 350–354
  changing demographics, 351, 353–354
  health professions workforce shortages, 351
  urban *vs.* rural health disparities, 351
  65-plus age group in, 353–354
Minnesota Area Health Education Center, 350, 355–356
Minnesota Department of Health, 351
Minorities. *See also* Ethnicity; Race
diabetes and, 265, 266
older adults, income disparities and, 95
Minority Youth Conference and Focus on Health Professions, 80
Missouri Bureau of Dental Health, 148, 150
Missouri Department of Family and Child Services, 151–152
Missouri Department of Health and Senior Services, 154
Missouri Department of Mental Health, 146, 147
Missouri Foundation of Health, 154
Missouri Primary Care Association, 153
Mobile telephones, promoting health-related behavior change via, 403
Modeling, 286
Models, 45
principles *vs.*, 142
Mole, L., 32
Montevideo, Minnesota, southern Minnesota Area Health Education Center, 360

Moose Lake, Northeast Minnesota Area Health Education Center, 359–360
Moose Lake Community Geriatric Project (Minnesota), 359–360
Moral development, service learning constructs measures and, 69*t*
Morris, D. M., 282
Mortality rates, for Native Americans, 250
Motives, service learning constructs measures and, 69*t*
MPE. *See* Multiprofessional education
Mu, K., 86
Multidisciplinary, 35*t*
defined, 48
Multimedia, promoting health-related behavior change via, 403
Multiprofessional education, 31, 34*t*
defined, 47
Mutual autonomy, interprofessional collaboration and, 244–245

N

NAPLEX, 90
National Academy of Sciences, 47
National Accrediting Agency for Clinical Laboratory Science, 36, 38*t*
National Advisory Committee on Interdisciplinary, Community-Based Linkages, 191
National AHEC Organization, 235
National Assessment of Adult Literacy, 394
National Assessment of Educational Progress, literacy levels, 395*t*
National Council on Aging, 98
National Health Service Corps, 79, 221

National Institutes of Health, Roadmap for Medical Research, 59–60
National League for Nursing Accrediting Commission, 36
National Library of Medicine, 117, 119, 120
National Network of Libraries of Medicine, 111, 116, 117, 118
National Review Board, 286
National Rural Health Association, 112, 249, 398, 416
Native American Church, 251, 252
Native American communities
interprofessional short-term immersions in, 84–85
understanding health challenges faced by, 87
Native American culture and health, service-learning-based elective courses on, 86
Native Americans, 201. *See also* Health Report Card Project; individual tribes
diabetes and, 250
disparities in health care for, 202
in four health care professions, 203*t*
geographical concentration of, in rural areas, 399
as healthcare providers in six healthcare professions, 204*t*
honoring words and promises made to, 413, 425
in New Mexico, 205
Nighthorse Campbell Building as homage to cultural heritage of, 439
public health challenges and, 413
reservation life in rural areas and, 249
respecting cultural responsibilities and rituals of, 210

rural, health gaps experienced by, 391
in rural America, 392
type 2 diabetes in, 265
unique health care needs of, 250
Native Canadians, nursing program for, 207
Native Hawaiians, 201
Nature factors, rural medical practice and, 78
Navajo Nation, 86, 206, 207, 209, 210, 214
Nebraska
ethnicity breakout of health professionals in, 301t
need for health care professionals in, 299–300
Omaha Tribe of, 251–253
"Nebraska Go Local" program, 121
Nebraska Health and Human Services, 253
Nebraska Healthy People 2010, 423
Nebraska Healthy People Goals, diabetes reduction and, 415
"Need a Library?" fact sheet, 116
Needs assessment, sustainable community partnerships and, 177
New Deal Resettlement program, 191–192
New Freedom Commission, 126
New Mexico, poverty level in, 205
New Mexico Occupational Therapy Graduate Program, 209
New York Public Library, 111
NHSC. See National Health Service Corps
No Man Is an Island (Donne), 156
Non-Hispanic whites
infant mortality and, 202
in New Mexico, 205
Norris, S. L., 269
North Carolina
"diabetes belt" in eastern coastal plain of, 268

eastern chronic care pilot project in, 274–277
therapist isolation in, 330, 331
North Carolina Department of Health and Human Services, 332, 342
North Carolina General Assembly, 331
Norton, D., 135
Nuclear medicine technology, accreditation standards in, 39t
Numeracy skills, 393
Nurses, ethnic/gender diversity among, 204t
Nursing liaison librarians, 122
Nursing students, reflections from rural, interdisciplinary training, 29
Nurture factors, rural medical practice and, 78
Nutrition, diabetes prevention and, 417
Nutrition and dietetics, accreditation standards in, 39t

O

Oandasan, I., 50, 312, 314
Obesity, 202
diabetes and, 416
increasing rates of, 3, 15
rural population and, 250, 281
type 2 diabetes and, 265
Observations research, in education and training, 60
Occupational justice, 384
Occupational therapists, ethnic/gender diversity among, 204t
Occupational therapy
accreditation standards in, 40t
ethnic diversity of students in, 203t
service-learning course immersion in, 86–88
Web-based health professions education in, 88–91
Occupational therapy students

educational interaction between physical therapy students and, 284
reflections from rural, interdisciplinary training, 293t
Office of eLearning and Academic Technologies, 88
Office of Interprofessional Scholarship, Service, and Education (Creighton University), 84, 118, 119
Health Report Card Project and, 413, 414, 415, 418, 419, 420, 422, 423, 424
student opportunities through, 289–290t, 291, 293
Office of Rural Health Policy's Rural Health Network Development Planning Grant Program, 128
OISSE. See Office of Interprofessional Scholarship, Service, and Education (Creighton University)
Older adults
addressing health needs of, 99
community-dwelling, 97–99
Omaha, Nebraska, demographics of, 299–300
Omaha, translation of word for, 249
Omaha Alcohol Program, 257
Omaha/Douglas County (Nebraska), health care professionals in, 300t
Omaha Indian Reservation (Nebraska), 417
Omaha Nation School, 253
Omaha Public Schools, 302
Office of Gifted Education, 302
Omaha Tribal Dialysis Center, 255
Omaha Tribe Diabetes Program, 253, 258, 291, 417–418
Omaha Tribe of Nebraska, 118, 119, 249–261, 288, 291
building community capacity and, 414–415

data collection, diabetes screening/education and, 420–421

demographic data from, 253–254

diabetes, community capacity building and, 413–414

diagnosing diabetes in members of, 415

diet, diabetes prevention and, 417

graduate student community and, 419–420

health care lessons learned and, 259–260

overview of, 251–253

overview of health care delivery system to, 254–258

alcohol program, 257

community services, 256–257

diabetes program, 258

dialysis unit, 255

long-term care services, 254–255

outpatient primary care services, 258

Valentine Parker Jr. Youth Prevention Center, 257

resource utilization by, 261

school communities and, 418

Ontology, of interdisciplinary learning, 53

Onwuegbuzie, A., 65

Open communication, 434

Organizational culture, in Appalachian region, 133

Organizational ethics framework, for analysis, 16–18

Organizational framework for ethics, realms or levels of, 17, 17–18

Organizational level, within organizational framework for ethics, 17, 17

Organizational processes, organizational theory and, 54

Organizational theory, processes related to, 54

Organization(s)

interprofessional education and, 21–22

people's programs and, 155

power and, 145, 156

rethinking learning for, in interprofessional education, 22–23

Osheroff, J. A., 112

O'Toole, T. P., 179

Outcomes

approaches and tools for measurement of, 67–72

health outcomes and IPE, 71–72

questionnaires, 70–71

self-assessment, 70

service-learning measures, 68, 69–70t

diabetes, 267–268

Health Report Card Project, 423–424

for interprofessional education, 65, 446

sustainable community partnerships and, 177

Overweight, defined, 421

Owen, N., 403

P

Pacific Islanders, 201

Parity, 35t

Parkinson's disease, 72

Parsell, G., 32

Participatory leadership, Appalachian culture and, 133–137

Partnerships

collaboration and, 59

defined, 167

long-lasting, 444

Partners in Information Access for the Public Health Workforce, 117

Part-time tracks, student lifestyles and, 208–209

Pathman, D. E., 79

Patient-centered care, 273, 282, 430

faculty role models and, 18–19

learning outcomes for students and, 19–20

providing, 7t

Patient registry, 271, 275

Patient safety, 5

PCAT. See Pharmacy College Admission Test

Peer review, 245

Peer-reviewed articles, 171, 182

Pellegrino, Edmund, 30, 47

definitions for interdisciplinary teaching and learning by, 31t

People's programs, 155

Peripheral neuropathy, diabetes and screening for, 269

Personality traits, effective leadership and, 126

Perspective, 442

Pew-Fetzer Task Force, 49

Pew Health Professions Commission, 29, 42, 282, 311

Pew Internet and American Life Project, 432

Pharmacy

accreditation standards in, 41t

ethnic diversity of students in, 203t

service-learning course immersion in, 86–88

Web-based health professions education in, 88–91

Pharmacy College Admission Test, 81

Pharmacy students, reflections from rural, interdisciplinary training, 292t

Phenomenon, defined, 45

Philadelphia Department of Public Health, 181

Phillips, M. A., 68

Physical therapists, ethnic/gender diversity among, 204t

Physical therapy

accreditation standards in, 41t

ethnic diversity of students in, 203t

Physical therapy services, James House Health Center and, 160

Physical therapy students
educational interaction between occupational therapy students and, 284
reflections from rural, interdisciplinary training, 292*t*

Physician assistants, accreditation standards and, 41*t*

Physicians, ethnic/gender diversity among, 204*t*

Physician shortages, rural settings and, 112

Pinon community, 87

Placement
Area Health Education Centers and, 227–228
of health professionals, root cause map for, 227, 229

Population-based assessment
HOPE consortium and, 145–147
James House Health Center (Missouri) and, 157–158

Porterfield, D. S., 268

Poverty. See also Disparities in health care; Socioeconomic status
in Appalachia, 378–379
disparities in health care, 202
Native Americans and, 249
in New Mexico, 205
Omaha Tribe and, 254
rural population and, 281
rural racial/ethnic culture and, 398–399
rural residents and, 250
in Washington County, Missouri, 145–146, 147

Powell, L. T., 70

Power
Alinsky on, 142
collaboration and, 59
dealing openly with, 383–384, 386, 389
integrative, 145

interactive models of care and, 276
organization, 156
sustainable community partnerships and, 178

Power approach, to professionalization, 243

Practice, 35*t*

Preceptor training, 286

Pre-Matriculation Program (Creighton University), 303, 306

Prescription drug costs, older adults and, 96

Primary teamwork competencies, 56–57*t*

Principles, models *vs.*, 142

Principles-based partnerships, 168
development of, 176–184

Print literacy ability, basic, 394–395

PRISYM
addressing justice and power at many levels, 383–384, 386, 389
challenges for staff and trainees in, 378–381
distance, weather, and technology challenges, 379–380
site development challenges, 380–381
systemic economic, service and education challenges, 378–379
development of, 370–372
feedback for future improvement of, 387–388
plan of study, 368*t*
student data related to interdisciplinary collaboration, 374*t*
success of training for team service to Appalachian at-risk youth, 386–388
take home lessons about, 388–389
training for services in Appalachia, 377–378

training for strong service team participation, 372–373
training objectives of, 367–368

PRISYM leadership team, story by member of, about own mental health, 369–370

PRISYM student performance, site supervisors' overall impression of, 388*t*

PRISYM training objectives, student data related to successful completion of, 387*t*

Problem-solving activities, 314

Process, collaboration and, 59

Professional culture, 277

Professionalism, renewed call for, 15

Professionalization, 243–245, 246
ethic of care and, 237–247
perspectives on, 243

Professional schools, habits of mind and, 24

Project ESCUELA, 211–215
description of, 211–212
evaluating graduates' impact on outcomes in children with disabilities, 213
financial support and individual students within, 214–215
increased recruitment of students from New Mexico native cultures, 212–213
percentage of students recruited for underrepresented cultures, 206

PROMISE Institute (University of Toledo), 100

Promotion
community-based work, faculty and, 286
community-engaged scholarship, faculty and, 183

Promotora, 274

Prose literacy scale, 394*t*

Protection of Human Subjects, 173

Provider bias, 202

Providing Rural Interdisciplinary Services for Youth with Mental Health Needs. *See* PRISYM

Public housing communities, 157–158

Public relations, effective health communication campaigns and, 402

Public service announcements, 402

PubMed, 116, 119, 120

Purtilo, Ruth, 441, 445

Q

Qualitative research methods, IPE assessment and, 73

Quality improvement, 430 applying, 7t

Quality of Health Care in America (IOM), 4

Quality of life, older adults and, 97

Quantitative literacy scale, 394t

Quantitative research methods, IPE assessment and, 73

Quentin N. Burdick Interdisciplinary Rural Health Training Programs, 72, 128, 285

budget cuts under Title VII of, 367

grants offered through, 85

removal of funding for, 429

Questionnaires, 70–71

Quiram, B., 112

R

Race. *See also* African Americans; Hispanics; Native Americans

disparities in health care and, 158, 202

type 2 diabetes and, 265

Racial communities, rural, health communication with, 391–410

Racism, 195

Radio, promoting health-related behavior change via, 402

Reciprocal learning, 169, 170

Reclaiming Mountain Futures, 381

Recreating Health Professional Practice for a New Century, 311

Recruitment, 215

Area Health Education Centers and, 226–227

increasing diversity and, 207–208

of students from New Mexico native cultures, 212–213

Redesigned systems of care, 268–270, 277

Reeves, S., 314

Reflections, 170, 175, 176, 291

student, from rural, interdisciplinary training, 292–293t

Reflective practitioner, educating, 53

Regional accreditation, 36

Regional culture, in Appalachia, 133

Registry, patient, 271, 275

Reliability, 71

Report of the Surgeon General's Conference on Children's Mental Health: A National Action Agenda, 126, 127

Research teams, interdisciplinary, 60

Reservation life, Omaha Tribe and, 249–261

Resources

interprofessional education and, 33–34

sharing, 287

Respect

for community, 144

sustainable community partnerships and, 177

Responsibility, ethics and, 16

Retention

Area Health Education Centers and, 228–229

for health professions, root cause map for, 229

Rink, E., 32

Risky behaviors, rural residents and, 250

Ritzer, G., 243

Rivalry, professional, overcoming barriers of, 246, 247

Robert Wood Johnson Health Professions Partnership Initiative, 80

Role and reward structure, of department, school, and educational institution, 21

Role models, 286

Roles, sustainable community partnerships and, 178

Ronald E. McNair Scholars Program (University of New Mexico), 212

Rose, M. A., 71

Royeen, C. B., 72

Rural, interdisciplinary training, student reflections from, 292–293t

Rural America

Area Health Education Centers in, 224–226

public perception of, 392

Rural areas

addressing needs of practice in, 432–435

shortages of health services in, 190

Rural best practices, 72

Rural career selection, factors related to, 77–78

Rural communities

integration of practitioner/practitioner's family into, 80

practitioner shortages in, 77

value of engagement in, 195–196

Rural concept, defining, 190

Rural employment, student data related to, 382t

Rural health care, Area Health Education Centers and reform of, 233–236
Rural health care professionals, information needs of, 112–114
Rural health issues, students and, 284
Rural health outreach, librarian's role in, 111–122
Rural health training, interprofessional, 85–86
Rural medical practice, nature and nurture factors and, 78
Rural patients, diabetes outcomes in urban patients *vs.*, 267*t*
Rural Physician Associate Program (University of Minnesota Medical School), 356–358, 361, 363, 364
Rural population, diabetes in, 266–267
Rural practice career, PRISYM and learning experiences focused on consideration of, 381, 383
Rural racial/ethnic communities, health communication with, 391–410
Rural racial/ethnic culture, 398–400
Rural racial/ethnic populations effective communication and, 410
  factors shared by, 400
  health communication strategies and, 408–410
Rural /underserved communities strategies for promoting practice in, 80–91
  interprofessional pre-matriculation program, 80–84
  interprofessional rural health training, 85–86
  interprofessional short-term immersions, 84–85
  interprofessional structured cultural immersions, 84

service-learning course immersion in pharmacy and occupational therapy, 86–88
Web-based education in pharmacy and occupational therapy, 88–91
Russian enclaves, in Minnesota, 353

S

Sacred circle (Huthuga), 252
Sacred tobacco smoking, 251
Sage burning, 251–252
Saint Louis University, 147, 148, 153, 161
  interprofessional education and mission of, 317–318
  School of Nursing, 150, 157
Sanchez, Matthew, 206, 210
Sandmann, L. R., 64, 181
Scammon, D. L., 79, 84
Scarce resources, stewardship for, 24
Scholarship, Boyer's four dimensions of, 181
Scholarship of engagement, interprofessional education and, 64, 73
Scholarship opportunities, community-engaged, for faculty in interprofessional education, 180–182
School communities, Omaha Tribe and, 418
School of Pharmacy and Health Professions (Creighton University), 80
  Pre-Matriculation Program admission into, 81–82
  description of, 82–83
  scholarship funds for, 83–84
Screenings, diabetes, Omaha Tribe and, 258
Self and self-concept, service learning constructs measures and, 69*t*

Self-assessment, 70
Self-knowledge, 442
Self-management support, chronic care model and, 270
Self-reflection, by students, 20–21, 292–293*t*
Self-reliance, in Appalachian culture, 129, 130
Sempowski, I. P., 79
Senge, P., 49
Senior centers, 97, 167
Service challenges, in Appalachia, 378–379
Service learning, 168, 169–171, 176, 182
Service learning constructs, measures of, 69–70*t*
Service-learning course immersion, in pharmacy and occupational therapy, 86–88
Service-learning measures, 68
Sharecropping, 191
Shared leadership, 35*t*, 435
Sharing, collaboration and, 59
Shije, Marie, 208, 210
Shojania, K. G., 269
Shortages of health care practitioners
  demographics and, 63
  informatics and, 431–432
  in Minnesota, 351
  older adults and, 99
  rural populations and, 77, 249, 250
  rural racial/ethnic culture and, 399
Short-term immersions, interprofessional, 84–85
Shulman, Lee, 441
Sifneos, P. E., 30
"Silo culture," of health professions education, 4
Silos, 237
Simpson, G., 250, 251
Sinusitis, older adults and, 96
Site development challenges, PRISYM and, 380–381

Skill competencies, primary teamwork competencies and,
56–57t
Slave-holding plantations, 191
Slavery, 191
Smith, C., 284
Smith, P., 71
Smoking, rural population and,
250, 281
Sobriety Powwow (Omaha Tribe),
256
Social contract, 445
Socialization
interprofessional, 53
during professional education,
246
Social justice, 189, 191, 442–443, 444
defined, 384
as theme within Doisy College
of Health Sciences cur-
riculum, 320, 321t
in Tillery, North Carolina,
191–195
Social learning, 53
Social marketing, 402
Social responsibility, understanding meaning of, 24
Societal level, within organizational framework for ethics,
17, 17, 18
Society, interprofessional education and, 23–24
Society of Jesus, 297
Socioeconomic status, 282
disparities in health care and,
202
older adults and, 95, 99
type 2 diabetes and, 266
Sociomedical model, biomedical
model vs., 281–284
Solidarity, James House Health
Center and, 156–162
Somali enclaves, in Minnesota,
353
Southern Association of Colleges
and Schools, 36
SPAHP. See School of Pharmacy
and Health Professions

Spalding, R., 32
Speech/language pathologists,
ethnic/gender diversity
among, 204t
Spirituality, Native American, 252
St. Cyr, Wehnona, 259
St. Louis Behavioral Medicine
Institute, 148
St. Louis Fire Department, 161
St. Louis Housing Authority
(Missouri), 157, 159, 161
St. Louis University, Edward and
Margaret Doisy College of
Health Sciences at, 312
Stanley, E. E., 114
Steinert, Y., 19, 103
Stereotypes, communication pro-
grams for diverse popula-
tions and, 409
Stone, N., 65
Streaming technology, 89
Stritter, F., 103
Student lifestyles, curriculum ad-
justed to, 208–209
Student loan repayment benefits,
rural community service
and, 79
Students
interprofessional teams of, at
University of South
Dakota, 284–285
Omaha Tribe and recruitment
of, 260
opportunities for, through
Office of Interprofessional
Scholarship, Service, and
Education, 289–290t
rural settings and preparation
for, 284
social justice and, 442–443
Substance abuse
Native Americans and, 249
Omaha Tribe and prevention
of, 256
Suicide
Native Americans and, 250
rural population and, 281
Sullivan, William, 24, 445

Summer Health Careers Institute,
227
Sundances, 251
Sustainability
community involvement in de-
cision making and, 155
James House Health Center
(Missouri) and, 162
Sustainable community partner-
ships, principles for, 177–179
Sweat lodges, 251, 252, 257
Systems, parts of, 55
Systems integration, collaboration
and, 127–128
Systems of care
process of redesigning, 268–269
redesigned, 277
in rural practices, 269–270
Systems theory, 54–55

T

Talking Circles, 257
Teaching, scholarship and, 181
Teams, successful, 433–434
Team treatment, 35t
Team work, 277
Technology, rural populations
and lack of, 249
Technology challenges, in
Appalachia, 379–380
Teen birth rate, 202
TelAbility Training Allied
Health
description of, 332–333, 337,
341
examples of multiple choice
knowledge questions in-
cluded on the pre- and
posttests, 340t
outcomes for, 341–342
racial diversity of faculty and
student participants, 337t
sample questions from pre- and
postprogram student sur-
veys, 338–339t
Telecommunication technologies,
329

Telehealth training plan, interprofessional, 334–336t
Television, promoting health-related behavior change via, 402
Tembladurani community (La Paz, Bolivia), 143–145
Tenure
community-based work, faculty and, 286
community-engaged scholarship, faculty and, 183
Theoretical models
for interprofessional health care education, 52–54
for interprofessional health care practice, 54–55
Theorizing, continuous process of, 45, 46
Theory(ies), 45
grounding instructional design models in, 45–54
practice informed by, 58
Thomas Jefferson University (Philadelphia), eHealth Summer Institute at, 119
Tillery, North Carolina, interprofessional rural health work in, 191–195
Tillery People's Health Clinic, 194
Tillery Plantation, 191
To Err Is Human: Building a Safer Health System, 4, 5, 52
Torres, Eliseo, 209
Tradition, interprofessional education and sense of, 33
Training
Area Health Education Centers and, 227–228
health communication and, 408–410
of health professionals, root cause map for, 227
in justice, power, and participatory action research, 386

for PRISYM service team participation, 372–373
for services in Appalachia, 377–378
team, 55, 58
for team service to Appalachian at-risk youth, 386–388
telehealth endeavors and, 329, 343
Transdisciplinary, defined, 48–49
Translational research, 60
Translations, communication programs for diverse populations and, 409
Transportation, 282
nutrition, diabetes prevention and, 417
older adults and, 97
rural populations and, 249, 281
TrendBender groups, 404
health literacy program, six-stage process and, 407
Tribal Connections Four Corner project, 117
Trust
building with Appalachian people, 131–132
mutual, collaboration and, 434
sustainable community partnerships and, 177
Tsaile community (Navajo Nation), 86, 87
Tuberculosis
in Brownsville, Texas, 406
Native Americans and, 250
Tuberculosis clinic, in Tembladurani (Bolivia), 144
Turnstall, S., 32

U

UK Prospectus Diabetes Study Group, 265
Ulian, J., 103
Underrepresented cultural groups, financial aid for students from, 214–215

Unemployment
Native Americans and, 250
Omaha Tribe and, 254
Unidisciplinary, defined, 48
Uninsured population
adults within, 23
in America, 429
growth in, 31–32
Native Americans and, 250
Uniprofessional education, 34t, 48
United States
Area Health Education Centers in, 220
diabetes mellitus in, 265
key events for interprofessional education in, 4–6
Unite for Sight, 120
University of Alaska (Anchorage), 91
University of Colorado
Health Sciences Center, 9
2006 conference and book creation: key events, 9–11
Medical Sciences Center, Nighthorse Campbell Building of, 439
University of Minnesota
Academic Health Center, 350, 354–362
challenges and opportunities for interprofessional education projects at, 360–362
Faculty Leadership Council, 358–359
Fergus Falls—Central Minnesota Area Health Education Center, 359
Hibbing—Northeast Minnesota Area Health Education Area, 359
Minnesota Area Health Education Center, 355–356

Montevideo—Southern
  Minnesota Area Health
  Education Center, 360
Moose Lake—Northeast
  Minnesota Area Health
  Center, 359–360
Rural Physician Associate
  Program, 356–358
building next generation of
  community-campus part-
  nerships at, 362–363
community attitude toward,
  361
Medical School, Rural
  Physician Associate
  Program, 356–358, 361,
  363, 364
University of Minnesota
  Extension, 356
University of Nebraska Medical
  Center, 121
University of New Mexico
  cultural diversity in occupa-
  tional therapy program at,
  205–207
Medical School, 208
Occupational Therapy
  Ambassador Program,
  207
Occupational Therapy
  Graduate Program, 211
employment of graduates
  from, 213, *213*
University of North Carolina
  (Chapel Hill), 332, 333
University of South Dakota, inter-
  professional teams of stu-
  dents at, 284
University of Toledo, PROMISE
  Institute, 100
University of Utah
  Health Sciences Center, 117
Spencer S. Eccles Health
  Science Library outreach
  program, 117, 118
University System of West
  Virginia, 168, 179

UPE. *See* Uniprofessional
  education
Urban patients, diabetes outcomes
  in rural patients *vs.*, 267*t*
U.S. Census Bureau, 201, 405
U.S. Department of Health and
  Human Services, Health
  Resources and Services
  Administration, Bureau of
  Health Professions, 219, 221
U.S. Public Health Service, 72
Utah Department of Health, 117

V

Valentine Parker Jr. Youth
  Prevention Center (Omaha
  Tribe), 253, 257, 258, 418
Validity, 71
Values
  service learning constructs
    measures and, 69*t*
  sustainable community part-
    nerships and, 177
Vegetables and fruits, diabetes
  prevention and, 417
vFellowship (Creighton Cardoner
  program), 419
Video cassette recorders, promot-
  ing health-related behavior
  change via, 403
Videoconferencing, 329, 332, 341,
  342, 343, 344
Vietnamese enclaves, in
  Minnesota, 353
Virtual clinics, 329, 332
Vision, shared, interprofessional
  education and, 22–23
Vision screening, for Omaha Tribe
  children, 421
Visual images, communication
  programs for diverse popu-
  lations and, 409
Vocational fellowship (Creighton
  University), 419
Volunteerism, service learning *vs.*,
  169

W

W. K. Kellogg Foundation, 103,
  104
Wagner, E. H., 270
Wake Area Telehealth
  Collaborative Helping chil-
  dren with special needs,
  342
Wakonda, 251, 252
Walesa, Lech, 156
Walking program, Omaha Nation
  and, 252, 253
Walthill, Nebraska, Omaha Tribe
  community in, 417
Washington County Community
  Partnership (Missouri), 153,
  154
Washington County Health
  Department (Missouri), 148
Washington County Memorial
  Hospital (Missouri), 148
WATCH. *See* Wake Area
  Telehealth Collaborative
  Helping children with spe-
  cial needs
Weather challenges, in
  Appalachia, 379–380
Web-based chats, 89
Web-based health professions ed-
  ucation, in pharmacy and
  occupational therapy, 88–91
Wenger, E., 330, 343
"We Shall All Be One," 156
Western medicine, Native
  American medicine and, 251
West Virginia Rural Health
  Education Partnership, 168,
  179
Whites
  as healthcare providers in six
    healthcare professions,
    204*t*
  type 2 diabetes in, 265
Williams, A. M., 190, 191
Winnebago Public Health Service,
  258

Winnebago Public Service
    Hospital (Nebraska), 288
Winnebago Tribe, 258, 288, 291
Wireless communication methods,
    promoting health-related be-
    havior change via, 403
Wittman, Peggy, 194
Women, Infant, and Children pro-
    gram, 417

Workforce
    health care, creating more cul-
        turally diverse, 205–207
    recruitment and diversity in,
        207–208, 215
Work load, rural careers and,
    78
World Health Organization, 30,
    31, 47

Z

Zia Pueblo community, 208, 210
Zoorob, R. J., 267
Zulkowski, K., 267
Zuni Pueblo community, 205–206,
    212
Zwarenstein, M., 71